Principles of Surgical Practice

Principles of Surgical Practice

Edited by

Andrew Kingsnorth, BSc, MBBS, MS, FRCS, FACS

Honorary Consultant Surgeon
Derriford Hospital, Plymouth
Professor of Surgery, Plymouth Postgraduate Medical School
External Undergraduate Examiner, Oxford, London and Kuala Lumpur; Member, Court of
Examiners, Royal College of Surgeons of England

Aljafri Abdul Majid, MBBS (Monash), BMedSc (Hons), FRCSEd, FRCSEd (Cardiothoracics)

Consultant Cardiothoracic Surgeon
University Hospital, Kuala Lumpur, Malaysia
Professor, Department of Surgery, Faculty of Medicine, University of Malaya
Member, Panel of Examiners, Royal College of Surgeons of Edinburgh

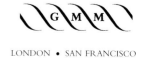

LONDON • SAN FRANCISCO

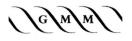

© 2001

GREENWICH MEDICAL MEDIA LIMITED
137 Euston Road
London
NW1 2AA

870 Market Street, Ste 720
San Francisco
CA 94109

ISBN 1 84110019 6

First published 2001

Apart from any fair dealing for the purposes of research or private study, or criticism or review, as permitted under the UK Copyright Designs and Patents Act 1988, this publication may not be reproduced, stored, or transmitted, in any form or by any means, without the prior permission in writing of the publishers, or in the case of reprographic reproduction only in accordance with the terms of the licences issued by the appropriate Reproduction Rights Organisations outside the UK. Enquiries concerning reproduction outside the terms stated here should be sent to the publishers at the London address printed above.

The rights of Andrew Kingsnorth and Aljafri Majid to be identified as editors of this work has been asserted by them in accordance with the Copyright, Designs and Patents Act 1988.

The publisher makes no representation, express or implied, with regard to the accuracy of the information contained in this book and cannot accept any legal responsibility or liability for any errors or omissions that may be made.

A catalogue record for this book is available from the British Library.

Visit our website at:
www.greenwich-medical.co.uk
Distributed worldwide by Plymbridge Distributors Ltd and in the USA by JAMCO Distribution

Illustrations by Bryony Kingsnorth and David Gardner

Typeset by Phoenix Photosetting Ltd

Printed in China by RDC

Contents

Contributors   vii

Preface   ix

Foreword   xi

Section 1:   Operative Surgery

1. **Basic principles**   3
   W.E.G. Thomas

2. **Radiology**   23
   Simon Jackson

3. **Breast and soft tissue surgery**   39
   Roger Watkins

4. **Abdominal wall and gastrointestinal tract**   51
   Andrew Kingsnorth

5. **Anal and perianal diseases**   71
   Richard Welbourn

6. **Common urological operations**   85
   Mark Fordham

7. **Head and neck**   99
   Denis Wilkins

8. **Vascular surgery**   107
   Denis Wilkins

9. **Thoracic surgery**   119
   Aljafri Majid

10. **Orthopaedic surgery**   135
    Godfrey Charnley

11. **Neurosurgery**   145
    Terry Hope

12. **Plastic surgery** 153
Loshan Kangesu

Section 2:   Critical care and applied physiology

13. **Fluid balance** 175
Andrew T. Raftery

14. **Blood and reticuloendothelial system** 191
Adrian Copplestone, A.L.G. Peel

15. **Gastrointestinal system** 215
Craig W. Vickery, Derek Alderson

16. **Neuromuscular system** 231
Chris J. R. Parker

17. **Endocrine emergencies** 249
Devasenan Devendra, Terence J. Wilkin

Section 3:   Surgical pathology

18. **General concepts** 261
Paul Newman

19. **Cell growth, differentiation and degeneration** 273
Frances McCormick

20. **Handling of specimens** 289
Hannah Monaghan

21. **Cell damage and response to injury** 297
Mark E. F. Smith

22. **Blood and circulation** 309
Neil Robertson

23. **Infection in surgery** 323
Richard Cunningham, David Dance

Index 339

Contributors

Derek Alderson FRCS
Professor of Gastrointestinal Surgery
Division of Surgery
University of Bristol
Bristol Royal Infirmary
Bristol, UK

Godfrey Charnley FRCS (Ed), FRCS, Orth
Consultant Surgeon, & Honorary Senior Lecturer in Orthopaedics
  & Traumatology
Derriford Hospital
Plymouth, UK

Adrian Copplestone MB, BS (Hons), FRCP, FRCPath
Consultant Haematologist
Derriford Hospital
Plymouth, UK

Richard Cunningham BA, MB, BCh, BAO, MRCPath
Consultant Microbiologist
Department of Pathology
Derriford Hospital
Plymouth, UK

David A. B. Dance MB, ChB, MSc, FRCPath, DLSHTM
Consultant Microbiologist
Public Health Laboratory
Derriford Hospital
Plymouth, UK

Devasenan Devendra MBChB (Liverpool), MRCP (UK)
Clinical Lecturer in Medicine and Honorary Specalist Registrar in
  Diabetes Medicine & Endocrinology
University of Medicine
Derriford Hospital
Plymouth, UK

Mark Fordham FRCS
Consultant Urologist
Royal Liverpool University Hospital
Liverpool,UK

Terry Hope FRCS
Consultant Neurosurgeon
University Hospital
Queens Medical Centre
Nottingham, UK

Simon Jackson MBBS, FRCS (Eng), FRCR
Consultant Radiologist
Derriford Hospital
Plymouth, UK

Loshan Kangesu FRCS
Plastic Surgery Unit
St Andrews Centre at Broomfield Hospital
Chelmsford, UK

Andrew Kingsnorth BSc, MS, FRCS, FAS
Postgraduate Medical School
University of Plymouth
Derriford Hospital
Plymouth, UK

Aljafri Majid MBBS (Monash), BMedSc (Hons), FRCSEd,
FRCSEd (Cardiothoracics)
Professor, Department of Surgery
Faculty of Medicine
University of Malaysia
Kuala Lumpur, Malaysia

Hannah Monaghan MBBS, BSc, (Hons), MRCP
Specialist Registrar in Histopathology
Department of Pathology
University of Edinburgh Medical School
Medical School
Edinburgh

Frances McCormick MB BCh, MSc, MRCPath
Consultant Hisopathologist
Department of Histopathology
Derriford Hospital
Plymouth, UK

Paul Newman MB BS, DipRCPath (Dermatopathology),
  MRCPath, FRCPath
Consultant Pathologist
Head of Department
Department of Histopathology
Derrriford Hospital
Plymouth, UK

Christopher J. R. Parker MA, MB BChir, FRCA, MD
Consultant Anaesthetist
Department of Anaesthetics
Royal Liverpool University Hospital
Liverpool, UK

Anthony L. G. Peel MA, M Chir, FRCS, FRCS (ed)
Chairman of the Court of Examiners of The Royal College
  of Surgeons of England
Consultant Surgeon
North Tees General Hospital
Stockton-on-Tees, UK

Andrew T. Raftery FRCS
Consultant Surgeon
Sheffield Kidney Institute
Northern General Hospitals NHS Trust
Sheffield, UK

Neil J. Robertson BMed, Sci (Hons), BM, BS, MRCPath
Consultant Histopathologist
Derriford Hospital
Plymouth, UK

Mark E. F. Smith PhD, FRCPath, MRCP
Consultant Histopathologist
Derriford Hospital,
Plymouth, UK

W.E.G. Thomas FRCS
Consultant Surgeon
Royal Hallamshire Hospital
Sheffield, UK

Craig W. Vickery BM BCh, FRCS
Specialist Registrar in General Surgery
Bristol Royal Infirmary
Bristol, UK

Roger MalcolmWatkins MChir, FRCS
Consultant Surgeon
Derriford Hospital
Plymouth, UK

Richard Welbourn MD, FRCS
Consultant Gastrointestinal Surgeon
Taunton and Somerset Hospital
Taunton
Somerset, UK

Denis C. Wilkins MD, FRCS
Consultant General & Vascular Surgeon
Derriford Hospital
Plymouth, UK

Terence J. Wilkin FRCS
Professor of Medicine
Department of Medicine
Derriford Hospital
Plymouth, UK

Preface

This is the second in a series of textbooks designed to meet the needs of Basic Surgical Trainees as they undergo training and prepare for the MRCS examinations. The first book, *Fundamentals of Surgical Practice* was created to provide an overview for candidates undergoing Basic Surgical Training (BST). This second book is meant to complement *Fundamentals of Surgical Practice* by providing more information on basic operative surgery, critical care and surgical pathology.

Trainees undergoing Basic Surgical Training (BST) rotate within a preset time frame through a series of surgical postings designed to provide them with the necessary exposure to surgical conditions. They will need to very rapidly gain a good understanding of the nature of the diseases they are treating and to build a repertoire of surgical operations. Basic Surgical Trainees must also pass the very searching MRCS examinations and thus there is pressure on them to obtain not only experience and training but also a considerable amount of factual and practical knowledge in a limited space of time.

The examinations for the MRCS consist of two parts. The first barrier is the MCQ component and the second barrier is the Final Assessment which consists of three *vivas* and a clinical examination. The three *vivas* test the candidate's knowledge of the principles and details of Operative Surgery, Critical Care and Surgical Pathology. Candidates will need to demonstrate (in the short period of time given to them for the *viva*) that they have a firm grasp of the principles and are focused and ready for Higher Surgical Training.

We have thus prepared this book to assist the trainees as they go through their training posts as well as to help them prepare for the *vivas*. Whilst the information presented can be found separately in textbooks of operative surgery, intensive care and pathology, the problem for the trainee is to extract the information relevant to his level of experience and training. This can be very time consuming. We have therefore, as with *Fundamentals of Surgical Practice*, invited experienced specialists, surgeons and examiners to contribute to this book to provide their perspective on the various aspects of surgical management relevant to this level of training. The content of the book is based on the syllabus of the Royal Colleges of Surgeons and is divided into three sections corresponding to the three *vivas* in Operative Surgery, Perioperative/Critical Care and Surgical Pathology that make up the MRCS examinations. We have deliberately adopted a different format and style for each of these three sections in order to better handle the topics being covered.

It is hoped that this book will help fill the hiatus in the present literature available to Basic Surgical Trainees.

ANK
AAM
Plymouth and Kuala Lumpur
2001

Foreword

It is now three years since Aljafri and Andrew Kingsnorth's *Fundamentals of Surgical Practice* was published and it soon became a key textbook for trainees who were working for the Membership examinations of the British Colleges. It filled an important niche in the surgical library. It was aimed at the young doctors who embarked on the revamped surgical training that followed implementation of the Calman report. Their Senior House Officer posts became the real start of their surgical career. Traditional texts were found wanting and the very applied attitude of the new book was timely.

Now that the educational system has matured, there has been a new look at the continuum of experience. The examinations that lead to the MRCS diploma are the route to the Fellowship which marks the end of higher specialist training. This new book both supplements and complements its predecessor. Together they give an excellently comprehensive introduction to the generality of surgery. They give clear descriptions of diagnostic methods as well as operative procedures. The authors are all experts in their various fields and without exception have combined to give an insight into both principles and techniques.

Armed with these works, the SHO's will have a truly encyclopaedic companion to lead them on towards success in the Membership. The editors and authors can be congratulated in their achievement.

Patrick S Boulter D Univ, FRCSEd & Eng
FRCPEd & Lond FRACS
June 2001

Acknowledgements

The editors wish to acknowledge the following significant contributions to the production of this book. Dr Kathryn McLaren, Senior Lecturer in Pathology, University of Edinburgh for reading the chapters on Pathology and providing valuable constructive criticisms which helped in the editing process. Bryony Kingsnorth who was responsible for the majority of the art work with the help of David Gardner who was responsible for some of the more complex drawings including those of the limbs and their appendages. Nora Naughton who succeeded in not only directing the delivery of this book but also an addition to her own family. Finally, we would like to thank the publishers, Greenwich Medical Media, in particular Geoff Nuttall and Gavin Smith for making this project possible.

Section 1

Operative Surgery

1

Basic principles

Asepsis and sterilisation
  Definitions
  Asepsis
Handling tissue
  Connective tissue
  Muscle
  Tendons
  Cartilage
  Bone
  Bowel
Diathermy
  The principle of diathermy
  The effects of diathermy
  Complications of diathermy
Tourniquets
Suturing and suture materials
  Suture and ligature materials
  Suture techniques
  Alternatives to sutures
Dressings
  Types of dressing
  Cleaning agents

Drains
  Open drainage
  Closed drains
  Suction drainage
  Specialist use of drains
  Removal of drains
Bleeding
  Assessment of blood loss
  Correction of coagulopathy
  Replacement of blood loss
  Complications of blood transfusion
  Alternatives to blood for volume replacement
Microsurgery
  Principles of microsurgery
Surgical skills workshops
  Objectives
  Content
  Strategy for workshops

W. E. G. Thomas

ASEPSIS AND STERILISATION

Definitions

Asepsis: A process or procedure performed under minimal risk of contamination by microorganisms

Antisepsis: The removal or destruction of microorganisms, especially resident flora

Sterilisation: A process used to render an object free from viable microorganisms

Disinfection: A process used to diminish the number of viable microorganisms

Cleaning: A process that physically removes contamination but does not necessarily remove or destroy viable microorganisms

Asepsis

Lister was the first surgeon to introduce the concept of hand antisepsis when he poured carbolic acid over his hands prior to surgery and as a result dramatically reduced the incidence of surgical sepsis. A significant number of antiseptic agents are now in common use and the choice will depend on their characteristics and antibacterial activity (Table 1.1). In current practice, aseptic technique involves:

- preparation of the surgeon
- preparation of the patient
- preparation of the instruments and operative equipment.

Preparation of the surgeon

'Scrubbing up' involves hand washing (cleaning) which removes contaminants and transient flora from the hands, as well as the use of antiseptic handwash. The duration of 'scrubbing' has traditionally been five minutes although this will depend on the degree of contamination and the antiseptic agent employed.

Currently agents in common use tend to be based on chlorhexidine, iodophores or alcohol and the application of such agents has been shown to reduce the viable organism count by over 99%.

Frequent or vigorous scrubbing increases the bacterial yield above baseline counts due to desquamation. Care should therefore be taken to avoid desquamation when using a nailbrush on the skin. In normal circumstances jewellery, rings and nail varnish should be removed because bacterial counts are higher under rings than on normal skin. However, nail varnish does not appear to be a significant risk and some surgeons and nurses are unable to remove their wedding rings or other jewellery. Special care should therefore be taken during 'scrubbing' to ensure that maximal cleaning is undertaken at high-risk sites. The use of gloves is no substitute for careful 'scrubbing'. The moist warm atmosphere within latex gloves can encourage the proliferation of bacteria and therefore antiseptics with a long half-life should be used during 'scrubbing'. Puncture of gloves is a common occurrence and they should be changed immediately if such a perforation is detected. It is for this reason that many surgeons are now using the double-gloving technique in cases of high-risk cross-contamination both to and from the patient. Complications such as drying or cracking of the surgeon's skin or an allergic dermatitis may arise from the use of antiseptic agents. This is not only uncomfortable but also renders adequate cleaning of the skin more difficult. Similar allergies to the latex of the gloves can occur. Prevention of such complications may involve the use of barrier creams, non-allergenic handwash and latex-free gloves.

Preparation of the patient

The patient should be admitted to hospital before operation for as short a period of time as possible because a lengthy preoperative stay predisposes towards postoperative surgical sepsis due to the acquisition of antibiotic-resistant organisms. In certain high-risk procedures some surgeons advocate the use of preoperative hexachlorophene showering although this is not standard practice. Preoperative shaving of the operative site should also be undertaken as near to the time of surgery as possible using a disposable single-use razor. Clipping is deemed to be associated with a lower incidence of wound infection as is the use of depilatory cream. Skin preparation should be undertaken using standard antiseptic solutions such as 0.5% chlorhexidine in 70% spirit or 1% iodine in 70% alcohol and then allowed to dry. Care should be exercised

	Action	Safety	Speed of action	Persistence	Gram +ve	Gram −ve	Fungi	Viruses
Table 1.1 Antiseptic solutions								
Alcohols	Denaturation of protein	Safe but flammable	Rapid 1 minute scrub	Poor	Good	Good	Moderate	Moderate
Chlorhexidine	Disruption of cell wall	Safe but occasional allergic reactions	Moderate 3–5 minute scrub	Good	Good	Moderate	Poor	Moderate
Iodine/Iodophores	Penetrates cell wall and replaces contents with iodine	Skin dryness Moderate Irritation Allergies	Good 2–3 minute scrub	Moderate	Good	Moderate	Moderate	Moderate

with the use of diathermy when alcohol-based solutions are used; pooling can be the cause of diathermy burns.

Drapes are then applied to isolate the operative site. Currently there is a move to use disposable drapes that are water repellent. They are more expensive but do not absorb fluid and blood as cotton drapes do. When cotton drapes become sodden with blood and/or tissue fluid, they become more porous and provide an ideal culture medium that can predispose to infection. Furthermore, such sodden cotton drapes need very careful laundering and sterilisation and if soaked with infected blood, can prove a risk to laundry staff. The use of prophylactic antibiotics has served to further reduce the risk of surgical sepsis but should not be regarded as a substitute for scrupulous aseptic technique.

Preparation of the instruments and operative equipment

The preparation of instruments and operative equipment depends on the infection risk associated with their use. Operative instruments need full sterilisation as do all catheters and needles, while operating tables can be cleaned with antiseptic solutions. The method of sterilisation chosen depends on the nature of the equipment, the time available, the availability of the process, safety, cost and its suitability for wrapped items (Table 1.2). Some methods are only available as an industrial process, such as irradiation, while others are widely available such as glutaraldehyde, although its use is now being discouraged for the sake of the health and safety of staff. Certain processes are unsuitable for specific pieces of medical equipment, for example, autoclaving is inappropriate for fibreoptic endoscopes which are heat sensitive, and such factors must be taken into consideration when choosing

an appropriate method for each piece of equipment. Furthermore some processes sterilise, e.g. autoclaves, while others only disinfect, e.g. boiling. In patients in whom there is a high risk of transmissible spongiform encephalopathies such as Creutzfeld–Jacob Disease (CJD), the prions are remarkably resistant to heat, irradiation and chemical inactivation and in certain situations it is preferable to discard any potentially infected instruments. If this is not possible it is often recommended that items are autoclaved at temperatures of 134–138°C for not less than 18 minutes or for six cycles of three minutes.

HANDLING TISSUE

Each form of tissue in the body has its own characteristics and should therefore be handled appropriately. Knowledge of these handling characteristics is as much a part of good surgical technique as is suturing. Tissues that are handled carefully will heal more quickly because tissue damage is minimised, but an intimate knowledge of the different tissue characteristics is also required in order for the correct instruments and operative techniques to be employed.

Connective tissue

This term covers a wide spectrum of tissues from flimsy and filmy areolar tissue to strong and tough tendons and they vary not only with regard to strength but also as to blood supply, disposition of collagen fibres and the presence of fat. Flimsy areolar tissue can sometimes be separated by finger dissection but otherwise requires division with scissors. However, the most important

Table 1.2 Methods of sterilisation				
	Action	**Cost**	**Advantages**	**Disadvantages**
Autoclaves	Moist heat under pressure	Inexpensive	Rapid action Highly effective Suitable for wrapped items No toxic residue	Unsuitable for heat-sensitive items
Ovens	Dry heat Lengthy process	Inexpensive	Suitable for wrapped items	Unsuitable for heat-sensitive items
Ethylene oxide	Penetrates vegetative organisms	Expensive	Suitable for heat-sensitive items Highly penetrative Suitable for items with lumens Suitable for wrapped items	Toxic Irritant Carcinogenic Explosive and flammable Toxic residue
Glutaraldehyde	Sporicidal	Inexpensive	Suitable for heat-sensitive items Wide spectrum of activity	Toxic Irritant Not suitable for wrapped items Sensitising
Irradiation	Destroys by gamma rays or accelerated electrons	Expensive	Effective	Industrial process only Unsuitable for health service use

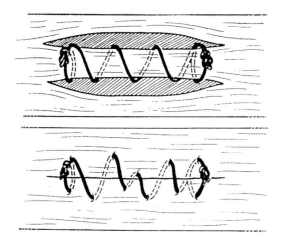

Figure 1.1 Closing an aponeurosis.

aspect of dissection of such tissue is to ensure that the dissection is undertaken in the correct plane. Areolar tissue rarely requires suturing but when condensations of such tissue form themselves into fascial layers they may be closed with fine absorbable sutures.

Tougher tissues such as aponeuroses need to be cut with firm scissors or a scalpel, preferably in the direction of the fibres. When closing such a defect the sutures should be placed at varying distances from the edge of the wound, unlike closing skin, in order to prevent the fibres parting (Figure 1.1). Tough connective tissue tends to heal slowly and therefore the suture material should be chosen with care to ensure that support for the closure is maintained for an adequate period of time. In abdominal closure of the rectus sheath, such support is usually deemed to be required indefinitely and many surgeons will therefore use non-absorbable sutures such as nylon.

Muscle

Muscle fibres run parallel to each other and therefore during dissection are either divided transversely or separated longitudinally. Separation of the fibres is always preferable where possible as this evokes minimal permanent tissue damage and afterwards the separated fibres can be approximated loosely with absorbable sutures. When muscle fibres are divided transversely the edges retract and any attempt to approximate them by simple sutures usually fails because the sutures cut through. When such approximation is required horizontal mattress sutures may be needed (see Figure 1.5C) although even these can cut out if too much tension exists. It is always preferable to close the muscle sheath, such as is done for the rectus abdominis muscle, rather than attempt to approximate the muscle fibres themselves, especially as the healing process will be by fibrosis and not by regeneration of the muscle fibres. Furthermore, if the nerve supply to one part of the divided muscle is damaged, that part will atrophy and be replaced by fibrous tissue.

Tendons

Tendons consist of aligned parallel collagen fibres that transmit the pull of muscles. When divided, the ends retract, especially that end attached to the muscle, and any repair will almost by definition be under a degree of tension. Initially materials like stainless steel were used for repair but currently suture techniques are used that employ non-absorbable suture material such as polypropylene. A tendon should be handled at all times with great care, often using a hypodermic needle rather than forceps that tend to crush the fibres (Figure 1.2A). The tendon ends should be trimmed square and neat and then sutured together using specially designed techniques such as the Kessler suture (Figure 1.2B). Once the suture has been suitably inserted, the tendon ends are approximated and the suture methodically tightened and ligated, burying the knot. A running suture can then be inserted around the paratenon (Figure 1.2C).

Cartilage

Cartilage may actually be divided by using a scalpel rather than a saw. It maintains a certain rigidity and thus closure is more an accurate approximation and suturing merely maintains the accuracy of the apposition. In certain situations cartilage may be sutured using firm needles but in other situations stitch holes may need to be drilled. Cartilage usually heals by the deposition of fibrocartilage and it is the intrinsic nature of the material that allows cartilage to be transplanted from one site to another within the body.

Bone

There is a tendency to regard bone as an inert tissue but in order to handle it correctly it must be recognised that it is dynamic and should be treated accordingly. Bone is remarkably strong and yet its characteristics change with age. In the young the bone consistency leads to fractures which have a particular characteristic, termed greenstick fracture, while in the elderly the cortical bone is thin and does not hold metal well and the cancellous bone is mainly replaced by fat.

Bone handling utilises the principle of 'minimal touch' to minimise infection risk, using instruments wherever possible rather than gloved hands. When it is necessary to handle bone with the hands, double gloving is recommended to protect against accidental glove puncture. Exposing a bone is a vital part of any orthopaedic procedure and care should be taken not to unnecessarily strip off the periosteum as the nutrient vessels reach the bone through this route and its deep layer is full of osteoblasts. The bone should be steadied with bone holders and, when required, division should be undertaken using a power saw. Hand saws or Gigli saws are still used in certain situations such as amputations but whatever instrument is used, it is important to ensure that the bone is cleanly divided and that the distal cortex is not fractured. Further shaping of bone may be achieved with

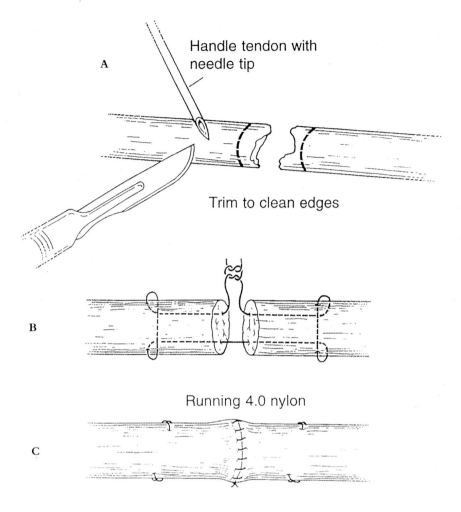

Handle tendon with needle tip

A

Trim to clean edges

B

Running 4.0 nylon

C

Figure 1.2 **A.** Handling the tendon. **B.** The Kessler suture. **C.** The running nylon paratenon suture.

osteotomes or chisels with the assistance of a mallet, while bone may be nibbled using rongeurs and ultimately smoothed using a file. External fixation requires specially designed external fixators and pin or screw insertion, while internal fixation depends on the use of screws, wiring, plates or intramedullary wires or nails and is beyond the remit of this chapter.

Whatever procedure is required, it is always essential to remember the dynamic nature of bone and it is this characteristic that also allows bone grafts, such as that from the iliac crest.

Bowel

Most of the intestine, except its mesenteric border, is enclosed on all surfaces by peritoneum. This serosal covering is tightly bound to the underlying muscular coat which is composed of longitudinal muscle (incomplete in the large bowel) and an inner circular muscle. Deep to this layer is the submucosa which is composed mainly of collagen. This layer is the most important for the surgeon because it holds sutures well and it is into this layer that the surgeon places sutures to form an anastomosis or a purse-string suture to bury an appendix stump. The mucosa deep to the submucosal layer does not hold suture material and hence many surgeons avoid placing sutures through this layer and adopt an anastomotic suturing method called extramucosal suturing. Because the collagenous submucosal layer is so tough, a single extramucosal interrupted anastomotic technique can be used for anastomoses throughout the length of the gastrointestinal tract.

When inflamed, the peritoneal covering of the bowel becomes thickened and oedematous and where it has been in contact with infected peritoneal fluid, plaques of granulation tissue form. Handling of bowel in this situation must be carried out with care because the serosal peritoneal covering is friable and easily torn and the tear may extend into the muscular coat and even breach the lumen, causing spillage of gastrointestinal contents with serious complications. Inflamed bowel is best handled with minimal traction and adherent loops are separated by blunt digital fracture.

Obstructed bowel must also be handled with care because the distension flattens out and thins the bowel wall, thereby weakening it and making it more vulnerable to rough handling. When delivering bowel into an abdominal wound, twisting of the base of the mesentery, which will occlude the blood supply and render loops of bowel ischaemic, should be avoided. Fluid-filled loops of bowel causing traction on the mesentery for the duration of the operation should be avoided for the same reason. If bowel is delivered into the wound for the formation of an anastomosis following resection, not only should surgeons ensure that the mesentery is not twisted, they should also ensure that exposed loops of bowel are kept warm and moist with packs placed over them.

The principles of good anastomotic technique are:

● ensure a good blood supply to the divided ends

● there should be no tension on the divided ends when they are approximated

● accurate apposition with evenly placed sutures, snugged down and not strangulating the tissues within the tied suture, i.e. approximation without strangulation.

DIATHERMY

For many years, short-wave diathermy has proved a most valuable and versatile aid to surgical technique. Its most common use is in securing haemostasis by means of coagulation; also, by varying the strength or waveform of the current produced, it can produce a cutting effect. Both these effects have been used in open surgery as well as in laparoscopic surgery or down intraluminal endoscopes, as in transurethral resection of the prostate. However, although diathermy is a valuable surgical tool, many accidents have occurred due to surgeons being unaware of or not fully conversant with the principles of its use. Most accidents are avoidable if the diathermy is used with care. It is therefore vital for a surgeon to have a sound understanding of the principles and practice of diathermy and how to avoid complications.

The principle of diathermy

When an electrical current passes through a conductor, some of its energy appears as heat. The heat produced depends upon:

● the intensity of the current

● the waveform of the current

● the electrical property of the tissues through which the current passes

● the relative sizes of the two electrodes.

There are two basic forms of diathermy in use: monopolar diathermy and bipolar diathermy (Figure 1.3). In monopolar diathermy, which is the most commonly used form, an alternating current is produced by a suitable generator and passed to the patient via an active electrode which has a very small surface area. The current then passes through the tissues and returns via a very

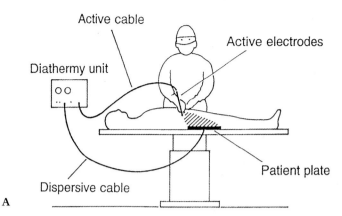

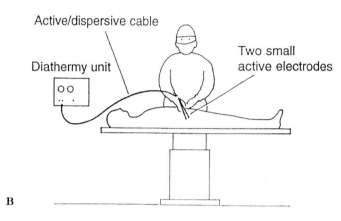

Figure 1.3 The principles of **A.** monopolar and **B.** bipolar diathermy.

large surface plate (the indifferent electrode) back to the earth pole of the generator. As the surface area of contact of the active electrode is so small by comparison to the indifferent electrode, the concentrated powerful current produces heat at the operative site. However, the large surface area electrode of the patient plate spreads the returning current over a wide surface area, so it is less concentrated and produces little heat.

In bipolar diathermy, the two active electrodes are usually represented by the tips of the limbs of a pair of diathermy forceps. The tips of the forceps are therefore active and current flows between them and only the tissue held between the limbs of the forceps heats up. This form of diathermy is used when it is essential that there is no risk of burning or passing current through the surrounding tissue.

The effects of diathermy

Diathermy can be used for three purposes.

1. Coagulation: the sealing of blood vessels.

2. Fulguration: the destructive coagulation of tissues with charring.

3. Cutting: used to divide tissues during bloodless surgery.

In coagulation, a heating effect leads to cell death by dehydration and protein denaturation. Bleeding is therefore stopped by a combination of the distortion of the walls of the blood vessel, coagulation of the plasma proteins, dried and shrunken dead tissue and stimulation of the clotting mechanism. In an ideal situation, intracellular temperature should not reach boiling during coagulation, because if it does an unwanted cutting effect may be experienced.

Cutting occurs when sufficient heat is applied to the tissue to cause cell water to explode into steam. The cut current is a continuous waveform and the monopolar diathermy is most effective when the active electrode is held a very short distance from the tissues. This allows an electrical discharge to arc across the gap, creating a series of sparks which produce the high temperatures needed for cutting.

In fulguration the diathermy matching is set to coagulation and a higher effective voltage is used to make larger sparks jump an air gap, thus fulgurating the tissues. This can continue until carbonisation or charring occurs. The voltage and power output can be varied by adjusting the duration of bursts of current as well as its intensity to give a combination of both cutting and coagulation. This is known as blended current and provides both forms of diathermy activity.

Complications of diathermy

Electrocution

Diathermy machines today are manufactured to very high safety standards and thus the risk of any part of the machine becoming live with mains current is minimised. However, as with any such instrument, there must be regular and expert servicing.

Explosion

Sparks from the diathermy can ignite any volatile or inflammable gas or fluid within the theatre. Alcohol-based skin preparations can catch fire if they are allowed to pool on or around the patient. Furthermore, diathermy should not be used in the presence of explosive gases, including those which may occur naturally in the colon, especially after certain forms of bowel preparation such as mannitol.

Burns

These are the most common type of diathermy accidents in both open and endoscopic surgery. They occur when the current flows in some way other than that in which the surgeon intended and are far more common in monopolar than bipolar diathermy. Burns may occur as a result of:

- faulty application of the indifferent electrode with inadequate contact area

- the patient being earthed by touching any metal object, e.g.

the Mayo table, the bar of an anaesthetic screen, an exposed metal armrest or a leg touching the metal stirrups used in maintaining the lithotomy position

- faulty insulation of the diathermy leads, either due to cracked insulation or instruments such as towel clips pinching the cable

- inadvertent activity such as the accidental activation of the foot pedal

- accidental contact of the active electrode with other metal instruments such as retractors, instruments or towel clips.

Channelling

Heat is produced wherever the current intensity is greatest. Normally this would be at the tip of the active electrode but if current passes up a narrow channel or pedicle to the active electrode, enough heat may be generated within this channel or pedicle to coagulate the tissues. This can prove disastrous; for example:

- coagulation of the penis in a child undergoing circumcision

- coagulation of the spermatic cord when the electrode is applied to the testis.

In such situations, diathermy should not be used or if it is necessary, then bipolar diathermy should be employed.

Interference with cardiac pacemakers

Diathermy currents can interfere with the working of a cardiac pacemaker with the obvious potential danger to the patient's life. Modern pacemakers are designed to be inhibited by high-frequency interference, so that the patient may receive no pacing stimulation at all while the diathermy is in use. Certain demand pacemakers may revert to the fixed rate of pacing and therefore it would be important for the anaesthetist to have a magnet available so that these can be reset if necessary. In most cases it is therefore wise to take precautions and to use bipolar diathermy wherever possible. If monopolar diathermy is required, then the patient plate should be sited as far away from the pacemaker as possible so that the path of the current does not pass through the heart or the vicinity of the pacemaker.

Monitoring of the heart rate should be undertaken throughout the operation and a defibrillator should always be available in case a dysrhythmia develops at any time.

Laparoscopic surgery

Diathermy burns are a particular hazard of laparoscopic surgery due to the nature of the visibility of the instrumentation and the actual structure of the instruments used. Such burns may occur because of:

- diathermy of the wrong structure because of lack of clarity of vision or misidentification

- faulty insulation of any of the laparoscopic instruments or equipment

- intraperitoneal contact of the diathermy with another metal instrument while activating the pedal

- inadvertent activation of the pedal while the diathermy tip is out of vision of the camera

- retained heat in the diathermy tip touching susceptible structures such as bowel

- capacitance coupling (Figure 1.4).

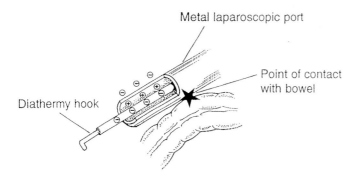

Figure 1.4 Capacitance coupling.

This is a phenomenon in which a capacitor is created by having an insulator sandwiched between two metal electrodes. This can be created in situations where there is a metal laparoscopic port and the diathermy hook is passed through it. The insulation of the diathermy hook acts as the sandwiched insulator and by means of electromagnetic induction, the diathermy current flowing through the hook can induce a current in the metal port, which can potentially damage intraperitoneal structures. In most cases this current is dissipated from the metal port through the abdominal wall but if a plastic cuff is used, this dissipation of current does not occur and the danger of capacitance coupling is significantly increased. Therefore, metal ports should never be used with a plastic cuff. The danger of capacitance coupling can be completely prevented by using entirely plastic ports.

TOURNIQUETS

For certain operations on the limbs, a bloodless field is essential for careful and safe surgery. In these situations it may be advisable to utilise a tourniquet. The principles behind its use include emptying the limb of blood by elevating it for five minutes and then applying a tourniquet around the proximal aspect of the limb over several layers of cotton wool padding or orthopaedic wool. Besides elevation, the limb can be exsanguinated by first applying a 3" Esmarch bandage, starting at the tips of the digits and over-

lapping each turn proximally, thus further emptying the limb of blood. Other sleeve-like appliances are now available to achieve the same purpose. The tourniquet is then inflated to just above systemic arterial blood pressure in the upper limb and to twice the systemic arterial blood pressure for the lower limb. The Esmarch bandage is then unwound. It is important to record the time at which the tourniquet was applied as it is conventional practice to limit tourniquet time to one hour. If necessary, the tourniquet may be released after one hour and subsequently reinflated if further operative time is required. At the end of the procedure the tourniquet is released before the wound is closed to ensure that all bleeding points have been secured.

The use of a tourniquet is contraindicated in limbs affected by vascular disease resulting in either ischaemia or venous thrombosis. Furthermore, tourniquets should be avoided in many cases of trauma in which there is soft tissue injury, infection or bony fractures.

The tourniquet principle is utilised in the technique of a Bier's block for the arm. This technique involves insertion of an intravenous cannula into a suitable vein of the proscribed limb and in addition, it is wise to have a similar cannula in the opposite limb for vascular access throughout the procedure. Once the cannulas have been sited a double cuff tourniquet is applied to the upper arm, the limb is then elevated and exsanguinated using an Esmarch bandage. The proximal tourniquet is then inflated to above arterial pressure and the Esmarch bandage removed. Thirty ml of a suitable local anaesthetic, e.g. 0.5% prilocaine, is then injected through the intravenous cannula. The second (distal) cuff should then be inflated to above arterial pressure. Some of the prilocaine will have by then infiltrated below the second cuff, producing a degree of anaesthesia at the cuff site and reducing discomfort for the patient. The double cuff technique is to ensure that if one cuff should fail, the prilocaine will not be allowed back into the circulation in a potentially dangerous bolus. Sufficient time must be given for the anaesthetic to become fixed within the tissues. Early release of the tourniquet can have disastrous effects, causing arrhythmias and even fits. Thus neither cuff should be deflated before 15 minutes and many surgeons prefer to keep the cuffs inflated for at least 30 minutes to avoid this situation.

SUTURING AND SUTURE MATERIALS

The suturing of any wound or anastomosis needs to take into consideration the site and tissues involved and the suture material and the technique should be chosen accordingly. There is no such product as the ideal suture and there is no universal suture technique that would be appropriate for all situations. Furthermore, the correct choice of technique and material will never compensate for inadequate operative technique and for any wound closure there should be a good blood supply and no tension.

The ideal suture for all situations has yet to be produced. However, many of the desired characteristics are listed in Box 1.1.

Box 1.1   The characteristics of an ideal suture

Ease of handling
Predictable tensile strength
Secure knotting ability
Pulls through tissues easily
Sterile
Inexpensive
No significant tissue reaction
Non-capillary
Non-allergenic
Non-carcinogenic
Non-electrolytic
Non-shrinking in tissues

Certain procedures require specific characteristics of the suture material; for example, vascular anastomoses require smooth, non-absorbable, non-elastic material while biliary anastomoses require an absorbable material that will not promote tissue reaction or stone formation. For absorbable material, the time for which wound support is maintained will vary according to the tissues into which it is inserted. Furthermore, certain tissues require wound support for longer than others, such as muscular aponeuroses as compared with subcutaneous tissues. It is therefore crucial for the surgeon to select the suture material and suture technique that will most effectively achieve the desired objective for each wound closure or anastomosis.

Suture and ligature materials

For any suture material, there are five specific characteristics to be considered.

1. Physical structure
2. Strength
3. Tensile behaviour
4. Absorbability
5. Biological behaviour

Physical structure

Suture material may be monofilament or multifilament. Monofilament suture material is smooth and tends to slide through tissues easily without any sawing action but requires greater skill in knot formation. Such material can be easily damaged by gripping it tightly with a needle holder or forceps and this can lead to fracture of the suture. Multifilament or braided sutures are much easier to knot but the suture material is not smooth. Such material has a surface area several thousand times that of monofilament sutures. In the interstices between the multifilaments bacteria may lodge and, together with capillary action, may be responsible for persistent infection or sinuses. In order to overcome some of these problems, certain materials are produced as a braided suture which is coated with silicone in order to make its surface smooth.

Strength

The strength of a suture material depends upon its thickness, the material it is made of and its behaviour in the tissues. Suture material thickness is classified according to its diameter in tenths of a millimetre (Table 1.3). However, the figure assigned to certain sutures also depends on the nature of the material – catgut and non-absorbable materials such as prolene differ in their designations. The strength of a suture can be expressed as the force required to break it when the two ends are pulled apart. This is known as tensile strength but is only a useful approximation of strength in the tissues, as what really matters is the strength of the material *in vivo*. Absorbable sutures show a decay of this strength with the passage of time and although a material may last in the tissues for the period stated in the manufacturer's data sheet, the tensile strength cannot be relied on for this entire period *in vivo*. Materials such as catgut last for several weeks. Even non-absorbable sutures do not maintain their strength indefinitely. Non-absorbable materials of synthetic origin, such as polypropylene, probably retain their tensile strength indefinitely and do not change in mass in the tissues. However, it is possible for them to fracture. Non-absorbable materials of biological origin such as silk will definitely fragment with time and lose their strength. Such materials therefore should never be used in vascular anastomoses because of the risk of late fistula formation.

Tensile behaviour

Suture materials behave differently depending on their deformability and flexibility. Some may be elastic and the material will return to its original length once the pull is released or it may be plastic in which case this phenomenon does not occur. Sutures may be deformable in that a circular cross-section may be converted to an oval shape or they may be more rigid or have the somewhat irritating capacity to kink and coil. Many synthetic

Table 1.3 Suture sizes

Metric number	Catgut	Non-absorbable (diameter of the suture in tenths of a millimetre)
0.1	–	–
0.2	–	10/0
0.3	–	9/0
0.4	–	8/0
0.5	8/0	7/0
0.7	7/0	6/0
1	6/0	5/0
1.5	5/0	4/0
2	4/0	3/0
3	3/0	2/0
3.5	2/0	0
4	0	1
5	1	2
6	2	3 + 4
7	3	5
8	4	6

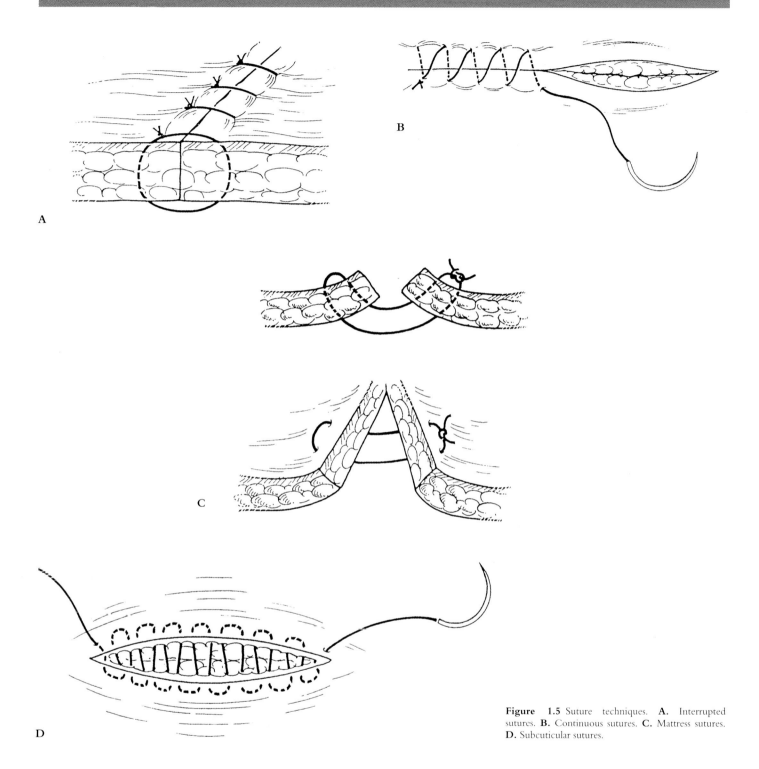

Figure 1.5 Suture techniques. **A.** Interrupted sutures. **B.** Continuous sutures. **C.** Mattress sutures. **D.** Subcuticular sutures.

materials demonstrate 'memory' so that they keep curling up in the pattern in which they were packaged. A sharp but gentle pull on the suture material helps to diminish this 'memory' but the more 'memory' a suture material has, the less dependable is the knot security. Therefore knotting technique also plays a significant role in the tensile strength of any suture line and it is important to recognise that sutures lose 50% of their strength at the knot.

Absorbability

Suture materials may be absorbable or non-absorbable and this property should be taken into consideration when choosing suture materials for specific sites. Sutures for use in the biliary tract or urinary tract need to be absorbable in order to minimise the risk of stone formation. However, a vascular anastomosis requires a non-absorbable material and it is wise to avoid braided material as platelet adherence may predispose to distal embolisation. Non-absorbable materials tend to be preferred where persistent strength is required and, as an artificial graft or prosthesis never heals fully or integrates into a host artery, a persistent monofilament suture material such as polypropylene is universally used.

Biological behaviour

The biological behaviour of suture material within the tissues depends on the origin of the raw materials. Biological or natural sutures such as catgut are proteolysed but this involves a process that is not entirely predictable and can cause local irritation. Man-made synthetic polymers are hydrolysed and their disappearance in the tissues is more predictable. However, the presence of infection, urine or faeces influences the final result and renders the outcome once again unpredictable. There is also some evidence that in the gut, cancer cells may accumulate at sites where sutures persist and this may be a cause of local recurrence. For this reason, synthetic materials that have a greater predictability and elicit minimal tissue reaction may be a preferable option in cancer surgery.

Suture techniques

There are four frequently used suture techniques (Figure 1.5).

Interrupted sutures (Figure 1.5A)

Interrupted sutures require the needle to be inserted at right angles to the incision and then to pass through both aspects of the suture line and exit again at right angles. It is important for the needle to be rotated through the tissues rather than to be dragged through in order to avoid an unnecessarily large needle hole. As a guide, the distance from the entry point of the needle to the edge of the wound should be approximately the same as the depth of the tissue being sutured and each successive suture should be placed at twice this distance apart (Figure 1.6). Each suture should reach into the depths of the wound and be placed at right angles to the axis of the wound. In linear wounds it is sometimes easier to insert the middle suture first and then to complete the closure by successively inserting sutures, halving the remaining deficits in the wound length.

Continuous sutures (Figure 1.5B)

For a continuous suture the first pass of the needle is in an identical manner to an interrupted suture but the rest of the sutures are inserted in a continuous manner until the far end of the wound is reached. Each throw of the continuous suture should be inserted at right angles to the wound and this will mean that the externally observed suture material will lie diagonal to the axis of the wound. It is important to have an assistant who will follow the suture, keeping it at the same tension in order to avoid either purse-stringing the wound by applying too much tension or leaving the suture material too slack. There is more danger of pro-

ducing too much tension by using too little suture length than there is of leaving the suture line too slack. Postoperative oedema will often take up this slack in the suture material. It has been estimated that for abdominal wall closure the optimal length of the suture material is four times the length of the wound to be closed.[1] At the far end of the wound, this suture line should be secured either by using an Aberdeen knot or by tying the free end to the loop of the last suture to be inserted.

Mattress sutures (Figure 1.5C)

Mattress sutures may be either vertical or horizontal and tend to be used to produce either eversion or inversion of a wound edge. The initial suture is inserted as for an interrupted suture but then the needle either moves horizontally or vertically and traverses both edges of the wound once again, as demonstrated in Figure 1.5C. Such sutures are very useful in producing accurate approximation of wound edges, especially when the edges to be anastomosed are irregular in depth or disposition.

Subcuticular sutures (Figure 1.5D)

This technique is used in skin where a cosmetic appearance is important and where the skin edges may be approximated easily. The suture material used may be either absorbable or non-absorbable. For non-absorbable sutures the ends may be secured by means of a collar and bead or tied loosely over the wound. When absorbable sutures are used the ends may be secured using a buried knot. Small bites of the subcuticular tissues are taken on alternate sides of the wound and then gently pulled together, thus approximating the wound edges without the risk of the cross-hatched markings of interrupted sutures.

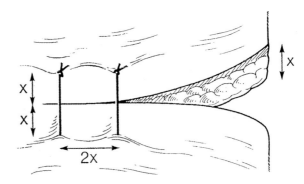

Figure 1.6 The positioning of interrupted sutures.

Alternatives to sutures

Several alternatives to standard suture materials are now available for the closure of wounds.

Self-adhesive tapes or Steristrips may be used for the skin, in situations where there is no tension or too much moisture.

Tissue adhesive or glue is also available based upon a solution of n-butyl-2 cyanoacrylate monomer. When applied to a wound, it polymerises to form a firm adhesive bond but once again the wound needs to be clean, dry and under no tension.

Staples of stainless steel may also be used, either applied individually for skin closure or as part of an integral device used to fashion anastomoses during either open or laparoscopic operative procedures. Such staples or devices have the advantage of being quick and easy to use but the disadvantage of being more expensive. Furthermore, it is vital for the surgeon to be familiar with both the principles and the practice behind each stapling device that is used. Devices are available for end-to-end anastomoses (EEA), transverse anastomoses (TA) and intraluminal anastomoses (IA) as well as those that will staple-ligate blood vessels. Almost all the stapling devices have now been modified and adapted to allow them to be used down a laparoscopic cannula for the purpose of intracorporeal stapled anastomoses during minimal access surgery.

DRESSINGS

The aim of any dressing is to promote and encourage wound healing and reduce the risk of infection. Dressings are therefore selected based upon the nature and site of the wound. During healing, a wound changes in characteristic and so should the dressings. Clean wounds require infrequent dressing changes while sloughy exuding wounds and cavities may require frequent changes. Wounds may heal by primary intention after suture closure or may be left open to heal by secondary intention. Open wounds that heal by secondary intention may also be subdivided into:

- healthy granulating wounds
- overexuberant hypergranulating wounds
- wounds containing slough
- infected wounds containing slough
- wounds that have a black, necrotic, dried eschar which may mask underlying sepsis.

Types of dressing

Conventional dressings

Conventional dressings consist of a non-adherent material covered by a more absorbent material such as gauze or wool. These may be kept in place with an adhesive tape or bandage, while some proprietary products have the adhesive and absorbent layers bonded together. Such dressings are indicated for wounds that are healing by primary intention after suturing and in situations where the infection risk is minimal and there is no slough or discharge. These dressings are easy to apply but are not indicated for moist wounds.

Polyurethane dressings

These are semiocclusive dressings that are permeable to vapour and gases but not to water or bacteria. They are often made with an adhesive backing and their main disadvantage is the accumulation of exudate or blood under the dressing. However, studies have shown that moist wounds heal faster than dry ones and furthermore, under such dressings the wound surface becomes hypoxic with an acidic pH. This encourages autolysis of slough and at the same time promotes angiogenesis, fibroblast proliferation and epidermal migration.

Hydrocolloid dressings

These dressings consist of an adhesive hydrocolloid with a semiocclusive foam and plastic film exterior. The hydrocolloid absorbs the exudate and forms a yellow liquefied gel that may easily be confused with pus. However, if the exudate is too heavy these dressings are inadequate. In addition, they are not ideal for deep cavity wounds. However, hydrocolloid paste and granules are available for such cavity wounds in situations where they can be easily removed; a secondary dressing is used to cover the paste or granules.

Osmotic agents

These agents work on the same principle as honey that was used in ancient times. By means of osmosis they help debride slough from the wound and create a moist wound environment. However, a secondary dressing is required on top of such agents.

Hydrogels

These are aqueous gels that contain a starch polymer matrix which absorbs excess exudate and once again produces a moist environment. As with osmotic agents, a secondary dressing is required. Such agents may be used on dry, sloughy or necrotic wounds but are unsuitable if the exudate is too heavy. If left too long in the wound, hydrogels dry and become difficult to remove and furthermore can cause maceration of the surrounding skin.

Alginates

These substances are derived from seaweed and release calcium ions on contact with wound fluid which exchanges with sodium ions in the exudate to form a fibrous gel. Release of calcium also activates the clotting cascade, thus assisting haemostasis. A secondary dressing is usually required. Alginates are useful for wounds that have a significant exudate.

Foams

These agents have an inner hydrophilic area and an outer hydrophobic layer. For cavity wounds silastic foam is available that will conform to the shape of the defect. This can be changed at regular intervals, allowing a smaller foam plug to be inserted as the defect closes.

Saline soaks

This very simple form of dressing is still favoured by many surgeons to encourage rapid desloughing but is only suitable for patients under regular nursing supervision because the dressing needs to be changed every 4–6 hours.

Cleaning agents

Normal saline (0.9% sodium chloride) continues to be the most suitable universal cleaning agent. It is not harmful to normal tissue and is readily available as well as being cheap. Most antiseptics are harmful to normal tissue and although EUSOL (Edinburgh University Solution Of Lime) has been popular in the past for infected and sloughy wounds, it has an adverse effect on granulation tissue and should not be used on clean granulating wounds. For infected wounds, solutions such as aqueous chlorhexidine (0.05%) and povidone iodine (10%) may be beneficial. 3% hydrogen peroxide may help dislodge small particles of debris as it effervesces but its use has fallen out of favour.

DRAINS

Drains are inserted to allow fluid or air that might collect at an operation site or in a wound to drain freely to the surface. The fluid to be drained may include blood, serum, pus, urine, faeces, bile or lymph. Drains may also allow wound irrigation in certain specific incidences. The adequate drainage of fluid collections prevents the development of cavities or spaces that may delay wound healing. Wounds may drain by gravity, by the pressure within a cavity such as an abscess or by means of suction applied to the drain. However, the value of drains in certain situations remains controversial. Protagonists suggest that the drainage of any fluid collection removes the potential for infection while the antagonists claim that the presence of drains increases the susceptibility to contamination and secondary infection. They also suggest that much of the fluid discharge is a reaction of the tissues to the presence of a foreign body. It is therefore important to have clearly defined objectives before placing any drain and to ensure that the most appropriate drain is used to achieve these objectives.

Drains may be superficial, e.g. in a wound, or deep, e.g. intraperitoneal, intracavity or intraluminal. In addition, they may be open, thus draining into a dressing or a bag open to the air, or they may be closed, draining into a sterile closed and self-contained system.

Open drainage

Simple wicks

The simplest form of drain is sterile cotton gauze inserted into an abscess cavity or laid in an open superficial fistula track. The gauze may be inserted dry but many surgeons prefer it to be moistened, either with isotonic saline or some other antiseptic solution. Such dressings need to be changed regularly but even so may become adherent to granulation tissue and delay wound healing. However, such regular changing will minimise the penetration of infecting organisms and daily changes are recommended.

Corrugated polyethylene drain

These drains may be used both to drain a superficial skin wound and for deep drainage. In the past rubber drains were used which caused significant tissue reaction and therefore the drain track left by such material persisted longer compared with more inert materials and erosion into neighbouring viscera was a significant risk. Corrugated drains manufactured from polyethylene are now the inert material of choice. The drain should be fixed in site by a suture that transfixes the drain and the skin. Convention dictates that a safety pin is placed through the outer end of the drain to prevent it slipping inwards. Should this happen, it is easily identified by means of X-ray.

Yeates drain (Figure 1.7)

This is a variant of a corrugated drain that is made up of a series of capillary tubes and is also usually made of polyethylene. Its indications are similar to the corrugated drain.

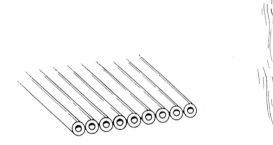

Figure 1.7 A Yeates drain.

Penrose drain

This consists of a piece of very thin-walled rubber tubing with a gauze wick threaded through the centre of the tube. Fluid then can track up to the gauze in the centre of the tubing or along the track once the drain has been removed. It is not as rigid as either a corrugated drain or a Yeates drain.

Closed drains

Silastic tube drain

Silastic drains are made of polymeric silicone and provoke very little tissue reaction. Therefore, once removed, the track closes rapidly. A closed silastic tube drain system is useful for intraperitoneal drainage such as for an anastomosis deep within the pelvis.

Red rubber tube drain

Such a drain may be required in certain specific situations such as draining a chronic abscess cavity, empyema or hepatic abscess where a strong fibrous reaction around the drain tract is required. In order to create a closed system of drainage, it would need to be connected to a sterile bag to drain the secretions.

Suction drainage

These systems consist of a fine tube with many holes, one end of which is attached to an evacuated container which provides the suction. This suction is constant and such systems are useful for draining blood after procedures such as a mastectomy or thyroidectomy. It may also be used to drain deep spaces such as around a vascular anastomosis but has little use in the peritoneal cavity as it will often suck omentum into the pores of the tubing.

Shirley sump drain (Figure 1.8)

This is a suction drain with a double lumen. The intake tube supplies air to the bottom of the main tube to which suction is applied. This system allows suction to be utilised while the flow of air prevents the tube from getting blocked.

Specialist use of drains

Chest drains

These are indicated for a pneumothorax, pleural effusion, haemothorax or to prevent the collection of fluid or air after thoracotomy. Once the drain has been inserted it should be connected to an underwater sealed drain (Figure 1.9). This system allows air to leave the pleural cavity but cannot draw it back in with the negative pressure that is created in the intrathoracic cavity. During the respiratory process it should be checked that the meniscus of the fluid is swinging to ensure that the tube is not blocked. Suction can be applied to the venting tube at the bottle whenever significant drainage of fluid or air is expected. 10–20 mmHg is adequate to obtain a gentle flow of bubbles from the chest cavity.

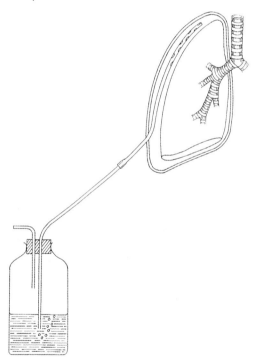

Figure 1.9 An underwater seal chest drain.

T-tube drains (Figure 1.10)

After exploration of the common bile duct, a T-tube may be inserted into the duct which allows bile to drain while the sphincter of Oddi is in spasm postoperatively. Once the sphincter relaxes bile drains normally down the bile duct and into the duodenum. To assist bile flow, the lumen of the limb of the T-tube which will lie within the duct can be converted into a gutter by removing a sliver of the circumference, which also facilitates removal.

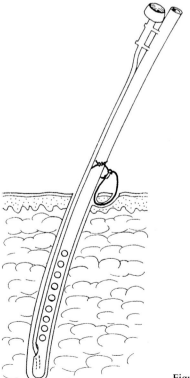

Figure 1.8 A Shirley sump drain.

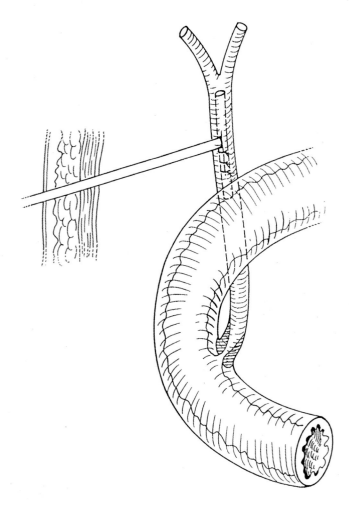

Figure 1.10 A biliary T-tube.

Guided drainage

For many intraabdominal collections or abscesses, drains may be inserted under ultrasound or CT control. In order for such drains to remain *in situ*, the end is often fashioned with a pigtail to discourage inadvertent removal.

Removal of drains

The drain should be removed when it is no longer required, as prolonged placement can itself predispose to fluid collections as a result of tissue reaction. Once again, it should be stressed how important it is to define the objective of each individual drain and to ensure that once that objective has been met, the drain is removed. The following principles are recommended.

- Drains put in to cover perioperative bleeding may usually be removed within 24–48 hours, e.g. thyroidectomy.

- Drains put in to drain serous collections can usually be removed after five days, e.g. mastectomy.

- Drains put in because of pus or contamination should be left until the infection is subsiding or the drainage is minimal.

- Drains put in to cover intestinal anastomoses should remain in for 5–7 days. However, it should be stressed that a drain does not prevent intestinal leakage; it will help any such leakage to drain externally rather than to produce life-threatening peritonitis.

- Common bile duct T-tubes should remain in for 10 days. However, once the T-tube cholangiogram has shown that there is free flow of bile into the duodenum and that there are no retained stones, some surgeons like to clamp the T-tube prior to removal. The 10-day period is required to ensure that the T-tube track is sealed off from the peritoneal cavity so that there is no danger of biliary peritonitis after removal.

- A suction drain should have the suction taken off prior to removal.

- During removal of a chest drain, patients should be asked to breathe in and hold their breath, thus doing a Valsalva manoeuvre. In this way no air is sucked into the pleural cavity during removal of the tube. Once the drain is out a previously inserted purse-string suture should be tied.

BLEEDING

Bleeding may either be part of the presenting features of a patient's condition, such as gastrointestinal haemorrhage, ruptured aortic aneurysm or trauma, or it may occur perioperatively as a result of the surgical procedure itself. Postoperative bleeding may be:

- primary haemorrhage, e.g. a slipped ligature or damaged vessel at the time of operation

- reactionary haemorrhage, which occurs within 24 hours of operation. It is caused either by a rise in blood pressure or a reversal of vasospasm, which results in ooze from blood vessels not secured at the time of surgery

- secondary haemorrhage, which may occur up to one week or more after operation and may be caused by infection or malignancy.

Assessment of blood loss

Careful monitoring of a patient's pulse, blood pressure, central venous pressure and haemoglobin may be helpful in indicating the degree of blood loss. However, the ability of the patient to compensate, which depends on age, makes this an imprecise science. Intraoperative blood loss may be assessed by collecting and weighing swabs. During lengthy procedures, intraoperative measurement of circulating haemoglobin may be appropriate. However, the true haemoglobin level will not be apparent until the changes in intravascular volume associated with the metabolic response to surgery are completed. Postoperative measurement of blood in drains is a notoriously inaccurate method for assessing blood loss.

Correction of coagulopathy

In those cases where coagulopathy exists in the presence of major haemorrhage, it is important wherever possible first to arrest the bleeding surgically and then to administer clotting factors and platelets. Fresh frozen plasma contains most of the required clotting factors but is deficient in fibrinogen and factor VIII. However, cryoprecipitate contains both factor VIII and fibrinogen and both may be required in some cases of disseminated intravascular coagulation (DIC). Platelets are available as concentrates and may be indicated in those patients with platelet deficiencies or DIC.

Replacement of blood loss

During surgery blood loss of less than 1.5 litres may be corrected by infusion of crystalloid solutions. However, in cases of preoperative anaemia or continued loss, blood transfusion is usually required. Whole blood is lost during intraoperative haemorrhage but whole blood is rarely available to replace it. Most blood for transfusion is provided as packed cells and each unit of 450 ml may be expected to raise the circulating haemoglobin by 1 g/dl in a stable patient. Transfused blood should be fully crossmatched and compatible, although in extreme emergency situations, there may be insufficient time for this to be accomplished. In such an emergency if the patient's ABO and Rhesus group is known, then grouped blood that has not been crossmatched may be used, but if an immediate transfusion is required then universal donor blood, which is O Rhesus negative, will have to be given.

Autologous blood transfusion, which is collected prior to surgery, is not possible for those patients requiring emergency operations. However, for elective surgery, because of the potential risks of blood transfusion this option is becoming more desirable. In those patients undergoing major procedures in which there is significant blood loss, it may be possible to salvage blood during the procedure and to reinfuse it. The cell-saver is a machine which allows such blood to be collected, the cells to be washed, resuspended and then reinfused. However, such equipment requires expertise to be used efficiently. Other systems may be simpler to use, including those in which surgical suction allows lost blood to be collected in a special container which has been primed with heparin. When the container is full the heparinised blood can be reinfused through a filter. This can apply to blood collected from the thoracic or abdominal cavities but is absolutely contraindicated if there is any contamination of the surgical field. Similarly, the technique should not be used when malignancy is present or suspected.

Complications of blood transfusion

Acute haemolytic transfusion reactions

These are the most severe complications of blood transfusion which are caused by the administration of incompatible blood. Regrettably, the most common cause is administrative failure resulting in blood being given to the wrong patient, rather than serological errors in the laboratory. As little as 5–10 ml of incompatible blood can cause hypotension, fever, pain and haemoglobinuria. Continued infusion of the incompatible blood can lead to shock, acute renal failure, DIC and even death. When an acute haemolytic reaction is suspected the transfusion should be stopped to exclude a clerical error and the blood returned to the laboratory, together with blood and urine samples from the patient for analysis and rechecking of compatibility. Careful monitoring should be undertaken to diagnose and treat any threatened or established renal failure and DIC.

Febrile non-haemolytic reactions

These are relatively common and affect up to 2% of all recipients of blood transfusion. They particularly affect those sensitised to leucocyte antigens by previous transfusions or pregnancy. The patient suffers from shivering and a pyrexia about 30–60 minutes after the start of the transfusion. Most patients can be managed by slowing the transfusion and administering an antipyretic such as paracetamol.

Infective complications

Donor screening has reduced the risk of infection by many organisms but the hazard still persists if donation occurs before seroconversion. The risks are also greater when products are prepared from pooled donations. Routine screening is undertaken for hepatitis B and C, human immunodeficiency virus (HIV) and *Treponema pallidum* (syphilis). More recently the risk of transmission of other viruses (cytomegalovirus and parvovirus) and the potential risk of transmitting prions, e.g. Creutzfeldt–Jakob disease (CJD) and new variant CJD, have caused concern.

Transfusion-related bacterial sepsis fortunately is uncommon due to the advent of closed sterile blood collecting systems. However, its incidence should not be underestimated as transfusion of bacterially contaminated blood components can produce severe septic shock and can lead to a mortality of up to 25%.

Massive blood transfusion (a transfused volume of greater than the patient's blood volume) is associated with a further spectrum of clinical problems. Fluid overload may occur when large volumes are administered, particularly to elderly patients, and careful monitoring of central venous pressure is required. A blood warmer should be used to prevent hypothermia and wherever possible, a filter should be utilised. Coagulopathy may develop because of the lack of clotting factors and platelets and fresh frozen plasma and platelet concentrate should be administered. Stored blood contains citrate and therefore large volume transfusions may be associated with hypocalcaemia as well as hyperkalaemia. Acidosis is a further risk but usually does not require specific correction with the administration of bicarbonate.

Alternatives to blood for volume replacement

If blood is not available or is unacceptable to the patient (e.g. a Jehovah's Witness), plasma expanders may be used as an alternative. Modified gelatine products (Haemaccel) can be used but may not be accepted by some patients because of their objection to beef products. Hydroxyethyl starch derivatives (Hespan) have a longer half-life and are acceptable to the majority of patients. The use of albumin as a plasma expander is extremely expensive and is no more effective than its cheaper synthetic alternatives. However, it may be of use in the treatment of the nephrotic syndrome and after drainage of massive ascites but it must be recognised that albumin solutions have a high sodium content. Chemically modified haemoglobin solutions present a potential alternative to the transfusion of red blood cells and have a theoretical advantage in that the oxygen delivered is potentially greater than that of conventional plasma expanders. Furthermore, it has a longer shelf life, an absence of pathogenic viruses and a universal compatibility. However, concern has been raised as to its safety, particularly with regard to renal toxicity, coagulopathies and vasoactivity. However, such solutions may be of value in the resuscitation of patients in haemorrhagic shock and during elective surgery.

MICROSURGERY

The operating microscope was first used for the treatment of otosclerosis in 1921 but since then technological advances, such as foot pedal zoom magnification, coaxial illumination to prevent hand shadowing and more flexibility of instrument control, have led to much wider use. The limited depth and field of vision remain unsolved problems but microscopes are improving all the time.

A double-headed microscope is required to allow for the help of an assistant; it also has advantages for training purposes. The instruments used are of necessity fine in calibre and many of them, such as needle holders and microscissors, are spring-handled to minimise sudden jerky movements. For microvascular surgery 9/0 or 10/0 monofilament nylon with a 3/8 circle taper-pointed atraumatic needle is used.

Principles of microsurgery

The surgeon should operate in a comfortable and stable position, with the forearm and hands or wrists supported. If an operating chair is available with arm or wrist supports, these can be covered with sterile drapes and the supports adjusted according to requirements. Fogging of the eyepieces can be prevented by taping the top of the mask to the nose and leaving the lower strings of the mask very loosely tied. The instruments tend to be held like a pen with the middle finger supporting the tip of the instrument for precision and stability.

The field of view should be kept clear at all times and all traces of blood, extraneous tissue or foreign material should be irrigated away using heparinised Ringer's solution; a 10 ml syringe with a carefully angled needle is useful in this situation. There should be meticulous atraumatic dissection of all tissues and this is assisted by binocular vision that provides depth perception. As in conventional surgery, when performing a microvascular anastomosis, there should be no tension, the tissues should be treated gently without grasping sensitive structures, such as the intima of a vessel, and sutures should be placed with accuracy. A small sheet of background material such as fine plastic may facilitate this process. The first two sutures inserted should be placed so as to clearly display the lumen of the vessel, thus acting not only as part of the ultimate anastomosis but also playing a role as stay sutures.

During microsurgery the forces of contact are often well below the threshold of human perception and so tactile feedback is minimal. Using modern technology this limitation can be minimised by the use of sound to indicate the amount of force the surgeon is both applying and receiving. This substitution of the sensory modality of touch by the different modality of sound is called synthesia and allows an enhancement of the surgeon's skills and capabilities. Furthermore, dexterity enhancement is now technically possible using computerisation to give the surgeon a more natural feel of the movements undertaken and also to enhance those movements which are normally beyond human perception. This provides a degree of accuracy, precision, sense of position and sensory input that is impossible for the unassisted human hand. Such technological abilities will be essential in the application of telepresence surgery which may feature widely for future generations of surgeons.

SURGICAL SKILLS WORKSHOPS

Surgical skills workshops have evolved dramatically over the last decade from an initial scepticism to the point where the Senate of Surgery of Great Britain and Ireland has stipulated that all basic surgical trainees (BSTs) should undergo a mandatory basic surgical skills course. This course is the first mandatory workshop of its kind and its content, programme, assessment materials and certification have been standardised throughout the UK. Furthermore, such courses are now being run internationally and form a bedrock upon which other skills courses can subsequently be built.

Objectives

In designing any skills course or craft workshop, it is essential to first define the objectives of such a course. The aim should be to 'teach, test and certify' trainees' abilities to use safe and sound surgical techniques within the sphere of surgery under consideration. A basic surgical skills course should seek to teach and inculcate safe operating techniques with the aim of producing surgeons who will be competent to perform the required procedures in whichever surgical discipline they ultimately choose. The course should emphasise that careful and sound aspects of technique are far more important than simple manual dexterity or speed, as well as defining and stressing the importance of universal precautions for safe theatre practice, especially in emergency situations.

In seeking to achieve this goal, BSTs are finding it increasingly difficult to acquire their skills solely within the operating theatre. The current reduction in junior doctors' working hours, the shortening of training and the pressure of maximising limited operating time have all served to limit the time available for operative teaching. Some may suggest that in the past such pure operative teaching never actually existed as surgical trainees learnt their operative skills by watching their seniors and then spent long hours within the operating theatre on their own learning from their own mistakes. Such apprenticeship learning is clearly not only unsatisfactory but also is an unjust reflection on those few dedicated and highly motivated surgeons who actually took operative teaching seriously. The old method of 'learning on the job' meant that many surgical trainees took on bad habits that were very difficult to correct. It is often said that 'old habits die hard' but with regard to surgery, we may well add that 'bad habits die even harder'. Therefore the aim of any skills workshop should be to introduce the trainee to good, sound and safe surgical technique before bad habits are allowed to take up residence in an otherwise budding surgical career.

The aim of any skills workshop should be to provide a hands-on practical and didactic course with a very high tutor-to-participant ratio. Operative surgery is a very practical skill and therefore needs to be taught in a practical manner with such a hands-on approach. Tying surgical knots or suturing wounds under the scrutiny of an instructor are the conditions under which the true craft of surgery is recognised. Furthermore, in the current era in which the risks of viral transmission are so prevalent, it is essential for both surgeons and assistants to be aware of the importance of universal precautions, particularly in relation to the handling of sharps.

Content

No course or workshop can provide a comprehensive coverage of all aspects of operative surgery. Furthermore, no course should seek to impose or promote any specific surgical technique as being the only safe and sound method of performing that procedure. However, it is wise to present one 'safe way' which is a recognised, tried, tested and accepted method, rather than introducing all the various possible options. The content will therefore depend on the seniority and expertise of the target audience, as well as the surgical speciality concerned.

For BSTs, the mandatory skills workshop includes such basic techniques as knot tying, suture technique, anastomotic principles

(both bowel and vascular anastomoses), wound debridement, plastering technique and the principles covering minimal access surgery. This includes such important and vital procedures as creating and maintaining a pneumoperitoneum, the use of instruments, diathermy and hand–eye coordination. There should be a strong emphasis on individual tuition with detailed personal feedback on performance. Assessment is crucial and a continuing assessment throughout the course is usually of more value as long as there is adequate feedback from instructors.

The role of trainers and instructors on such courses is crucial. 'Training the Trainers' courses form an important part of the delivery of such skills courses, with the principles and methods of adult education being emphasised. However, skills courses should not be regarded as a form of aptitude testing and instructors are encouraged to provide positive feedback and criticism that will help trainees develop their surgical skills and grasp the essential principles being demonstrated.

Strategy for workshops

Basic surgical skills workshops should not be regarded as an end in themselves. They are a platform upon which surgical trainees can develop their surgical skills and they should be encouraged to practise such techniques subsequent to the course. An accompanying handbook and video are of value in this respect and when trainees return to their place of work, hospitals are encouraged to provide a skills training centre or laboratory where trainees can go for an hour or so and practise using simulated materials. It is not appropriate for individuals to assume that because they have attended a basic skills workshop, they are now proficient in the art of surgical technique. Assiduous attention to the practice of good, safe and sound surgery will produce positive results and ensure that the next generation of surgeons will be firmly grounded in the philosophy and practice of safe surgery.

A basic surgical skills workshop should be regarded as the building block on which other skill workshops are developed. When BSTs have finished this potential period of surgical education, they will pass into higher surgical training in the speciality of their choice. It is anticipated then that an intermediate skills workshop should be developed for all the surgical specialities, concentrating on the core skills required. It is proposed that a strategy for the provision of skills courses should be developed across all surgical specialities. Each such skills course for specialist registrars should deal with the core skills required for that speciality, as well as address more advanced surgical techniques for both open and minimal access surgery. Such courses currently are not mandatory, although with the developing concern over clinical governance, certain courses may become compulsory in the future.

Following such an intermediate course, more advanced or master class workshops are becoming available. These are more focused and are relevant for both senior higher surgical trainees and consultants, for continuing medical education and continuing professional development. Modern teaching methods and multimedia communication systems allow for live operating sessions to be relayed not only across the country but also internationally. Master class demonstrations can therefore be disseminated to a very wide audience in different venues. There is also opportunity for live feedback and such workshops can cover the minutiae of specific operative detail rather than simply addressing overall principles of practice.

Starting with the basic surgical skills course and progressing through to the very focused procedure-based master classes, this range of courses will be able to impart safe and sound surgical techniques that have stood the test of time as well as address new and exciting surgical innovations.

Acknowledgements

The author gratefully acknowledges the assistance of Mr Pat Elliot in the production of the illustrations and the permission of the Royal College of Surgeons of England to reproduce Figures 1.1–1.6 from the Basic Surgical Skills Course participants manual.

REFERENCE

1   Jenkins TPN. The burst abdominal wound: a mechanical approach. *BMJ* 1976;**131**:130–140

FURTHER READING

1   *Basic Surgical Skills: The Intercollegiate Participants Manual.* London: Royal College of Surgeons of England, 1999

2   Dunn DC, Rawlinson N. *Surgical Diagnosis and Management.* Oxford: Blackwell Science, 1995

3   Kirk RM. *Basic Surgical Techniques.* Edinburgh: Churchill Livingstone, 1994

4   Thomas WEG. The place of basic skills workshops in surgical training. *Br J Postgrad Med* 1996; **55**: 346–348

2

Radiology

Introduction
  Minimising radiation dose
Diagnostic radiology
  Imaging techniques
  System-based imaging
Interventional radiology
  Percutaneous biopsy and drainage procedures
  Percutaneous interventional biliary procedures
  Interventional vascular procedures
  Interventional uroradiology
Further reading

Simon Jackson

INTRODUCTION

Since the discovery of the X-ray by Roentgen in November 1895, the range and complexity of imaging techniques have been expanding. This has become even more evident during the past 40 years when the speciality has undergone enormous technological advances, in part due to the rapid development of computing which has resulted in a doubling of computer power approximately every 18 months (Moore's Law). These advances have heralded the advent of digital-based imaging modalities which now offer a wide range of techniques to accurately image the anatomy of the body.

This chapter succinctly reviews basic diagnostic and interventional imaging techniques with particular reference to their principles of use. Wider reading is suggested and the Royal College of Radiologists' publication *Making the Best Use of a Department of Clinical Radiology* is recommended as a suitable starting point (see Further reading).

Minimising radiation dose

With the exception of ultrasound (US) and magnetic resonance imaging (MRI), radiological examinations result in exposure of the patient to a dose of ionising radiation. Whilst this dose is potentially harmful, the risks of adverse health effects are extremely small when compared to the clinical benefits of the examination.

Adverse effects can be broadly classified into two categories.

- *Stochastic effects*. These can be defined as effects in which the probability (but not necessarily the severity) of occurrence increases with the size or quantity of the radiation dose. Examples include genetic mutations and carcinogenesis.

- *Deterministic effects*. These are associated with a minimum threshold radiation dose. Below this level the effect will not occur although above the threshold the probability of an effect is almost 100%. In addition, the severity of the effect increases with the size of the dose. Examples include cataracts, haematopoietic damage and skin changes such as erythema.

To minimise the possible danger of hazards, statutory regulations (see Further reading) require persons using ionising radiation to reduce any unnecessary exposure to the patient. In practice, all examinations must be clinically justified in order to avoid undertaking inappropriate investigations.

Table 2.1 includes typical effective doses from diagnostic medical exposures in the United Kingdom during the 1990s. The effective dose provides a single dose estimate related to total radiation risk to the body. The table also compares each dose to an equivalent

Table 2.1 Typical effective doses of diagnostic medical exposures in the UK

Diagnostic procedure	Typical effective dose (mSv)	Equivalent number of chest radiographs	Approx. equivalent period of natural background radiation*
X-ray examinations			
Limbs and joints (except hip)	<0.01	<0.5	<1.5 days
Chest (single PA film)	0.02	1	3 days
Skull	0.07	3.5	11 days
Thoracic spine	0.7	35	4 months
Lumbar spine	1.3	65	7 months
Hip	0.3	15	7 weeks
Pelvis	0.7	35	4 months
Abdomen	1.0	50	6 months
IVU	2.5	125	14 months
Barium swallow	1.5	75	8 months
Barium meal	3	150	16 months
Barium follow-through	3	150	16 months
Barium enema	7	350	3.2 years
CT head	2.3	115	1 year
CT chest	8	400	3.6 years
CT abdomen or pelvis	10	500	4.5 years
Radionuclide studies			
Lung ventilation (Xe-133)	0.3	15	7 weeks
Lung perfusion (Tc-99m)	1	50	6 months
Kidney (Tc-99m)	1	50	6 months
Thyroid (Tc-99m)	1	50	6 months
Bone (Tc-99m)	4	200	1.8 years
Dynamic cardiac (Tc-99m)	6	300	2.7 years

*UK average background radiation = 2.2 mSv per year: regional averages range from 1.5 to 7.5 mSv per year.

number of chest radiographs and period of natural background radiation.

DIAGNOSTIC RADIOLOGY

Imaging techniques

Plain radiographs

Whilst other imaging modalities may yield more detailed anatomical information, the relatively inexpensive plain radiograph is often the first diagnostic examination performed on a patient. The two-dimensional image is acquired on photosensitive film following exposure of the relevant anatomy to an X-ray beam. The differential attenuation of the beam by the various tissues within the area examined results in the differences in density on the final image. Because both air and bone have marked inherent differences in density, many pathologies affecting, for example, the chest or musculoskeletal system can thus be demonstrated. In contrast, soft tissue anatomy is in general poorly defined.

Digital radiology

Recent advances in technology now allow the acquisition of plain radiographs in a digital format suitable for computer-based storage and processing. The technology is known commercially as computed radiography. This important advance eliminates the problem of 'the lost film' and allows the transmission of images to remote sites – teleradiology. Increasingly, radiology departments are embracing the benefits of digital radiology to become totally 'filmless'.

Contrast radiology

A variety of contrast media are currently available and their use can broadly be divided into:

- contrast media used to opacify specific structures (for example, the gastrointestinal tract, the urinary tract and blood vessels) in order to detect associated abnormalities.

- contrast media used to detect and characterise abnormal tissues (for example, inflammation or tumour) which enhance differently when compared to normal surrounding tissues.

The compounds contain molecules of a high atomic number which cause increased attenuation of the X-ray beam. This results in an increased radiographic density of the organ or tissue which they opacify. Although most compounds are relatively non-toxic, side effects can occur ranging from minor flushing or nausea to major anaphylactic reactions. More recently new types of contrast media have been developed for use in MRI (Figure 2.1) and ultrasound.

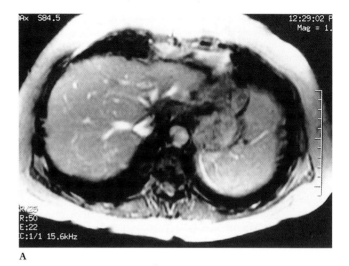

A

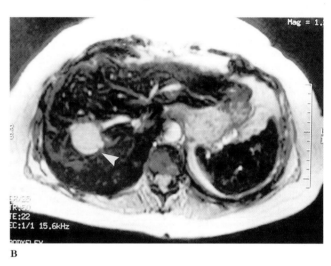

B

Figure 2.1 Liver metastasis. **A.** Precontrast MRI. **B.** Postcontrast MRI showing metastasis within right lobe of liver (arrow head).

Gastrointestinal contrast radiology

The use of contrast media to opacify the alimentary tract was introduced during the 1890's and remains in widespread use within the modern department of radiology. If there is no clinical suspicion of a bowel perforation, a suspension of barium sulphate is the contrast medium of choice. The combination of air with the barium allows better anatomical delineation of the bowel and is termed a double-contrast examination. The type of study depends on the clinical indication and the length of bowel which requires delineation.

- *Videofluoroscopy/modified barium swallow.* This is used for the evaluation of patients with dysphagia secondary to suspected swallowing dysfunction. The examination images the oropharyngeal region and is often performed in the presence of a speech therapist.

- *Barium swallow.* The study assesses both structure and function of the oesophagus and is recommended for patients with dysphagia prior to endoscopy.

- *Barium meal.* Whilst endoscopy is currently accepted as the first-line method of investigation, the double-contrast barium meal examination remains a useful technique to demonstrate pathology within the stomach and proximal duodenum.

- *The small bowel.* A variety of barium techniques are available for the assessment of the small bowel. These include both the antegrade and retrograde introduction of contrast into the jejunum or ileum. The most widely performed study is the small bowel meal (barium follow-through). During the examination the patient swallows a quantity of barium suspension and subsequent radiographs demonstrate the anatomy of the small bowel as the contrast passes to the colon. More detailed images are obtained using fluoroscopy (Figure 2.2). In contrast, the small bowel enema (enteroclysis) examination requires the initial passage of a nasojejunal feeding tube into the proximal jejunum. The small intestine is then directly distended with contrast pumped through the tube. This examination clearly demonstrates mucosal anatomy but the technique is both uncomfortable for the patient and time consuming for the radiologist. Indications for small bowel meal and small bowel enema examinations vary between centres.

- *The large bowel.* A double-contrast barium enema (DCBE) demonstrates both the mucosal surface and anatomical configuration of the colon (Figure 2.3). The examination is only accurate if the bowel is properly prepared. Although a DCBE offers the significant advantages of speed and safety as well as the ability to demonstrate the caecum during most examinations, in many centres colonoscopy is the primary investigation of colonic pathology. The direct endoscopic view is more

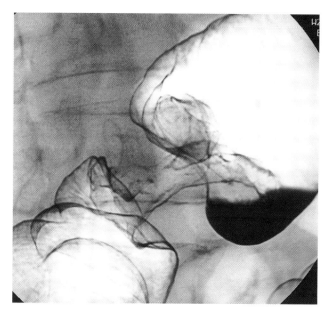

Figure 2.3 Double-contrast barium enema showing typical 'apple core' appearance of a carcinoma of the colon.

sensitive for the assessment of small mucosal abnormalities. In addition, therapeutic procedures (such as the removal of polyps) can be performed. Water-soluble contrast media examinations of the large bowel are used postoperatively for the assessment of colonic anastomoses and to demonstrate pathology in an unprepared colon (the instant enema). Other large bowel barium studies include evacuating proctography. This examination is a test of voluntary rectal evacuation and is used for the evaluation of patients with symptoms of intractable constipation or incontinence.

Renal contrast radiology

The intravenous urogram (IVU) examination is now performed less frequently for the primary diagnosis of urinary tract pathology. The major reason for the decrease is the development of alternative, less invasive imaging modalities, in particular ultrasound. The use of ionising radiation during the procedure and associated small risk of allergic reactions to the intravenous contrast medium have also contributed to the decline.

There is a wide variation in local policy between hospitals but current indications for an IVU include the investigation of:

- renal colic

- haematuria.

An IVU is *no* longer the primary imaging modality for the investigation of:

- hypertension

- prostatism

- renal failure

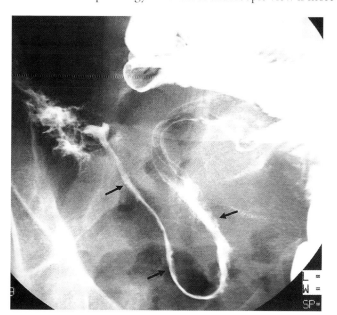

Figure 2.2 Crohn's disease. Small bowel meal showing active Crohn's disease narrowing terminal ileum (arrows).

- urinary tract infections (particularly in children)
- urinary retention.

Other contrast imaging techniques used to evaluate the renal tract include the following:

- *Antegrade pyelogram.* The examination is performed by the direct percutaneous injection of contrast medium into the pelvicalyceal system using either a needle or catheter. The technique is used as a specialised investigation for the diagnosis of urinary tract pathology.

- *Retrograde pyelogram.* Contrast medium is injected retrogradely into the ureter via a catheter usually placed cystoscopically in the operating theatre. The technique allows detailed imaging of the upper urinary tracts.

- *Micturating cystogram.* The study is usually performed for the investigation of reflux. A catheter is passed into the bladder and the bladder lumen is then opacified using a water-soluble contrast medium. Images are obtained during both initial filling of the bladder and voiding.

- *Loopogram.* The contrast study images both the ileal conduit (cutaneous uretero-ileostomy) and ureters of patients following urinary diversion surgery.

- *Urethrogram.* Water-soluble contrast is introduced into the urethra and is used for the assessment of patients with a suspected urethral stricture or urethral trauma.

Biliary contrast radiology

The biliary tree can be imaged by either the direct endoscopic retrograde or percutaneous antegrade injection of water-soluble contrast media. Antegrade studies are performed via a needle

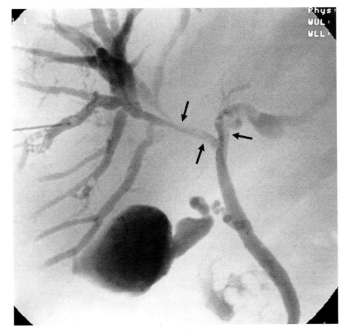

Figure 2.4 PTC performed for obstructive jaundice showing hilar stricture (arrows).

placed into the intrahepatic biliary tree – percutaneous transhepatic cholangiogram (PTC). These techniques offer the most accurate assessment of biliary anatomy (Figure 2.4). Other contrast studies include the oral cholecystogram and intravenous cholangiogram. These more invasive examinations are now no longer routinely recommended, having been largely replaced by ultrasound and MRI.

Vascular contrast radiology

The intravascular injection of contrast media remains the most accurate method for the demonstration of vascular anatomy. The technique of vascular cannulation was first described by Seldinger in 1953. This involves the placement of a catheter into the vascular tree over a guidewire following initial percutaneous puncture of the vessel with a needle. A water-soluble contrast medium is then injected through the catheter to obtain the final images. Most angiograms are performed using the technique of digital subtraction angiography (DSA). This method allows the subtraction of all anatomy except the contrast-filled vessel from the final image (Figure 2.5). The advantage of DSA is the increased image quality which allows examinations to be performed using smaller volumes of intravascular contrast media.

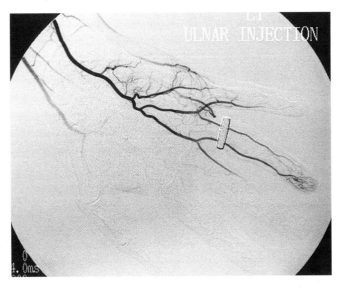

Figure 2.5 Digital subtraction angiogram following selective contrast injection into left ulnar artery.

Complications of angiography include:

- complications associated with catheter insertion and manipulation such as vessel occlusion, dissection, perforation, embolisation and haematoma formation at the puncture site.

- contrast media-related complications which include allergic reactions and renal toxicity. Overall diagnostic lower limb angiography has a complication rate of approximately 2–3%.

Ultrasound (US)

The technique utilises high-frequency sound waves to image tissues within the body. Sound waves are produced by applying a voltage across a piezoelectric crystal which is located within a handheld ultrasound transducer. The crystal resonates at a specific frequency, generating the ultrasound beam. The beam is transmitted into the body, being both absorbed by tissues as well as reflected at tissue interfaces. Only a small proportion of the beam is reflected at each tissue boundary, the remainder of the sound waves becoming progressively more attenuated as the depth from the probe increases. The various reflected waves return to the transducer and are used to generate the ultrasound image.

Soft tissues and fluid are particularly well demonstrated by this technique (Figure 2.6). However, the ultrasound beam cannot penetrate gas-containing structures or bone. The original scanners produced static (B–mode) tomograms but modern machines allow rapid real-time viewing of multiple images, enabling the demonstration of tissue movement. Because images are viewed in real time their interpretation is very much operator dependent.

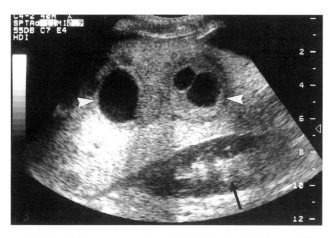

Figure 2.6 Cystic liver metastases (arrow heads). Longitudinal ultrasound image through right lobe of liver and right kidney (arrow).

Advances in scanner technology have led to other ultrasound techniques.

● *Doppler ultrasound.* The technique utilises the Doppler principle as the basis of a method to detect flow and quantify flow velocity within vessels. When combined with real-time images, a duplex scan is produced. Allocation of colour to the image (colour Doppler) provides information on the direction of flow.

● *Intraoperative and laparoscopic ultrasound.* Specific probes designed for use in the operating theatre allow a significant increase in image quality by their direct application to internal organs.

● *Intracavity ultrasound.* A multitude of transducers are now available including transvaginal, transrectal, oesophageal and intravascular probes. These use high-frequency transducers to produce high-resolution images.

● *Contrast-enhanced ultrasound.* Various contrast agents based on gas-filled microbubbles are under investigation to further enhance the accuracy of ultrasound examinations. Current areas of interest include echocardiography and the assessment of infertility disorders.

Computed tomography (CT)

As the name tomography or 'slice imaging' describes, this technique uses X-rays to generate cross-sectional two-dimensional images of the body.

Since the first CT scanner was developed by Sir Godfrey Hounsfield in 1972, the modality has become established as an essential radiological technique applicable in a wide range of clinical situations. Images are generated by rapid rotation of an X-ray tube and detectors around the patient. Mathematical reconstruction techniques are then performed to calculate different density or attenuation values of the X-ray beam at each point within the image slice. These values are then represented on the CT image as a regular matrix of picture elements or 'pixels'. The value of each pixel is compared with the attenuation value of water and displayed on a scale of arbitrary units (Hounsfield units). Water has an attenuation value of 0 Hounsfield units (HU) and the scale is 2000 HU wide. Other values include:

● air   −1000 HU

● fat   −70 to −100 HU

● soft tissues   +20 and +70 HU

● bone   greater than +400 HU.

More recently, spiral or helical CT has been developed. This significant advance in scanner technology combines movement of the CT table (and thus the patient) with the X-ray exposure. A much larger volume of the patient can thus be scanned during a single breathhold and image artefacts caused by patient breathing are eliminated. In addition, image data can be manipulated to produce multiplanar reconstructions of anatomical regions.

The use of contrast media to opacify bowel loops and vascular structures further improves the diagnostic information from a CT examination. This technique is now widely available but the modality is relatively expensive and each examination exposes the patient to a significant radiation dose (see Table 2.1).

Magnetic resonance imaging (MRI)

Although both CT and MRI provide a cross-sectional display of anatomy, the two techniques differ fundamentally because MRI does *not* use ionising radiation. The basic principle of image generation utilises a very strong magnetic field in order to align the protons of abundant hydrogen nuclei throughout the body. A radio frequency wave is then applied to disrupt this alignment. Upon cessation of the wave the protons return to their original axis of equilibrium. The latter process is called 'relaxation' and results in an emission of energy which is detected by the scanner, analysed and displayed as cross-sectional images.

A major advantage of MRI is that the images can be acquired not only in the axial but also in the coronal, oblique or sagittal planes. Specific contrast media, for example gadolinium-based compounds, can be used to opacify vascular structures which further increases the diagnostic information obtained from a study. The technique is, however, expensive and a significant proportion of patients cannot be imaged due to claustrophobia. A number of other contraindications to MR examination have also been published by regulatory bodies. These include patients with:

- cardiac pacemakers
- cochlear implants
- some prosthetic heart valves
- some brain aneurysm clips or coils
- periorbital metallic foreign bodies.

Examinations are currently contraindicated during early pregnancy.

Nuclear medicine – radionuclide radiology

Nuclear medicine can be defined as 'the medical speciality that utilises the nuclear properties of radioactive and stable nuclides to make diagnostic evaluations of anatomical or physiological conditions of the body and to provide therapy with unsealed radioactive sources'.

The technique requires the introduction into the body of a specific pharmaceutical labelled with a gamma-emitting radionuclide. The distribution of the compound is then detected using a gamma camera. The advantage when compared to other imaging modalities is the ability of the technique to measure organ function relatively non-invasively. However, the spatial resolution of the final images is limited and examinations expose the patient to ionising radiation (see Table 2.1).

System-based imaging

The abdomen

The logical use of imaging modalities for the diagnosis of abdominal pathology must be based on a limited differential diagnosis formulated from initial clinical history and examination of the patient. Appropriate imaging should then be directed towards this differential.

The plain abdominal radiograph is an important initial investigation in patients who present with symptoms or signs of an acute abdomen. Indications for this study include suspected:

- perforation of a viscus
- intestinal obstruction
- acute colitis/toxic megacolon
- colonic volvulus
- urinary tract calculi
- foreign body
- abdominal aortic aneurysm
- abscess
- biliary tract pathology.

Using good radiographic technique, as little as 1 ml of free intraperitoneal air can be demonstrated by an erect chest radiograph and supine abdominal film of patients with a suspected visceral perforation (Figure 2.7). The chest radiograph should be substituted for a left lateral decubitus film for patients who are too ill to move into the erect position.

If the initial radiographs are non-diagnostic a variety of other imaging modalities may be beneficial. Ultrasound is the simplest cross-sectional imaging technique and for the sick patient can be performed portably on the ward. Ultrasound is particularly useful for the assessment of intraperitoneal fluid collections and for the diagnosis of suspected biliary, gynaecological, hepatic, pancreatic and renal disease. Further information can be obtained from CT and, where available, MRI. These latter modalities are most commonly used for staging intraabdominal malignancies and imaging retroperitoneal anatomy.

The alimentary tract

As described earlier in the chapter, contrast imaging provides an accurate technique for the evaluation of alimentary tract pathol-

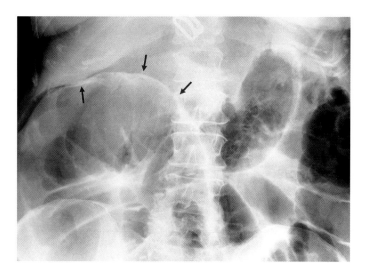

Figure 2.7 Supine upper abdominal radiograph demonstrating free intraperitoneal air. Note air outlining bowel wall (arrows) – Rigler's sign.

ogy and is complementary to endoscopy. Endoscopic ultrasound can also provide detailed anatomical information of the bowel wall and surrounding local anatomy.

Current indications for CT imaging of the alimentary tract include the following:

OESOPHAGUS

- The evaluation and staging of patients with oesophageal carcinoma (Figure 2.8).

- The evaluation of other intramural or extrinsic lesions diagnosed during endoscopy or contrast studies.

- The assessment of oesophageal perforations.

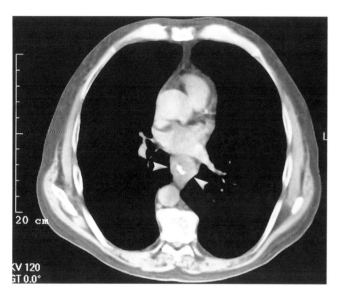

Figure 2.8 Carcinoma of the oesophagus. CT showing irregular oesophageal wall thickening (arrow heads).

STOMACH AND DUODENUM

- The evaluation and staging of tumours.

- The assessment of postoperative complications and tumour recurrence.

- Radiotherapy planning.

SMALL BOWEL

- A screening modality for patients with occult small bowel pathology.

- The evaluation and staging of tumours.

- The assessment of suspected small bowel trauma.

- The evaluation of patients with suspected small bowel obstruction. The technique is particularly valuable for the postoperative patient.

- The diagnosis of patients with suspected intestinal ischaemia.

- The evaluation of the complications of Crohn's disease.

LARGE BOWEL

- The preoperative staging of patients with known colonic carcinoma.

- The evaluation of recurrent malignant disease.

- The evaluation of inflammatory conditions involving the colon and appendix.

- CT-guided percutaneous drainage of pericolic abscesses.

- CT colography (virtual endoscopy) for the detection of colonic pathology. This exciting development challenges the role of barium enema and colonoscopy for the diagnosis of colonic lesions. The place of the technique has yet to be determined.

The exact role of MRI for the investigation of alimentary tract pathology remains to be defined but current indications include:

- the staging of rectal malignancy.

- the differentiation of tumour recurrence from postradiation fibrosis following colorectal surgery.

- the evaluation of perianal fistulas.

- the diagnosis and distribution of inflammatory bowel disease.

GASTROINTESTINAL HAEMORRHAGE

The diagnostic imaging approach to gastrointestinal bleeding depends on whether the haemorrhage is acute or chronic and if the suspected source of bleeding lies in the upper or lower gastrointestinal tract. The type of blood loss can then be subdivided according to whether the aetiology of the haemorrhage is arterial or venous.

Endoscopy is generally accepted as the initial diagnostic imaging investigation for patients with suspected acute or chronic gastrointestinal blood loss. Therapeutic manoeuvres can also be performed. Both upper and lower GI barium studies have little role in the diagnosis of acute haemorrhage. The barium enema and small bowel enema examinations, however, are useful screening procedures for patients with chronic gastrointestinal blood loss.

Indications for mesenteric arteriography include severe life-threatening haemorrhage or bleeding refractory to medical management. Arteriography requires a bleeding rate of 0.5–1.0 ml per minute for the accurate detection of haemorrhage (Figure 2.9). In cases where the source of haemorrhage is identified, either trans-catheter embolotherapy or intraarterial infusion of vasoconstrictive drugs can be used to facilitate haemostasis. For selected cases of intermittent, chronic GI blood loss and where other imaging has been negative, arteriography may also identify occult pathologies including tumours, angiodysplasia or a Meckel's diverticulum.

When available, radioisotope imaging using technetium-99m radio-labelled red blood cells can also diagnose GI haemorrhage. These studies are more sensitive than arteriography (bleeding rates as low as 0.1 ml per minute can be detected) but are not as specific. Similar studies can also diagnose a Meckel's diverticulum as an occult source of blood loss.

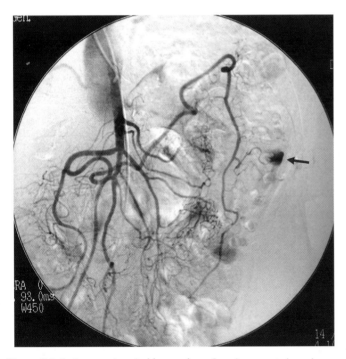

Figure 2.9 Active gastrointestinal haemorrhage. Superior mesenteric angiogram showing extravasation of contrast from wall of descending colon (arrow).

The liver and biliary tract

Plain films, contrast imaging, cross-sectional techniques and radionuclide studies are all used to image the anatomy of the liver and biliary tract. The choice of modality will depend on an appropriate differential diagnosis. Ultrasound is usually the initial investigation because of a high sensitivity for the detection of focal and diffuse liver pathology as well as biliary tract abnormalities. The technique is also highly accurate for the diagnosis of bile duct dilatation and can demonstrate the level and cause of biliary obstruction.

Contrast-enhanced CT and MRI studies are the most sensitive methods for the diagnosis of both focal and diffuse liver pathology (Figure 2.10). The techniques also provide an accurate method for staging local and distant malignant disease. The indications for each modality depend on local availability and expertise.

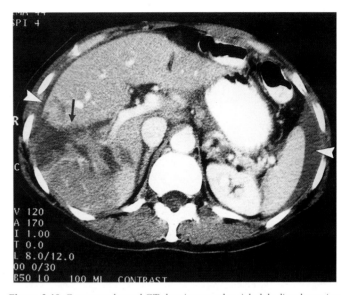

Figure 2.10 Contrast-enhanced CT showing complex right lobe liver laceration following trauma (arrow). Note free fluid around both liver and spleen (arrow heads).

The pancreas

Plain abdominal radiographs are not routinely indicated for patients presenting with suspected pancreatic disease. They may, however, demonstrate evidence of pancreatic calcification in cases of chronic pancreatitis. Ultrasound can accurately image the pancreas although because of the retroperitoneal position of the gland, overlying bowel gas may obscure views. Endoscopic ultrasound allows closer approximation of the transducer to the area of interest but requires a skilled operator. Similarly if the technical expertise is available laparoscopic ultrasound is also a sensitive modality for staging pancreatic neoplasms.

CT and more recently MRI offer the most sensitive non-invasive techniques for pancreatic imaging. Spiral CT and endoscopic ultrasound offer equal accuracy in the local staging of pancreatic neoplasms. Contrast-enhanced CT can diagnose pancreatic necrosis in patients with complicated acute pancreatitis as well as detect and stage pancreatic tumours (Figure 2.11). The definitive role of magnetic resonance cholangiopancreatography (MRCP) has yet to be determined although MRI can accurately demonstrate pancreatic pathology and image both the pancreatic and bile ducts using specific sequences (Figure 2.12).

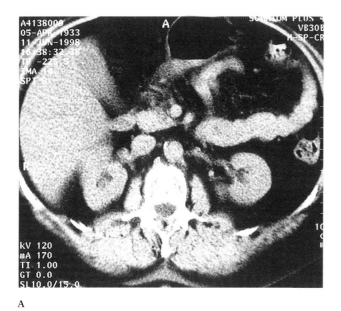

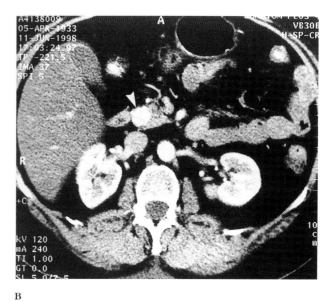

A

B

Figure 2.11 Pancreatic insulinoma. **A.** Precontrast CT. **B.** Arterial phase of dynamic contrast-enhanced CT showing hypervascular tumour within head of pancreas (arrow head).

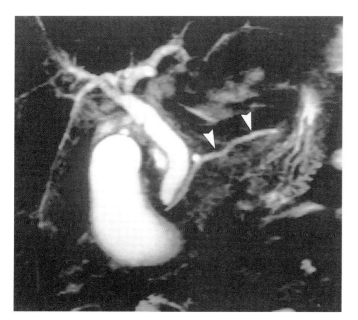

Figure 2.12 MRCP showing anatomy of biliary tree and pancreatic duct (arrow heads).

The urinary tract

Approximately 90% of renal calculi are radioopaque and therefore plain radiographs usually demonstrate renal tract calcification. The other modalities routinely used to image the urinary tract, including contrast studies, cross-sectional techniques and radionuclide studies, are covered in Chapter 00.

The vascular system

Conventional diagnostic arteriography has for many years been regarded as the 'gold standard' investigation of the vascular tree. By definition, however, the investigation is an invasive procedure and the development of other less invasive imaging modalities has reduced the overall number of arteriograms performed. These other techniques include the following.

- *Ultrasound.* Duplex ultrasound can provide information on both the anatomy and variations of flow velocity within a vessel. The technique is accurate for the assessment of vascular disease in both peripheral and central vessels. Intravascular ultrasound (IVUS), where available, provides more detailed high resolution images of vascular anatomy. Ultrasound is also widely accepted as the initial investigation for patients with suspected lower limb deep venous thrombosis.

- *CT.* Contrast-enhanced CT and in particular CT angiography (CTA) is used for the investigation of thoracoabdominal vascular disease. The technique allows three-dimensional reconstructions of the vascular tree.

- *MRI.* Magnetic resonance angiography (MRA) can assess both vascular anatomy and function. The role of this imaging modality for the assessment of vascular disease continues to evolve with an increasingly wide number of applications.

The thorax

Despite the numerous imaging modalities currently available, the plain radiograph is an extremely valuable technique for the assessment of chest pathology. The chest radiograph is also recommended as a preoperative screening test in patients undergoing cardiopulmonary surgery and in cases of suspected malignancy or possible TB. Anaesthetists may also request a preoperative chest radiograph for the assessment of dyspnoeic patients, the very elderly and patients with known cardiac disease.

Ultrasound is used for the identification of pleural fluid collections and for the guidance of chest aspirations. Whilst complementary, CT is more sensitive than the chest radiograph for the assessment of thoracic anatomy and indications for this technique include:

● diagnosis of chest pathology in patients with a normal chest radiograph (Figure 2.13). For example, detection of occult pulmonary or mediastinal masses and interstitial pulmonary disease.

● confirmation or exclusion of pathology suspected on the chest radiograph. For example, focal pulmonary masses.

● evaluation of abnormalities demonstrated on the chest radiograph. For example, staging of pulmonary or mediastinal neoplasms and the demonstration of vascular pathology within the chest.

A variety of techniques are available for the assessment of the pulmonary arteries in cases of suspected pulmonary embolism. Although a chest radiograph remains the initial investigation, radionuclide imaging and in particular a ventilation/perfusion (V/Q) scan offer a sensitive screening test. Pulmonary angiography is the most accurate technique for the detection of small emboli but is relatively invasive. CT angiography is now performed in many centres, offering a less invasive alternative. The role of MRI for the diagnosis of pulmonary embolism is currently under investigation. Both MRI and radionuclide studies are also routinely used for the imaging of both the heart and thoracic vessels.

The musculoskeletal system

Plain radiographs are the initial investigation of choice for the assessment of suspected skeletal trauma, skeletal neoplasia and joint arthropathies.

Ultrasound is performed for the evaluation of soft tissue masses and tendon abnormalities. CT is routinely used for the imaging of complex musculoskeletal trauma and for the detection and staging of tumours. MRI, however, offers a number of advantages over the other imaging modalities and indications also include the staging of both bone and soft tissue tumours. Radionuclide studies and in particular a bone scan offer highly sensitive screening techniques for the diagnosis of occult skeletal metastases in patients with a known primary malignancy. In addition, radio-labelled white cell studies can help in the detection of osteomyelitis (see *Fundamentals of Surgical Practice*, Chapter 20).

The head and neck

Both CT and MRI now offer the widest clinical applications for imaging this region which includes the central nervous system. The use of these techniques is covered in Chapter 19 of *Fundamentals of Surgical Practice*. Plain radiographs are useful for the initial assessment of trauma, the demonstration of radio-opaque foreign bodies and focal bony abnormalities secondary to tumour infiltration. Ultrasound is routinely indicated for the initial evaluation of masses involving the soft tissues of the neck and duplex ultrasound can accurately image the anatomy of the carotid vessels.

INTERVENTIONAL RADIOLOGY

The subspeciality of interventional radiology is currently undergoing a period of rapid expansion and the distinction between this area of radiology and minimal access surgery is becoming increasingly blurred. Thus some techniques previously performed exclusively by radiologists are now also being practised by other clinicians. The principles of interventional radiology require the use of various imaging modalities to perform invasive diagnostic and therapeutic procedures. These modalities allow the accurate placement of needles, guidewires, catheters and stents within the body, significantly reducing tissue trauma. This reduction in trauma minimises patient discomfort and in general lowers the overall morbidity and mortality of the procedures.

The use of imaging techniques during a therapeutic minimally invasive procedure can be divided into four phases.

● Phase 1: localisation of the relevant anatomy.

● Phase 2: guidance for the introduction of instruments.

● Phase 3: treatment.

● Phase 4: documentation and follow-up of the effects of treatment.

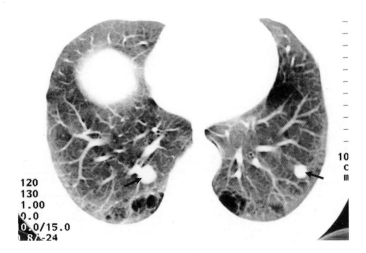

Figure 2.13 CT showing occult pulmonary metastases (arrows).

Percutaneous biopsy and drainage procedures

Image-guided techniques allow the safe percutaneous biopsy and drainage of many inaccessible lesions and collections within the body. The choice of technique will depend on local availability and which modality best depicts the pathology. Complex biopsy and drainage procedures may require more than one technique.

Percutaneous biopsy is routinely performed using either ultrasound or CT guidance. Ultrasound can offer a number of advantages over CT including multiplanar imaging and portability but some lesions may be obscured by air or bony structures and thus are better imaged using CT. Types of percutaneous biopsy include the following:

- *Fine needle aspiration cytology (FNAC).* This is performed using a small-calibre needle (usually 21 gauge) and a 10 or 20 ml syringe. A cytological aspirate is obtained by repeatedly passing the needle through the lesion with suction applied to the syringe either by hand or with the use of a special aspiration gun. The needle is then withdrawn from the lesion and the contents of the needle and syringe transferred to slides before being sent for cytological analysis.

- *Histological biopsy.* If a biopsy is required for histological examination then a tissue sample can be obtained using a large biopsy needle (most commonly 18 gauge). Although this technique is slightly more invasive than FNAC, complications are still rare.

Percutaneous drainage techniques have now replaced more invasive open surgical procedures for the management of pathological collections within the body. In particular, most abscesses within the abdomen and pelvis are now drained percutaneously. Small collections can be aspirated but larger collections require the placement of a temporary drainage catheter. Catheter size is determined by the complexity of the collection. Catheters are introduced into the body using either a 'one-stick' method, in which the collection is punctured directly by the catheter containing a central needle stylet, or as a two-stage procedure following initial image-guided placement of a guidewire into the collection. The choice of technique will depend on a number of factors although deeply placed collections are usually more safely drained by the latter method.

Complications are rare and include haemorrhage, septicaemia and damage to adjacent structures.

Percutaneous interventional biliary procedures

Percutaneous procedures and endoscopic retrograde cholangiopancreatography (ERCP) are complementary for the imaging of biliary tract disease. The main advantage of ERCP is that the biliary tree can be accessed without trauma to the liver parenchyma. However, when the endoscopic approach is not possible, for example following gastric surgery, or ERCP is unsuccessful, then percutaneous techniques are indicated.

Percutaneous techniques include the following.

- *Percutaneous transhepatic cholangiogram (PTC).* This procedure is performed by the image-guided introduction of a small (22 gauge) needle into the biliary tree under aseptic conditions. A water-soluble contrast medium is then injected through the needle to demonstrate bile duct anatomy.

- *External biliary drainage.* The technique is performed for patients with biliary obstruction. A catheter is placed into the intrahepatic bile ducts above the level of the biliary obstruction. Bile drains externally into an attached catheter bag. The enterohepatic bile circulation is, however, not restored.

- *Internal/external biliary drainage.* During the procedure a guidewire is manipulated across the level of biliary obstruction. A specifically designed catheter is then placed into the biliary tree with side holes both above and below the obstructing lesion. Bile can drain into both the duodenum and attached catheter bag, restoring the enterohepatic circulation.

- *Internal biliary drainage or biliary stenting.* Stents can be placed by an endoscopic, a combined endoscopic and percutaneous or percutaneous approach. The choice of technique will depend on the type of pathology and local expertise. Two types of stent are available – plastic and metallic. Metallic stents are more expensive but due to their large internal diameter (8–10 mm), long-term patency is increased when compared to plastic prostheses (Figure 2.14).

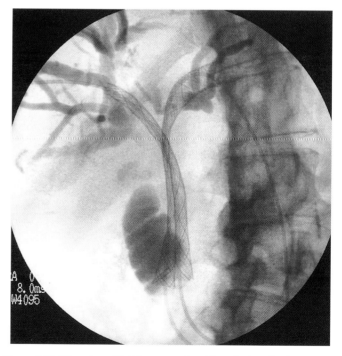

Figure 2.14 Bilateral metallic biliary stents placed for palliation of malignant hilar obstruction. Temporary catheters have been inserted within the stents following the procedure.

The Gallbladder

Ultrasound-guided percutaneous drainage of the gallbladder is performed for the sick patient with acute gallbladder pathology who is unfit for emergency surgery. A catheter is placed by either a transhepatic or subhepatic image-guided approach. The subhepatic approach is more direct but carries a higher risk of intraperitoneal bile leak.

Interventional vascular procedures

The arterial system

Most interventional procedures are performed for patients with occlusive arterial disease secondary to atheroma. Due to the overlap between the specialities of interventional radiology and vascular surgery, the optimal management of patients will depend on local expertise, availability of equipment and close collaboration between the disciplines.

● *Percutaneous transluminal angioplasty (PTA)*. This is the most frequently performed procedure and outcome is most successful for short, non-calcified concentric stenoses or short occlusions. The standard technique is well established.
Following initial percutaneous access via a Seldinger technique, the stenosis is crossed using a guidewire with a floppy or tapered tip. A balloon catheter is passed over the guidewire and centred on the lesion prior to inflation. Heparin is administered to prevent thrombosis at the angioplasty site. A postdilatation angiogram is then performed to evaluate technical success. A new technique utilising the subintimal tissue plane is currently under investigation. Complications develop in approximately 8% of procedures although only 2% require further intervention.

● *Intravascular stents*. Specifically designed metallic stents can be used to maintain or restore vascular patency. Indications include failed angioplasty or complications of the procedure such as a local dissection. Stents are most commonly placed in the iliac and coronary arteries (Figure 2.15). Recent advances in technology have resulted in the development of 'stent grafts'. These devices combine a metallic stent with synthetic arterial graft material. Their exact role has yet to be determined.

● *Thrombolytic therapy*. The therapeutic technique uses thrombolytic agents which accelerate the natural fibrinolytic system of the body to restore patency of an occluded artery, vein or surgical bypass graft (see *Fundamentals of Surgical Practice*, Chapter 13).

● *Embolotherapy*. The procedure utilises image guidance to therapeutically embolise either blood vessels or vascular spaces. The variety of embolic materials can be classified into temporary, semipermanent or permanent in nature. The technique has a number of clinical applications:

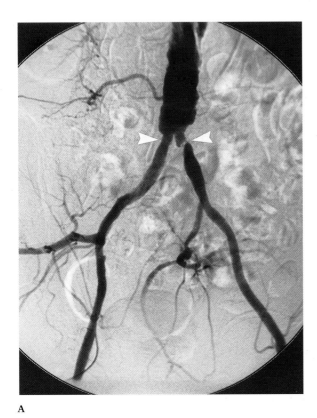

A

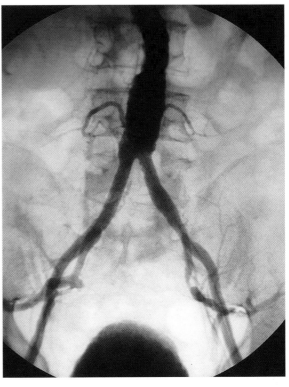

B

Figure 2.15 Digital subtraction angiograms pre (**A**) and post (**B**) metallic iliac stent placement for vascular disease involving the aortic bifurcation (arrow heads).

– the management of uncontrolled arterial haemorrhage, for example, into the gastrointestinal tract.

– the preoperative devascularisation of lesions to reduce intra-operative bleeding.

– the therapeutic or palliative treatment of vascular tumours

– the occlusion of aneurysms.

Complications of the procedure vary with the type of embolic agent, the technique of administration and site of embolisation. They include postembolisation syndrome, non-target embolisation, migration of embolic material and abscess formation.

The venous system

The various procedures use the same principles of catheter intro-duction and manipulation as previously described for the arterial system. Percutaneous angioplasty is used for the dilatation of venous stenoses and intravascular stents can be placed for the pal-liation of malignant superior vena caval obstruction. Other proce-dures include the following.

Placement of inferior vena caval filters for patients who are at high risk of pulmonary embolism (Figure 2.16). Absolute indications for the technique include:

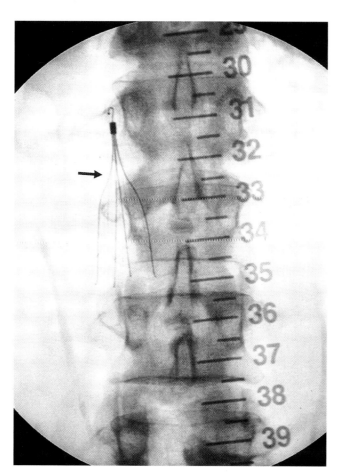

Figure 2.16 Inferior vena caval filter (arrow).

● pulmonary embolism with a contraindication to anticoagula-tion.

● recurrent pulmonary emboli despite adequate anticoagulation.

● extensive deep venous thrombosis with a contraindication to anticoagulation.

● following a complication of anticoagulation, necessitating ces-sation of anticoagulant therapy.

Transjugular interventional procedures of the liver.

● *Transjugular liver biopsy.* The procedure is performed where transcutaneous biopsy techniques are contraindicated, for example, in patients with blood-clotting abnormalities or ascites. After initial ultrasound-guided catheterisation of an internal jugular vein, liver biopsies are obtained through a catheter placed within a hepatic vein.

● *Transjugular intrahepatic portosystemic stent shunt (TIPSS).* During the procedure a metallic stent is placed into the liver parenchyma to create an intrahepatic portacaval shunt. The technique offers a minimally invasive alternative to open surgery for patients with complicated portal hypertension.

Interventional uroradiology

Commonly performed image-guided procedures include the fol-lowing.

● *Percutaneous nephrostomy.* The technique has completely replaced surgical nephrostomy and is performed by the image-guided insertion of a drainage catheter into the pelvicalyceal system of the kidney. The most common indication is for the relief of ureteric obstruction. Ultrasound is initially used to guide a needle into the lower pole collecting system of the kidney. A water-soluble contrast medium is then injected through the needle to opacify the collecting system prior to the introduction of a catheter over a guidewire into the renal pelvis. The technique is successful in over 98% of cases.

● *Percutaneous nephrolithotomy (PCNL).* The technique is an alternative to open surgery for the management of renal stone disease. A common indication is for patients who are unsuit-able for lithotripsy. The procedure is performed under general anaesthesia and requires the image-guided placement of a large sheath into a suitable calyx prior to endoscopic extraction of stone material by a urologist. PCNL can be associated with significant haemorrhage, requiring transfusion in approxi-mately 5% of cases.

● *Angioplasty.* Benign ureteric strictures can be treated by bal-loon dilatation. The procedure is successful in approxi-mately 80% of cases. The technique is particularly useful in the transplant kidney where open surgery is hazardous.

● *Stents.* Ureteric stents can be used for the management of both benign and malignant ureteric strictures and can act as a conduit for the passage of stone fragments following lithotripsy. They are also inserted for the management of urinary fistulas. Using image guidance, stents can be placed by either an antegrade or retrograde ureteric approach. The antegrade technique is successful in approximately 90% of cases.

Acknowledgements

Table 2.1 is adapted from an illustration in *Making the Best Use of a Department of Clinical Radiology – Guidelines for Doctors*, with advice from B.Wall, National Radiological Protection Board.

The author is grateful to Mrs Anita Radford for secretarial assistance.

FURTHER READING

1   RCR Working Party. *Making the Best Use of a Department of Clinical Radiology – Guidelines for Doctors,* 4th edn. London: Royal College of Radiologists, 1998

2   *The Ionising Radiation (Protection of Persons Undergoing Medical Examinations and Treatment – POPUMET) Regulations.* London: HMSO, 1988

3   Sutton D, ed. *Textbook of Radiology and Imaging,* 6th edn. London: Churchill Livingstone, 1998

3

Breast and Soft Tissue Surgery

Needle aspiration of a breast cyst
Fine needle aspiration cytology (FNAC) of a
  breast mass
Needle core biopsy (NCB) of breast tissue
Needle aspiration of a breast abscess
Incision and drainage of a breast abscess

Excision of a palpable breast mass
Management of superficial skin wounds
Management of superficial skin infections
Lymph node biopsy
Excision of skin lesions

Roger Watkins

NEEDLE ASPIRATION OF A BREAST CYST

Indications

This diagnostic and therapeutic procedure is normally performed in the outpatient clinic. It is indicated for the following reasons:

● Confirmation that a palpable breast mass is indeed a cyst.

● Therapeutic drainage to eliminate a palpable cystic mass within the breast.

Patient preparation

Patients over the age of 35–40 would normally undergo preliminary mammography. Ultrasound examination of the breast can be used to distinguish between cystic and solid masses if required. Ultrasound may also suggest the presence of atypical features within the cyst. The procedure is fully explained to the patient in order to allay her anxiety.

Anaesthesia

Local anaesthetic is not used routinely but in selected patients either local anaesthetic cream is applied to the overlying skin or 1–2 ml of 1% plain lignocaine is injected into the skin at the site of proposed aspiration.

Operative procedure

The patient is positioned supine with the head well supported by a few comfortable pillows. The skin overlying the cyst is usually cleaned with isopropyl alcohol.

● The cyst is fixed using the index finger and thumb of the non-dominant hand (Figure 3.1).

● A 21 (green) or 23 (blue) gauge needle attached to a 10 ml or 20 ml syringe is inserted through the skin into the breast cyst. As the needle is advanced through the cyst wall, a slight loss of resistance is felt.

● As suction is applied, the fluid contents of the cyst are aspirated into the syringe.

● The amount and colour of breast cyst fluid varies markedly. It may be a relatively clear, yellowish colour or a darker green, even almost black colour (Figure 3.2). If the patient is lactating or has recently finished breast feeding the cyst may be a galactocoele containing milky fluid.

● During the course of aspiration the needle tip may need to be repositioned in order to guarantee that the cyst is aspirated completely.

● Once no more fluid is seen to enter the syringe, the suction is released, the needle withdrawn and local pressure applied to prevent bleeding.

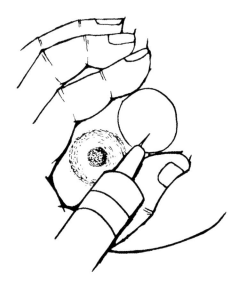

Figure 3.1 The cyst is immobilised between the thumb and index finger of the non-dominant hand and the aspirating needle inserted through the overlying skin into the cyst.

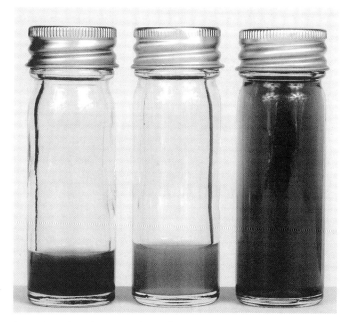

Figure 3.2 The volume and colour of breast cyst fluid are very variable.

● Palpation of the breast tissue following aspiration is required to ensure there is no residual palpable abnormality. If the cyst has been completely aspirated and the cyst fluid is not uniformly bloodstained, cytological examination of the fluid is not required.

- If uniformly bloodstained fluid is aspirated cytology is mandatory. Similarly, if a residual mass is palpable, the cyst fluid is examined cytologically. Fine needle aspiration cytology (FNAC) of the residual mass should also be performed.

Hazards

Bleeding may occur into the breast tissue if a vessel is traumatised by the aspirating needle. This is not normally a significant problem and any haematoma will normally resolve spontaneously over the following 1–2 weeks. Damage to the pleura with resultant pneumothorax is an extremely rare complication following breast cyst aspiration and can be prevented by carefully controlling the point of the aspirating needle at all times.

Postoperative management

If the cyst does not recur, no further action is required. Recurrence of the cyst will call for further aspiration and cytological examination of the fluid. If the fluid contains suspicious or malignant cells or the cyst continues to recur, formal excision will be required.

FINE NEEDLE ASPIRATION CYTOLOGY (FNAC) OF A BREAST MASS

Cytological diagnosis of discrete breast masses is an important part of triple assessment (clinical, radiological and cytological) and is normally performed in the outpatient clinic, once clinical examination and mammography and/or ultrasound examination have been performed and the results assessed.

Patient preparation

The procedure is explained to the patient. The patient lies supine on the clinic couch with the head supported by pillows.

Anaesthesia

No anaesthetic is usually employed. Occasionally, local anaesthetic cream or direct local anaesthetic infiltration will be requested by a particularly anxious patient.

Operative procedure

- A 21 (blue) or 23 (green) gauge needle attached to a 10 ml or 20 ml syringe is normally used.

- Some operators are able to obtain more control over the needle and the plunger of the syringe by using a syringe holder as illustrated in Figure 3.3.

- Prior to inserting the needle into the breast mass, a small volume of air is drawn into the syringe.

- The skin overlying the breast mass is cleaned, normally with isopropyl alcohol.

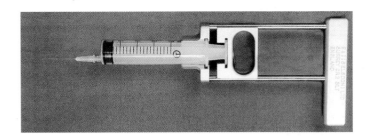

Figure 3.3 Syringe holder used to facilitate control of the needle tip and syringe plunger when performing fine needle aspiration cytology.

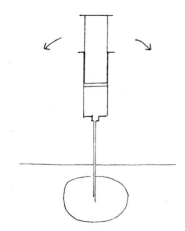

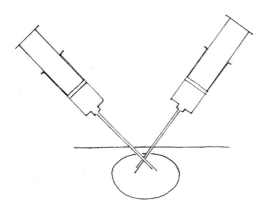

Figure 3.4 The fine needle is moved in and out through the mass whilst suction on the syringe is maintained. The direction of each needle passage is varied to reduce the possibility of sampling error.

- The breast mass is immobilised between the thumb and index finger or middle and index fingers of the non-dominant hand.

- The needle is inserted through the overlying skin into the centre of the breast mass and the syringe plunger withdrawn while steadying the syringe and needle. With the suction maintained, the needle tip is moved in and out through the lesion and the direction of each passage varied so that wide sampling of the lesion is obtained (Figure 3.4).

- Prior to removing the needle and syringe from the breast tissue, traction on the plunger is released to prevent aspiration of the needle contents into the barrel of the syringe.

- Having removed the needle from the breast tissue, the syringe is detached from the needle, filled with air and reattached. The contents of the needle are then expelled onto the surface of two or three clean microscope slides. The aspirate is then spread carefully to form a thin layer using either the aspirating needle or another slide. Excessive pressure on the aspirate during spreading may produce artefactual appearances which in turn may mean that reporting accuracy is impaired.

- The aspirate is normally air-fixed prior to staining. Slides are then stained by the Papanicolaou or Giemsa technique. Immediate reporting by an experienced cytopathologist will determine the need for repeat aspiration if the preparations are non-diagnostic due to inadequate cellularity or excessive spreading artefact.

Hazards

Injury to blood vessels within the breast tissue may lead to aspiration of blood. Significant aspiration of blood into the needle and syringe normally indicates that a non-diagnostic aspirate will be obtained. As soon as a significant amount of blood is drawn into the needle and syringe, it is best to abandon the procedure with a view to repeating it later if necessary.

Some bruising normally occurs after even an apparently atraumatic needle aspirate. Occasionally a large haematoma or significant bruising occurs but this normally settles spontaneously. Entry of the needle tip into the pleural cavity may lead to a pneumothorax but the overall incidence of this complication should be less than 0.1%. Careful control of the needle tip, especially for lesions situated near to the chest wall, should avoid this complication.

Postoperative management

Once the results of the cytological examination are available, they can be discussed with the patient.

NEEDLE CORE BIOPSY (NCB) OF BREAST TISSUE

The Super-Core (Manan Medical Products, Northbrook, IL, USA) biopsy needle is a disposable guillotine soft tissue needle that can be used for obtaining percutaneous histological samples of breast tissue (Figure 3.5). It is an automatic device which is easier to use than the Tru-Cut (Travenol) needle. It facilitates a one-handed biopsy technique thus allowing the operator's other hand to stabilise the breast lesion. The device will retrieve a core of tissue approximately 15 mm long with a diameter of 1 mm.

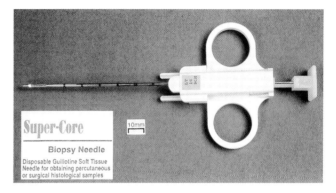

Figure 3.5 Super-Core biopsy needle used to obtain histological samples of breast tissue.

Patient preparation

The procedure is carefully explained to the patient before starting, in particular the action of the biopsy needle when fired. The patient lies supine with the ipsilateral arm positioned away from the biopsy site.

Anaesthesia

The skin surface overlying the lesion is cleaned with an antiseptic solution and 2 ml of 1% lignocaine is inserted into the skin and underlying subcutaneous tissues.

Operative procedure

- A 3 mm skin incision is made with a pointed scalpel blade to allow entry of the biopsy needle into the breast tissue.

- The biopsy needle is charged by pulling back on its plunger until a firm click is felt, indicating that the needle spring is engaged. The stylet of the biopsy needle is fully retracted so that the specimen notch is completely covered by the cannula.

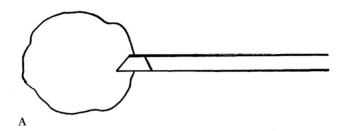

A

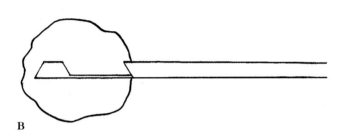

B

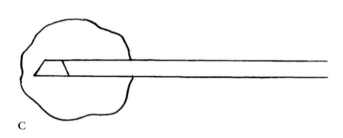

C

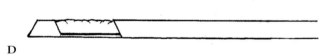

D

Figure 3.6 Mechanism of action of Super-Core biopsy needle. **A.** With the stylet retracted, the core biopsy needle is advanced to a point adjacent to the breast tissue to be biopsied. **B.** By pressing the plunger, the stylet is advanced into the breast tissue. **C.** The plunger is pressed fully which triggers the cannula to close, trapping tissue within the specimen notch. **D.** Having removed the biopsy needle from the breast, the stylet is again advanced to expose the specimen notch containing the core of breast tissue.

- The tip of the biopsy needle is inserted through the skin incision up to a point adjacent to the area of breast tissue to be sampled (Figure 3.6A).

- The plunger is pressed with the thumb, advancing the stylet into the breast tissue to be sampled, thus exposing the specimen notch (Figure 3.6B). The biopsy needle is then moved a few millimetres to allow the specimen notch to fill with tissue. The plunger is pressed, automatically triggering

the cannula to close, trapping tissue within the specimen notch (Figure 3.6C).

- The biopsy needle is withdrawn from the breast and the instrument recharged, advancing the stylet and exposing the specimen notch (Figure 3.6D). The tissue sample is retrieved and placed into formalin whilst firm pressure is applied to the biopsy site for 2–3 minutes to prevent excessive bleeding.

- Cores of breast tissue which float in formalin are likely to be composed mainly of fatty tissue and therefore unlikely to be diagnostic. In contrast, cores which sink rapidly in formalin are likely to be diagnostic.

- The procedure can be repeated to obtain two or three cores suitable for histological examination.

- Once adequate cores of tissue have been obtained and excessive bleeding has been dealt with, the skin incision is closed using a single Steristrip.

Hazards

Bleeding and haematoma formation can occur especially if vascular lesions are biopsied. Large vessels, particularly veins within the breast tissue, may also be injured leading to significant haemorrhage and bruising.

Advancement of the biopsy needle between the ribs and through the pleura might lead to pneumothorax or haemothorax. These are rare complications and can be prevented by ensuring that the biopsy needle is advanced into the breast tissue in a direction parallel to the chest wall.

Postoperative management

Once the formal histological diagnosis is obtained the results can be discussed with the patient. The biopsy site is reviewed at that stage.

NEEDLE ASPIRATION OF A BREAST ABSCESS

The distinction between cellulitis of the breast and a localised breast abscess can usually be resolved by means of ultrasound examination. Diagnostic needle aspiration can also be used to confirm the presence of pus. Therapeutic needle aspiration of a breast abscess is only indicated if the skin overlying the abscess is relatively healthy. Formal surgical incision and drainage is indicated if the overlying skin appears very thin or non-viable.

Patient preparation

The procedure is described and explained to the patient. If she has a lactational breast abscess, discussions about breast feeding following the procedure should take place. The patient lies supine. The surgeon usually stands on the side of the abscess. If the abscess is situated in the lateral half of the breast, abduction of the ipsilateral arm to 90° may be necessary. Alternatively the patient's hand on that side can be rested behind her head.

Anaesthesia

Aspiration of a breast abscess can be performed following topical application of a local anaesthetic cream such as EMLA (lignocaine/prilocaine) or Ametop (amethocaine) to the overlying skin. The full local anaesthetic effect is only obtained one hour after application of the cream. Conventional local anaesthetic such as 1% lignocaine injected into the skin can also be used.

Operative procedure

- Aspiration is performed using a 20 ml syringe and a white (19 gauge) needle.

- The aspirating needle attached to the syringe is inserted through the anaesthetised skin overlying the abscess at the point of maximal fluctuance or erythema.

- The needle tip is advanced towards the centre of the abscess cavity and the pus aspirated.

- The pus is sent for microscopy, culture and sensitivity of the pathogenic organism(s).

Hazards

If the abscess is multiloculated, further aspiration may be required. Even after successful aspiration, repeated aspiration may be required if the abscess recurs. Formal surgical incision and drainage may also be necessary in a few cases.

Postoperative management

The patient is usually treated with oral antibiotics and reviewed on a daily basis. Flucloxacillin, or erythromycin in penicillin-sensitive patients, is used for lactational abscesses as these are nearly always due to staphylococcal infection. Co-amoxiclav is used for non-lactational abscesses as these are more likely to be due to a mixed growth of organisms often including anaerobic bacteria. Erythromycin with metronidazole would be used in penicillin-sensitive patients. Ultrasound examination can be used in addition to clinical examination to monitor progress of the infection within the breast and detect the presence of any further localised collection of pus.

INCISION AND DRAINAGE OF A BREAST ABSCESS

Patient preparation

Having explained the procedure to the patient, routine preparations for general anaesthetic are carried out. The patient is placed supine with the arm on the affected side abducted to 90° and supported on an armboard attached to the operating table.

Anaesthesia

A general anaesthetic is usually employed although muscle relaxation is not required.

Operative procedure

- A small incision, usually about 2–3 cm long, is made over the point of maximal fluctuation.

- Once the abscess cavity has been entered, any loculi are broken down either by digital pressure or insertion of sinus forceps.

- Pus that is drained is sent for microscopy, culture and sensitivity.

- A small biopsy from the wall of the abscess cavity is taken to exclude any significant underlying pathology in those cases presenting with atypical features.

- A small corrugated drain may be inserted into the abscess cavity if it is situated deeply. It is secured with a single suture at the skin surface.

- An absorbent dressing is applied to the wound.

Hazards

Damage to lactiferous ducts, especially in the periareolar tissues, can be reduced by performing a small radial incision. Significant duct damage may lead to temporary discharge of milk through the drainage site in cases of lactational abscess or a mamillary duct fistula. An established mamillary duct fistula will require further definitive surgical treatment.

Postoperative management

Antibiotics are given if there is significant surrounding inflammation and cellulitis of the breast tissue. Patients who have had a lactational breast abscess drained may continue to breast feed on the unaffected side. Manual expression or use of a breast pump is normally required on the side where the abscess has been drained. If a mother with a lactational abscess wishes to discontinue breast feeding, lactation can be suppressed using bromocriptine 2.5 mg once daily for three days then 2.5 mg twice daily for 14 days. Any residual breast engorgement can be reduced by manual expression. Oral fluid restriction, diuretic therapy, firm binding of the breast tissue and oestrogen therapy are no longer used for suppression of lactation.

If used, the small wound drain can be shortened at 24–48 hours and removed at 72 hours. The wound is allowed to heal by secondary intention and delayed closure is not normally required. If a drain has not been inserted the wound should be irrigated daily using normal saline.

EXCISION OF A PALPABLE BREAST MASS

With information from preoperative triple assessment (clinical examination, imaging and needle aspiration cytology or needle core biopsy), the nature of a palpable breast mass is usually known prior to its removal. In those cases where a preoperative diagnosis is not available, it is important that only a limited amount of breast tissue is removed for diagnostic purposes. Excision of more than 20 g of breast tissue for a lesion later shown to be benign is regarded as unacceptable.

If a lesion is shown to be a fibroadenoma and excision is required, the procedure is as follows.

Patient preparation

The procedure is explained to the patient, indicating the site and direction of the proposed incision. The site of the palpable mass is marked with the patient lying in the position to be used during the operative procedure.

The patient is positioned supine on the operating table with the ipsilateral arm abducted to 90°. The surgeon stands on the same side as the palpable mass.

Anaesthesia

Local anaesthesia may be appropriate for superficial breast masses. Otherwise a general anaesthetic is employed.

Incision

For lesions within 4 cm of the nipple, a circumareolar incision is used as this produces the best cosmetic result (Figure 3.7A). Fibroadenomas situated more peripherally are removed through a curved circumferential incision directly overlying the palpable mass (Figure 3.7B). Radial incisions can be used as an alternative for lesions situated directly medial or lateral to the nipple (Figure 3.7C).

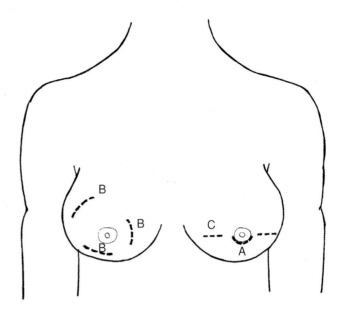

Figure 3.7 Skin incisions used for excision of palpable breast masses. **A.** Circumareolar incision. **B.** Circumferential incisions. **C.** Radial incisions.

Operative procedure

- Following incision of the skin, the wound is deepened and a small self-retaining retractor inserted. Haemostasis is achieved.

- Careful palpation within the wound identifies the lesion.

- By sharp dissection, the capsule of the fibroadenoma is entered and the lesion enucleated.

- A vascular pedicle supplying the fibroadenoma may require specific ligation or diathermy to achieve haemostasis.

- The weight of the breast tissue excised should be recorded prior to its placement in formalin fixative solution.

- Haemostasis is checked and a small suction drain may be inserted if required.

- The breast tissue of the biopsy site is closed using 2/0 absorbable sutures and the skin wound closed using a subcuticular suture.

Hazards

Fibroadenomas are well-defined lesions but are often situated in rather dense fibrotic tissue, especially in younger women. In addition, they are often readily mobile and may prove elusive once the skin incision has been made. It is important not to remove the normal breast tissue surrounding a fibroadenoma as removal of such tissue may produce a rather poor cosmetic result. Movement of the fibroadenoma during dissection can be limited by preoperative percutaneous insertion of a 21 gauge needle such that its tip rests within the fibroadenoma.

Haemostasis of fibrotic breast tissue may be difficult. Inadequate haemostasis may lead to haematoma formation. Especially if the breast tissue is lax, bleeding at the operative site may produce a large haematoma requiring formal evacuation.

Postoperative management

If a suction drain has been inserted it can normally be removed at some stage within the first 24 hours. If a non-absorbable subcuticular suture has been used, it is removed at 10 days.

MANAGEMENT OF SUPERFICIAL SKIN WOUNDS

Patient preparation

Prior to exploring and suturing a traumatic skin wound, it is essential to check the integrity of underlying structures, particularly neurovascular structures, muscles and tendons. Any impaired function indicates the need for thorough exploration of the wound, normally under general anaesthetic and, if appropriate, using a limb tourniquet.

The patient is positioned comfortably with the traumatic wound exposed. The surgeon stands or sits close to the wound.

Anaesthesia

Most superficial skin wounds can be sutured under local anaesthetic providing the patient is cooperative.

Operative procedure

- The skin around the wound is cleaned. The wound itself is irrigated using normal saline and the wound edges infiltrated with local anaesthetic.

- The wound is explored and all foreign material removed. Any necrotic or non-viable tissue should also be removed and haemostasis secured.

- If the wound edges are significantly traumatised, excision may be required. In this case, some undermining of the skin edge may be necessary to effect primary closure.

- The dead space within the wound should be closed using absorbable sutures. Interrupted skin sutures using monofilament nylon or prolene are usually recommended for traumatic skin wounds as accurate apposition at the skin edges may prove difficult, especially if excision of the wound edges has been necessary.

Hazards

Failure to remove all foreign material and non-viable tissue will predispose to wound infection. Haematoma formation is also a significant risk factor. Wound edges opposed under excessive tension are unlikely to heal satisfactorily.

Postoperative management

Adequate tetanus immunisation is necessary and a booster dose of tetanus toxoid is given if required. The rate of healing depends on the site of the wound and sutures will be removed in 5–10 days accordingly.

MANAGEMENT OF SUPERFICIAL SKIN INFECTIONS

Staphylococci and streptococci are the main organisms responsible for superficial skin and soft tissue infections. Infections caused by streptococci tend to be cellulitic in nature. Such infections normally respond rapidly to benzylpenicillin.

In contrast, superficial infections caused by staphylococci are associated with localised abscess formation which will often require surgical treatment. Folliculitis is a staphylococcal infection of a hair follicle and will often resolve spontaneously. With the development of a furuncle the follicular infection also involves the subcutaneous layers of the skin. A carbuncle is an even deeper, more extensive lesion which always requires formal surgical incision and drainage.

Patient preparation

The planned procedure is explained to the patient and informed consent obtained.

The position of the patient is dictated by the site of the abscess to be drained and the surgeon is positioned adjacent to the lesion.

Anaesthesia

Small cutaneous abscesses or furuncles can normally be drained under local anaesthetic by using either ethyl chloride spray on the overlying skin or direct infiltration of local anaesthetic. A carbuncle is normally drained under general anaesthetic as it is usually extensive, tends to involve the deeper layers of subcutaneous tissue and also contains multiple loculi of pus.

Operative procedure

- A 1–2 cm skin incision is made at the point of maximal fluctuation.

- The pus is drained and sent for microscopy culture and sensitivity.

- The abscess cavity is entered with a pair of sinus forceps and all loculi broken down. A small wick of ribbon gauze can be inserted to hold open the incision and aid postoperative drainage.

Hazards

When draining a localised collection of pus, it is important not to incise through the pyogenic membrane surrounding the abscess cavity. This membrane is a natural barrier and if breached, local spread of the infection may occur.

Postoperative management

Appropriate antibiotic therapy with either flucloxacillin or erythromycin in the first instance is usually given to those patients who show signs of local spread of infection or evidence of systemic disturbance. Multiresistant *Staphylococcus aureus* may require treatment with vancomycin.

If a small wick has been inserted into the abscess cavity, it is removed within 24 hours. The drainage site then heals by secondary intention.

LYMPH NODE BIOPSY

Common sites for open biopsy of a pathologically enlarged lymph node include the neck, axilla and inguinal regions. Prior to biopsy of any lymph node, full clinical examination of the other lymph node regions, along with the liver and spleen, are undertaken. In addition, the drainage area of the enlarged node is examined carefully for any regional pathology.

The main principles of lymph node biopsy apply to all nodal areas and are illustrated by a description of cervical lymph node biopsy.

Patient preparation

The procedure is explained to the patient and fully informed consent obtained.

With the patient supine and the head of the operating table elevated 15° to reduce venous congestion, the patient's head is rotated away from the operative side and supported by a head ring.

Anaesthesia

Cervical lymph node biopsy is usually performed under general anaesthetic. Use of an endotracheal tube or laryngeal mask airway is recommended, as this will allow unhindered access to the operative field. If the patient's condition precludes general anaesthetic and the lymph node is situated superficially, local anaesthetic infiltration may be used as an alternative to general anaesthetic.

Operative procedure

- Following skin preparation and towelling, a skin crease incision is made directly over the enlarged lymph node extending 1 cm either side of it.

- 5–10 ml of 1:200 000 adrenaline in normal saline can be infiltrated subcutaneously prior to the skin incision being made, in order to reduce bleeding from the skin edges.

- The incision is deepened through the fibres of the platysma muscle and haemostasis achieved using bipolar diathermy.

- A small self-retaining retractor is inserted into the wound.

- The investing layer of the deep cervical fascia is incised to expose the surface of the enlarged lymph node.

- In some cases neighbouring muscles such as the sternocleidomastoid or trapezius need to be retracted to allow access to the lymph node.

- Having reached the capsular surface of the lymph node, blunt dissection using scissors or an artery forcep can be used to mobilise the lymph node. Careful sharp dissection may also be required but any vessels supplying the node should be diathermised or ligated prior to division.

- Enlarged lymph nodes are often quite friable and gentle handling is required to prevent damage to them. Direct handling of the node should be kept to a minimum.

- A main vessel supplying the lymph node is often identified on its deep aspect. It should be ligated or diathermised prior to removal of the node.

- Once dissected free, the node is removed and divided into two equal halves. One half is sent for culture, including for acid- and alcohol-fast bacilli, and the other is also sent fresh for histological examination. An unfixed sample for histology allows imprint cytology to be taken and also facilitates immunohistochemistry. Both these techniques are useful in diagnosing lymphomas and determining the appropriate histological subtype.

- A small suction drain may be required postoperatively if the biopsy site is not completely dry.

- 3/0 absorbable sutures such as plain catgut can be used to close the platysma muscle.

- The skin wound is closed with a subcuticular suture such as 4/0 PDS or prolene.

- An occlusive dressing is applied.

Hazards

Enlarged lymph nodes are often quite vascular and careful haemostasis is required. Failure to achieve adequate haemostasis may lead to haematoma formation, which predisposes to subsequent wound infection.

Neighbouring nerves may be at risk during lymph node biopsy. Of particular risk in the neck is the accessory nerve in the posterior triangle of the neck supplying the trapezius muscle. Nerve damage can be avoided by awareness of the site and course of the nerve. All dissection must be performed carefully and under direct vision.

Postoperative management

If a drain has been inserted it can normally be removed after 24 hours; otherwise the patient can be discharged home soon after surgery and is reviewed with the results of histological examination in a few days time.

Any non-absorbable sutures can be removed from the cervical incision at five days.

EXCISION OF SKIN LESIONS

Many small benign skin lesions, such as seborrhoeic keratoses, skin tags and papillomata, benign pigmented naevi, dermatofibromas and sebaceous cysts, can be excised with an ellipse of surrounding skin following local anaesthetic infiltration. The resultant cutaneous defect can usually be closed primarily.

Patient preparation

The procedure is explained to the patient, who lies on the operating table in a position which is comfortable but which allows adequate exposure of the area of skin where the lesion is situated. Prior to local anaesthetic infiltration, an ellipse is marked around the lesion using a skin marker.

Anaesthesia

Local anaesthetic such as 1% lignocaine is infiltrated into the skin and subcutaneous tissues around the lesion as a field block (Figure 3.8). In areas of significant vascularity the local anaesthetic solution should contain adrenalin at a concentration of 1:200 000.

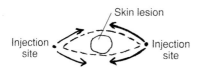

Figure 3.8 Local anaesthetic field block is achieved by infiltration around the lesion to be excised. The sites of injection are indicated along with the directions of local anaesthetic infiltration.

Incision

The long axis of the skin ellipse should be in the line of a natural skin crease wherever possible. In the head and neck, the skin creases are at 90° to the direction of pull of the muscles of facial expression. In the region of joint flexures the skin creases are easily seen. Outside these areas the direction of the lines of skin tension should be followed but the shape and position of the skin lesion may also have some influence on the siting of the skin ellipse. The skin ellipse should be at least three times longer than it is wide to allow satisfactory closure of the wound and to produce a good cosmetic result (Figure 3.9).

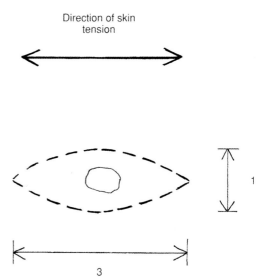

Figure 3.9 Elliptical skin incision used for excision of small cutaneous lesions. The long axis is ideally placed in the direction of the line of skin tension and should be at least three times longer than the short axis.

Operative procedure

- The skin is incised along the previously marked line and the ellipse of skin mobilised from the underlying subcutaneous fatty tissues. If appropriate, the lesion is sent for histological examination.

- Haemostasis is achieved by fine absorbable ligatures or diathermy.

- For small elliptical skin excisions the natural plasticity of the skin may allow primary direct closure without undue tension. In other cases the skin edges will require mobilisation by undercutting. The skin edges can be undermined by scissor or scalpel dissection.

- Wound drainage is not usually required and the wound can be closed by either interrupted non-absorbable skin sutures, such as prolene or nylon, or a subcuticular suture.

Hazards

Damage to underlying structures can be avoided by careful attention to anatomical detail. Haematoma formation may predispose to wound infection. Hypertrophic scarring and keloid formation may occur particularly in those individuals at risk. In those areas of the body where the process is common it is important that patients are warned of this possibility and fully informed consent obtained preoperatively.

Postoperative management

Non-absorbable skin sutures are removed at 5–10 days depending on the site of excision.

FURTHER READING

1   Dixon JM, ed. *ABC of Breast Diseases* London: BMJ Publishing Group, 1995

2   Hughes LE, Mansel RE, Webster DJT. *Benign Disorders and Diseases of the Breast: Concepts and Clinical Management.* London: Baillière Tindall, 1989

3   Trott PA, ed. *Breast Cytopathology. A Diagnostic Atlas.* London: Chapman and Hall, 1996

4

Abdominal wall and gastrointestinal tract

Abdominal incisions
   Upper midline incision
   Lower midline incision
   Paramedian incision
   McEvedy's incision
   Kocher's incision
   Pfannenstiel incision
   Gridiron and Lanz incisions
Appendicectomy
   Patient preparation
   Procedure
   Hazards
   Postoperative management
Perforated duodenal ulcer
   Patient preparation
   Procedure
   Hazards
   Postoperative management
Small bowel resection
   Patient preparation
   Procedure

Anastomosis
   Hazards
   Postoperative management
Colostomy
   Loop colostomy
Inguinal hernia repair
   Patient preparation
   Anaesthesia
   Procedure
   Hazards
   Postoperative management
Femoral hernia repair
   Procedure
   Hazards
   Postoperative management
Umbilical hernia repair
   Patient preparation
   Anaesthesia
   Procedure
   Hazards

Andrew Kingsnorth

ABDOMINAL INCISIONS

Selection of an appropriate incision is important for both the surgeon and the patient. The most important concept is to provide the best exposure of the area to be operated upon in order to give the surgeon ready and direct access to the viscera to be investigated and to perform the operation with adequate exposure and the minimum of difficulty. Access is then maximised by carefully placed retractors and positioning of the operative table and operative lights. In the upper abdomen, access can be impaired due to the presence of the costal margin and the diaphragm. An incision should provide the option for extension should the scope of the operation enlarge and additional access be required.

Abdominal incisions are vertical, transverse or oblique. Vertical incisions have a more profound effect on pulmonary function but the widespread use of epidural anaesthesia, patient-controlled anaesthesia and local anaesthetic wound infiltration has minimised these effects. For the surgeon, a vertical incision often provides quicker and easier access to the abdominal cavity and is therefore used more frequently. However, if the surgery is confined to viscera in the upper abdomen such as the liver, pancreas and cardia, transverse or oblique upper abdominal incisions are preferred.

The skin incision is made with a scalpel and the deeper layers may be incised with the diathermy on 'blend' (combined cutting and coagulation) until the fascial layers of the abdominal wall are reached. Haemostasis in the skin and subcutaneous layers is then obtained with diathermy forceps or fine ties to larger vessels. The fascial aponeurosis is then incised with a scalpel or cutting diathermy to expose the peritoneum. The peritoneum is then picked up with tooth dissecting forceps and the tented portion gripped between two artery forceps. Care is taken to ensure that only peritoneum is gripped by these artery forceps by releasing and reapplying them to the peritoneum alone. The peritoneum is now incised, at first by a small 'nick', and once air has entered the peritoneal cavity, the viscera fall away and the peritoneum can be incised with scissors under direct vision to the full length of the skin and aponeurotic incision.

The full range of popular abdominal incisions is shown in Figure 4.1.

Upper midline incision (Figure 4.2)

This incision may be extended upwards to remove the xiphoid process. A terminal branch of the internal mammary artery should be coagulated or ligated prior to incision of the xiphoid with cutting diathermy scissors or double-action bone shears. The upper midline incision is quick, relatively bloodless, transects neither nerves nor muscles and is relatively easy to close. Before entering the abdominal cavity the falciform ligament is clamped, divided and ligated.

The incision is best closed with a No. 1 non-absorbable running suture approximating the linea alba and peritoneum in a single layer (Figure 4.3). A tissue bite of at least 1 cm from the edge of the linea alba and a stitch interval of 1 cm will achieve a suture length to wound length of 4:1, which is the optimal ratio to achieve maximum bursting strength in the wound and to prevent wound failure and incisional hernia.

Lower midline incision (Figure 4.4)

This incision gives good access to the pelvic viscera, the left colon and rectosigmoid colon. A urinary bladder catheter should be

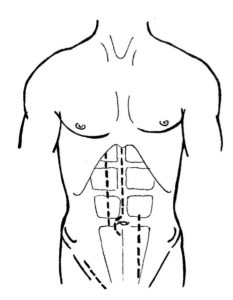

A

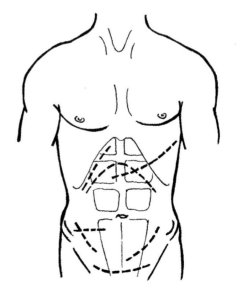

B

Figure 4.1 Abdominal incisions. **A.** Vertical. **B.** Transverse and oblique.

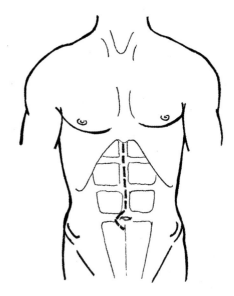

Figure 4.2 Upper midline incision.

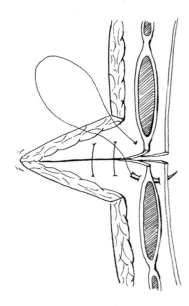

Figure 4.3 Linea alba closure.

placed before making the incision to prevent injury to the bladder. The linea alba is narrower below the umbilicus and its situation in the midline may be difficult to find in an obese patient with a flabby lower abdomen. A good tip is to find the linea alba just inferior to the umbilicus and then to continue inferiorly to the symphysis pubis. As with the upper midline incision, this incision may be extended superiorly around the umbilicus.

The lower midline incision is closed in a similar fashion to the upper midline incision with a No. 1 absorbable suture in a continuous manner.

Paramedian incision (Figure 4.5)

The use of strong non-absorbable suture materials has diminished the need for this incision which provides the extra protection of the rectus muscle overlying the closure of the posterior rectus sheath. Proponents claim that the incision gives slightly better access to one or other side of the abdomen. Some advocate placement of the incision in the posterior rectus sheath 2–3 cm lateral to the incision in the superficial layers and anterior rectus sheath – the so-called lateral paramedian incision. The rectus splitting incision cannot be recommended on the basis that incisional hernia after this method of opening the abdomen is frequent.

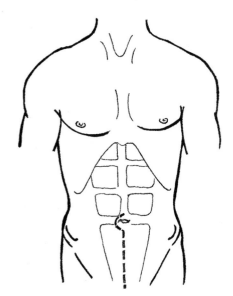

Figure 4.4 Lower midline incision.

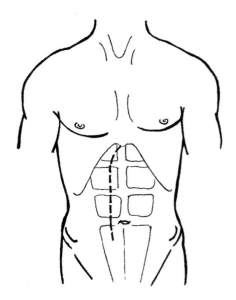

Figure 4.5 Paramedian incisions.

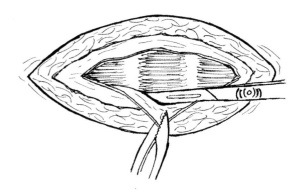

Figure 4.6 Dissection of rectus sheath.

The technique of paramedian incision is the same in the upper and lower abdomen, except that below the arcuate line, the posterior sheath is deficient. Once through the fat and subcutaneous tissues, the anterior rectus sheath is divided vertically in the line of the incision. Holding the medial flap up with artery clips, the rectus muscle is separated from the rectus sheath as far as the linea alba with particular attention to sharp dissection where the tendinous intersections are adherent to the rectus sheath (Figure 4.6). The rectus muscle can then retract laterally on its posterior sheath where there are no vascular pedicles or tendinous insertions. With the surgeon's non-dominant hand or a retractor placed to hold the rectus laterally, the posterior rectus sheath is tented between artery forceps, 'nicked' and then incised along its length with the closely adherent, underlying peritoneum, to expose the abdominal cavity.

Posterior and anterior rectus sheaths are closed separately with a No. 1 non-absorbable suture in a continuous method with a 1 cm bite and a 1 cm stitch interval.

McEvedy's incision

The classic McEvedy incision is a lower midline pararectal skin incision. This incision is now obsolete because of the high incidence of incisional hernia which follows its use. The 'modified' transverse McEvedy incision is 'half' a Pfannenstiel incision, i.e. placed two fingers breadth above the symphysis pubis extending from the midline laterally. Once through the skin and subcutaneous tissues, the anterior rectus sheath is divided horizontally, the rectus muscle is retracted medially and the transversalis fascia (there being no posterior rectus sheath below the arcuate line) is incised to enter the preperitoneal space. This incision gives access to Hesselbach's triangle, through which groin hernias protrude and can subsequently be reduced. Additionally, should the need arise, the peritoneal cavity can be entered by incising the peritoneum cephalad, which may be required to deal with strangulated bowel.

Kocher's incision (Figure 4.7)

A right subcostal or Kocher's incision gives good access to viscera in the right upper quadrant of the abdomen in a patient with a wide costal margin. When placed more obliquely, it can be extended across the midline and across the left costal margin into the chest to create a thoracoabdominal incision.

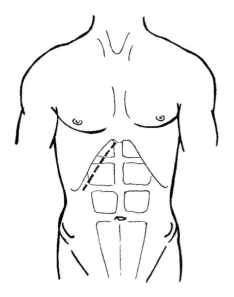

Figure 4.7 Kocher's incision.

The incision is placed 2 cm below and parallel to the costal margin with its medial end in the midline and extending laterally beyond the lateral margin of the rectus sheath. After division of the skin, subcutaneous tissues and anterior rectus sheath, the rectus muscle is encountered. This muscle is lifted clear from the posterior rectus sheath with a sling, swab or large artery clamp and incised with cutting diathermy whilst securing branches of the superior epigastric artery when these vessels are exposed between muscle bundles. Laterally the external oblique, internal oblique and transversus abdominis muscles are split or divided in the line of the incision as far as necessary to gain adequate exposure to the abdominal cavity. Peritoneum is then opened in the usual manner.

The author's preferred closure is in layers to the posterior and anterior rectus sheath with a continuous No. 1 non-absorbable suture taking 1 cm bites with a 1 cm stitch interval. Others prefer a mass closure with tissue bites of 1–2 cm and a stitch interval of 1 cm. A bilateral subcostal incision (gable incision or chevron incision) is generally utilised for major surgery in the upper abdomen including liver, pancreas, spleen and cardia of the stomach.

Pfannenstiel incision (Figure 4.8)

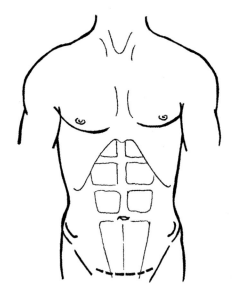

Figure 4.8 Pfannenstiel incision.

A popular incision for surgery on the female pelvic organs, bladder and prostate. The skin incision is made in a slightly curvilinear fashion, two fingers breadth above the pubic symphysis. Once through the skin and subcutaneous layers, the anterior rectus sheaths are divided horizontally in the same line to their lateral margins (Figure 4.9). The rectus muscles are separated from the anterior rectus sheath with sharp dissection, retracted laterally and then the linea alba is split vertically in the midline with the scalpel. A retractor is placed to maintain lateral retraction of the rectus muscles and underlying transversalis fascia is exposed in the lower part of the incision which, after division, allows entry to the preperitoneal space or if desired more superiorly the peritoneum may be opened to enter the lower abdominal cavity.

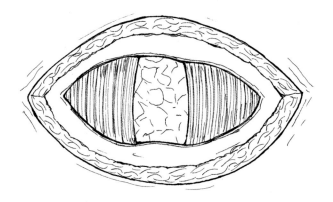

Figure 4.9 Horizontal incision in rectus sheaths.

Closure is obtained first by approximating the posterior rectus sheath/peritoneum and the rectus muscles then approximate themselves in the midline. The anterior rectus sheath is now closed with a continuous No. 1 non-absorbable suture using 1 cm bites and a 1 cm stitch interval.

Gridiron and Lanz incisions (Figure 4.10)

These incisions are centred on the junction of the middle and outer thirds of a line joining the umbilicus to the anterior superior iliac spine. The skin crease curvilinear Lanz incision provides a good cosmetic result. The incision may be placed more medially overlying the rectus muscle in which case the anterior rectus sheath is divided in the line of the incision, retracted medially and the peritoneum incised behind the rectus muscle.

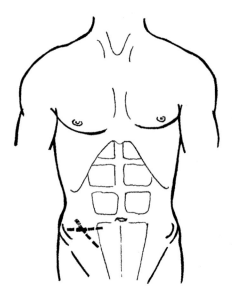

Figure 4.10 Gridiron and Lanz incisions.

With the more lateral incision, after incising the skin and subcutaneous tissues, the external oblique is split in the line of its fibres to expose the internal oblique and transversus muscles which are then split in the line of their fibres (Figure 4.11). The peritoneum is now exposed and opened in the usual manner. This incision can easily be extended laterally or medially to increase exposure.

The muscle and fascial layers of this incision are closed in layers with interrupted or continuous sutures of slowly absorbed absorbable suture materials such as polyglycolic acid or polydioxanone.

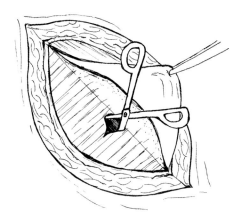

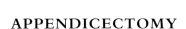

Figure 4.11 External and internal oblique are split in the line of their fibres.

APPENDICECTOMY

Patient preparation

- Antibiotic prophylaxis: metronidazole suppository with pre-medication (adult 1 g, children 500 mg).

- Parenteral antibiotics in the presence of generalised peritonitis.

- Consider thromboembolic prophylaxis in the 50+ age group and those with generalised peritonitis (the operation will take longer).

- Establish intravenous access for fluid administration in the presence of dehydration or peritonitis or for antibiotic administration.

- Consider nasogastric intubation if vomiting has been a marked feature of the illness.

- General anaesthesia is induced and maintained with endotracheal intubation.

- Supine position on the operating table.

- Gridiron or Lanz incision (see above).

Procedure

- If there is free fluid or pus, take a specimen for culture and aspirate excess fluid.

- The site of the appendix is variable. The commonest positions are: paracolic, retrocaecal, pelvic, in front of or behind the terminal part of the ileum (Figure 4.12).

- Theoretically the appendix is identified by following the taenia coli distally and the caecum and the appendix are then both delivered into the wound by gentle traction.

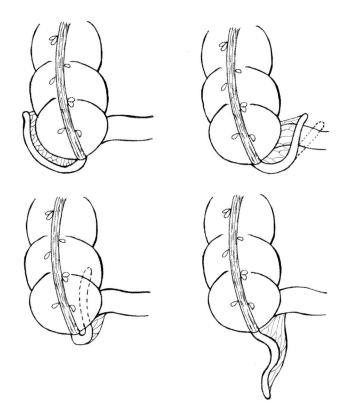

Figure 4.12 Positions of the appendix.

- In practice, inflammatory adhesions will bind the appendix to adjacent viscera or visceral peritoneum and the appendix will need to be freed before it can be delivered to the surface of the wound. The lateral peritoneal reflection of the caecum may also require division to improve mobility of the caecum. In some cases it may be easier to deliver the caecum to the surface initially and then by gentle traction deliver the appendix, base-first, through the incision.

- Grasp the appendix tip with a Babcock's tissue forceps (Figure 4.13).

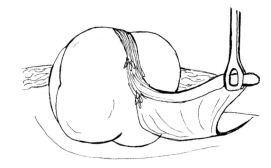

Figure 4.13 Grasp the appendix tip with a Babcock's tissue forceps.

- Identify the mesoappendix and clamp, divide and ligate appendicular arteries. If the mesoappendix is thickened and oedematous, take small bites with artery clamps and transfix the mesoappendix on the mesenteric side.

- The appendicular stump created by resection of the appendix can be treated by either inversion or simple ligation.

- Inversion: a seromuscular purse-string suture of 2/0 absorbable polymer is inserted 1 cm from the base of the appendix (Figure 4.14).

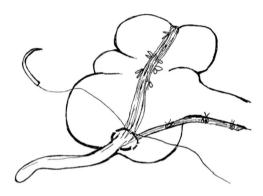

Figure 4.14 Purse-string suture.

- The appendix is crushed at its base with a straight artery forceps; the crushed area is ligated with a No. 1 absorbable polymer suture.

- A clamp is applied above the suture ligation and the appendix divided with a scalpel below this clamp and removed (simple ligation method).

- If desired, the stump may be inverted into the caecum using the previously placed purse-string suture which is snugged down above the stump as it is pushed inwards by the assistant.

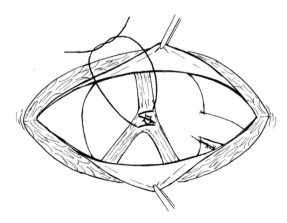

Figure 4.15 The Z-stitch.

- Oedema may prevent purse-string inversion in which case a z-stitch distal to the base of the appendix can be utilised (Figure 4.15).

- If the appendix is not inflamed, viscera in the right side of the abdomen should be palpated and visualised as far as possible, and in the female scrutinise the pelvic organs.

- Exclude a Meckel's diverticulum, Crohn's disease and a tumour of the appendix or right colon.

Hazards

- If the appendix cannot be localised within an abscess cavity, drain the abscess through a separate stab incision, leave the appendix and close the incision.

- If Crohn's disease is found, only perform an appendicectomy if the caecum is healthy.

- Postoperative faecal fistula may develop after a blown appendicular stump from insecure ligature or sepsis.

- Unidentified and residual abscesses, particularly in the pelvis, will result in signs of sepsis and a prolonged ileus and require further intervention to drain the abscess cavity either radiologically or surgically.

Postoperative management

- Most patients require 2–3 days hospitalisation and quickly progress to oral fluids and diet and rapid mobilisation.

- Antibiotics may need to be continued in a minority of patients for 24 hours, 48 hours or even five days in cases of peritonitis.

- Analgesics and antiemetics should be administered as required.

- Swinging fever in the absence of chest infection or urinary tract infection suggests an intraabdominal abscess which should be excluded by rectal examination and ultrasound or CT examination.

PERFORATED DUODENAL ULCER

Not all patients with perforated duodenal ulcer require operative treatment. In patients with typical symptoms of short duration and with a confident diagnosis who respond well to minimal resuscitation with intravenous fluids and in whom the signs of peritonitis are localised to the upper abdomen, conservative treatment may be instituted after ultrasound examination has demonstrated the absence of intraabdominal abscess. Therapy consists of nasogastric suction, intravenous fluids, systemic antibiotics and chest physiotherapy together with vigilant observation. Any signs of sepsis or generalised peritonitis signify failure of conservative treatment and should be acted upon immediately to convert to an operative treatment.

Patient preparation

- Provide adequate analgesia.

- Establish intravenous access and administer an intravenous infusion of fluid and electrolytes adequate to resuscitate the patient.

- Initiate broad-spectrum intravenous antibiotic treatment.

- Initiate thromboembolic prophylaxis.

- Supine position on the operating table.

- Upper midline incision (see above).

Procedure

- A specimen of free fluid is taken and sent for culture.

- Any excess free fluid or pus is aspirated.

- The subphrenic spaces, the paracolic gutters and the pelvis should each in turn be explored manually and fluid evacuated.

- Insert a self-retaining retractor into the wound.

- Identify the perforation which is usually on the anterior aspect of the duodenum and easily identifiable. Some mobilisation of the duodenum may be required by incising the peritoneum along the lateral border of the second part of the duodenum (Kocher's manoeuvre) to bring the perforation more clearly into view, most notably if the perforation is posterior.

- To close the perforation, sutures of 2/0 absorbable polymer are passed through all layers of the duodenal wall, sufficiently far from the margin of the perforation so that they do not tear through friable tissue. The needle is brought through the perforation then reinserted through the perforation and through all layers of the duodenal wall on the other side. Usually no more than three sutures are required.

- After insertion, the sutures are left long and held in the tips of artery forceps (Figure 4.16).

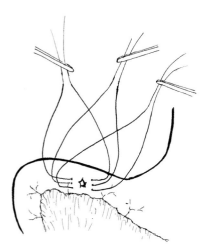

Figure 4.16 Sutures in a perforated duodenal ulcer.

- A tongue of convenient adjacent omentum is brought up anterior to the perforation and laid over it and held in place by the assistant (Figure 4.17).

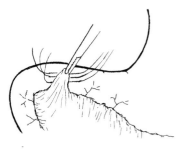

Figure 4.17 Omental patch laid over perforation.

- The previously placed sutures are tied over the omental patch, sufficiently tightly to retain the patch snugly in position and oppose the edges of the perforation (Figure 4.18).

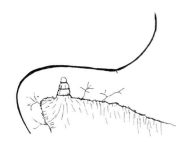

Figure 4.18 Sutures tied over the omental patch.

- The peritoneal cavity is washed out with 2–3 litres of saline with or without an antibiotic.

- Drainage of the peritoneal cavity is not necessary.

Hazards

- A large perforation or one associated with duodenal stenosis may result in duodenal obstruction after closure and this may require gastroenterostomy.

- When perforation and bleeding occur simultaneously (the bleeding is usually from a snail-tract ulcer extending over the posterior surface of the duodenum and eroding the gastroduodenal artery), it is advisable for an experienced surgeon to perform gastrectomy. Vagotomy and a drainage procedure or partial gastrectomy are rarely performed nowadays for perforated duodenal ulcer.

Note: Simple closure of an apparently benign perforated gastric ulcer is carried out in a similar fashion to the procedure for duodenal ulcer, with the exception that generous four-quadrant biopsies should be taken before closure to exclude microscopic malignancy. Perforated gastric ulcers that are obviously malignant at the time of surgery should be treated with gastrectomy by an experienced surgeon.

Postoperative management

- Most patients require 2–3 days hospitalisation and quickly progress to oral fluids and diet with mobilisation.

- Antibiotics may need to be continued in a minority of patients for 24 hours, 48 hours or even five days in cases of peritonitis.

- Analgesics and antiemetics should be administered as required.

- Swinging fever in the absence of chest infection or urinary tract infection suggests an intraabdominal abscess which should be excluded by rectal examination and ultrasound or CT examination.

- Haematemesis, melaena or suction of blood through the nasogastric tube suggests perforation has been complicated by peptic ulcer bleeding and this generally requires gastrectomy by an experienced surgeon.

- Upon recovery all patients should be given a course of *Helicobacter pylori* eradication therapy.

- Maintenance proton pump inhibitors should be given for one year in the first instance and persistent dyspeptic symptoms should be investigated by upper gastrointestinal endoscopy.

SMALL BOWEL RESECTION

The decision to resect small bowel may be taken for a variety of reasons including benign or malignant tumours, traumatic perforation, ischaemia, Crohn's disease, stricture or intussusception. The description below assumes that a length of approximately 40 cm requires resection.

Patient preparation

- Establish intravenous access to replace fluid loss if required.

- Preoperative blood transfusion to correct anaemia associated with bleeding lesions of the small bowel may be required.

- A nasogastric tube is inserted to decompress the stomach and small bowel if obstruction is present.

- Obstructed small intestine is often colonised by pathogenic bacteria and broad-spectrum intravenous antibiotics should be commenced preoperatively.

- Thromboembolic prophylaxis should be commenced preoperatively.

- Supine position on the operating table.

- Midline incision centred on the umbilicus (see above).

Procedure

- A self-retaining retractor is inserted into the abdominal wound.

- The affected loop of small bowel is delivered through the incision onto the anterior abdominal wall, together with sufficient length proximal and distal to the area to be resected.

- The exposed segment is protected with warm packs.

- Non-crushing clamps are applied across the lumen of the bowel not including mesenteric vessels and at a distance of approximately 5–10 cm from the segment to be resected (Figure 4.19).

- The length of intestine to be resected is now accurately determined and straight crushing clamps are placed across the bowel lumen at these points (Figure 4.20).

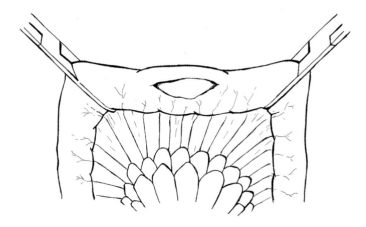

Figure 4.19 Non-crushing clamps applied.

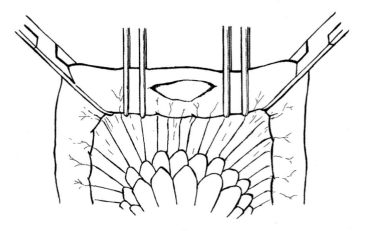

Figure 4.20 Crushing clamps applied.

● The bowel loop is now held up by the surgeon with the operating light shining over his shoulder onto the mesentery so that it may be examined to determine the vascular pattern (Figure 4.21).

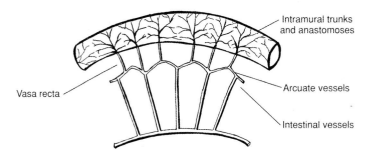

Figure 4.21 Mesenteric vasculature.

● A V-shaped incision is made in the peritoneum overlying the mesentery on both surfaces, superimposed in order to expose the intestinal vessels and their branches. After making a 'nick' in the visceral peritoneum by tenting up a small area with forceps and then incising with scissors, the V-shaped incision is achieved with a scissor slit.

● Each individual arcuate branch of the intestinal vessels in the line of the V-shaped incision is isolated, clamped, divided and ligated with fine absorbable ligatures (Figure 4.22).

● The bowel on the outer side of each of the crushing clamps is now cut with a scalpel and the affected segment of small intestine with its mesentery is removed.

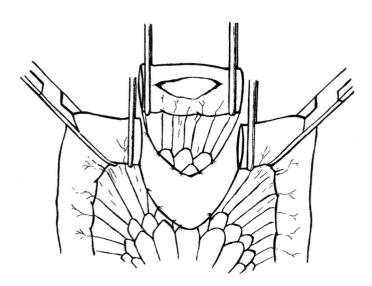

Figure 4.22 Mesenteric vessels ligated.

Anastomosis

An extra mucosal technique with interrupted sutures of 3/0 absorbable polymer incorporating all layers except the mucosa will be described.

● The first two anastomotic sutures to be applied are those on the mesenteric and antimesenteric borders. The needle is inserted in the easily visible cleavage between the mucosa and subserosa which is a tough collagenous layer adjacent to the submucosa. A 3–4 mm bite of tissue is taken on each side. These sutures will not be tied until the back layer is complete (Figure 4.23).

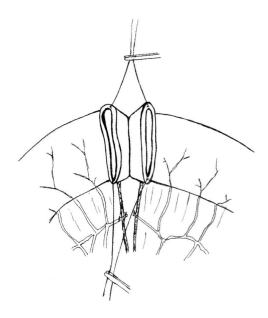

Figure 4.23 Mesenteric and antimesenteric stay sutures.

● The posterior layer of sutures are now placed extramucosally (as described above) approximately 2–3 mm apart (Figure 4.24). When the row of sutures is complete they are tied sequentially progressing from the antimesenteric to the mesenteric border. The stay sutures are now tied to complete the posterior layer; they are not cut but retained as stay sutures.

● The anterior layer is now completed in a similar manner by insertion of sutures in the extramucosal layer sequentially from antimesenteric to mesenteric border.

● The defect in the mesentery is closed with interrupted sutures to the visceral peritoneum taking care not to damage the intestinal arcades (Figure 4.25). The lumen should be tested for patency by gentle invagination with finger and thumb of small bowel either side of the anastomosis through its lumen.

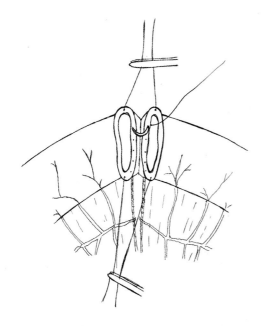

Figure 4.24 Posterior layer complete.

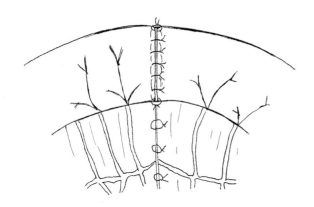

Figure 4.25 Completed anastomosis.

Hazards

- A technically unsatisfactory or ischaemic anastomosis may result in intestinal obstruction and require refashioning.
- Anastomotic failure may result in formation of an intraabdominal abscess, sepsis or an enterocutaneous fistula.

Postoperative management

- Most patients require 4–5 days hospitalisation and quickly progress to oral fluids and diet with mobilisation.
- Antibiotics may be discontinued within 24–48 hours unless the resection was performed in the presence of peritonitis.

- Analgesics and antiemetics should be administered as required.
- Swinging fever in the absence of chest infection or urinary tract infection suggests an intraabdominal abscess which should be excluded by rectal examination and ultrasound examination.

COLOSTOMY

There are a number of types of colostomy.

- *Loop* colostomy is usually sited in the transverse colon but any loop of the colon may be brought to the surface of the anterior abdominal wall provided this is achieved without tension.
- *Terminal* colostomy is either permanent, when a segment of or the entire distal colon/rectum has been removed; or temporary, when a diseased distal segment has been removed (either with internal closure of the distal stump or a mucous fistula) and colonic continuity will be reestablished at a later date.
- *Double-barrelled* colostomy is now of historical interest and was termed the Paul-Mikulicz operation in which the spur between two limbs of colon was slowly necrosed by application of a crushing enterotome.
- *Divided* colostomy, in which the two ends of the colon are separated by a skin bridge of varying size, is infrequently performed.

Loop colostomy

The loop colostomy of the transverse colon will be described. The indications are:

- *emergency*, to defunction an obstructed colon due to stenosing carcinoma, anastomotic dehiscence or in children with Hirschsprung's disease or imperforate anus
- *elective,* to protect the anastomosis of a low anterior resection, to defunction the left colon in patients with colonic fistulas usually secondary to diverticular disease, and to defunction the anorectum in patients undergoing surgery for complex anorectal fistulas.

Patient preparation

This will depend on the indication. In emergency cases the patient will require fluid resuscitation, decompression of the stomach and upper small bowel by nasogastric intubation, intravenous antibiotics and thromboembolic prophylaxis.

In elective cases:

- mechanical bowel preparation is advisable
- counselling by a stoma therapist is essential

- an indelible mark on the anterior abdominal wall should indicate the most convenient anatomical site for the stoma where it can be managed by the patient without interference from clothing or body folds

- urinary bladder catheter should be inserted to monitor postoperative urine output.

Anaesthesia

- Supine position on the operating table.

- A transverse incision is sited midway between the umbilicus and the costal margin overlying the lateral part of the rectus muscle extending laterally beyond its margin (Figure 4.26).

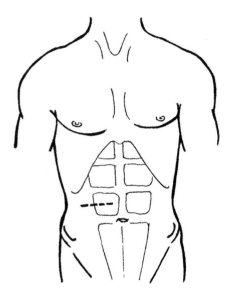

Figure 4.26 Site of incision for transverse colostomy.

The utilisation of the proximal transverse colon allows subsequent mobilisation of the splenic flexure when definitive surgery is required for pathology in the left colon.

Procedure

- After division of the skin and subcutaneous tissues, the anterior rectus sheath is incised followed by a portion of the rectus abdominis muscle in the line of the incision which is achieved by elevating the muscle over a large artery clamp and dividing the muscle bundles with cutting diathermy and coagulating branches of the superior epigastric artery with diathermy as the muscle bundles are cut (Figure 4.27).

- The posterior rectus sheath is divided with cutting diathermy.

- The peritoneum is grasped and tented with tooth dissecting

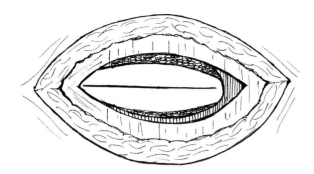

Figure 4.27 Deepening of incision to posterior rectus sheath.

forceps to which two small artery clamps are applied and then reapplied to ensure viscera are not trapped on its undersurface. The peritoneum is then 'nicked' and opened with scissors in the line of the incision.

- The transverse colon immediately below the incision is grasped with Babcock forceps and delivered through the abdominal wound (Figure 4.28).

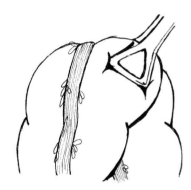

Figure 4.28 Delivery of colon through abdominal wall.

- At the selected site for opening of the colon the greater omentum on the inferior border is separated from it for a distance of approximately 5 cm by clamping, dividing and ligating individual vessels or strands of fat to create a window.

- A site is selected between the vasa recti where a hole may be made in the mesocolon close to the bowel wall at the apex of the loop (Figure 4.29).

- A soft rubber tube is placed through this hole to deliver and retain the loop on the anterior abdominal wall.

- The rubber tubing may now be replaced by a plastic rod to form a bridge for the colostomy (Figure 4.30).

- The skin at each side of the colon is closed with interrupted sutures to provide a snug aperture for the colostomy.

- The colon is opened transversely along a taenia at the apex of

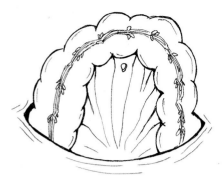

Figure 4.29 Hole in the mesentery.

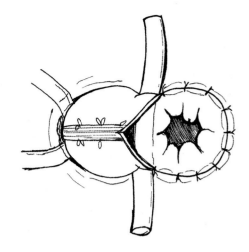

Figure 4.31 Anastomosis between skin and colon.

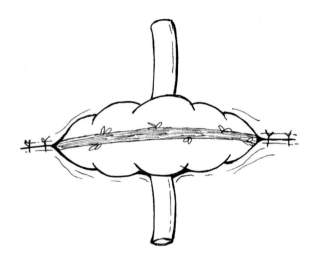

Figure 4.30 A rod forms a bridge for the colostomy.

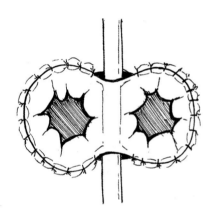

Figure 4.32 Anastomosis completed.

the loop for half the intended aperture and then secured with sutures between the skin and all layers of the colon excluding the mucosa with interrupted sutures of 3/0 absorbable polymer (Figure 4.31).

- The other half of the intended aperture is then opened and sutured to the skin by a similar technique (Figure 4.32).

- Gentle digital exploration of the lumen can now be performed to ensure patency of the proximal and distal colon.

- A suitable colostomy bag is applied over the stoma including the plastic rod within the bag.

Hazards

- Inadequate mobilisation of the colon may cause retraction, leading to later stenosis or difficulty in application of the colostomy bag.

- Ischaemia of the colon due to damage to the blood supply of the apex of colon can result in a dusky appearance which may recover or permanent ischaemia can result in later stenosis or even possibly early necrosis, which will require revision by an experienced surgeon.

- Paracolostomy hernia and colostomy prolapse are relatively common late complications.

Postoperative management

The postoperative recovery is generally dependent on the primary condition for which the loop colostomy was performed and will include management of that specific condition. Once intestinal function has returned and the stoma is active, the most important aspect of postoperative care is for the patient to be able to manage the stoma at home. This will be achieved by adequate counselling, coaching and encouragement from a trained stoma therapist.

INGUINAL HERNIA REPAIR

Inguinal hernia is the most common general surgical operation performed. The vast majority of hernias present as a reducible swelling in the groin. The repair of complex or recurrent hernias will not be described nor will the management of strangulated hernia be dealt with. Most elective inguinal hernias are now repaired by the Lichtenstein technique utilising a sheet of prosthetic mesh and this is the operation that will be described. Experienced surgeons will have learnt the multilayered suture technique of Shouldice but for the trainee surgeon, the Lichtenstein technique is simple, easy to learn and effective.

Patient preparation

- The peak age of incidence is 55–85 years and thus many of these patients are elderly men with other significant co-morbidity. Local anaesthesia is therefore a valuable option but should be administered by an expert and full cardiorespiratory monitoring must take place during the operation.

- If general anaesthesia is to be used, the patient should be prepared accordingly.

- Shave the inguinal region on the side to be operated upon on the day of operation.

- Mark the affected side so there is no mistake when the patient is asleep or sedated.

- Obtain intravenous access whether the patient is operated on under LA or GA.

- Administer rectal non-steroidal antiinflammatory drug with the premedication to assist in postoperative pain relief.

- There is no evidence to support the use of prophylactic antibiotics when prosthetic mesh is utilised, although the majority of surgeons give this as a precaution.

- Thromboembolic prophylaxis is not required for the repair of a straightforward hernia.

Anaesthesia

- The patient lies supine on the operating table.

- If the operation is under LA, have an expert apply an inguinal field block to anaesthetise the sensory nerves: ilioinguinal, iliohypogastric and genital branch of the genitofemoral, together with the subcutaneous and fascial layers of the groin.

- There are two choices of incision: one placed 1 cm above and parallel to the medial half of the inguinal ligament and extending for 1 or 2 cm medial to this to expose the pubic tubercle or one lying in a transverse direction in a skin crease at the level of the internal ring.

Procedure

- The external oblique aponeurosis is exposed and opened along the axis of the spermatic cord, beginning at the external ring (Figure 4.33).

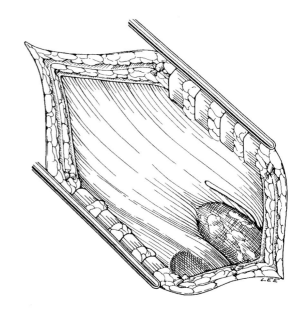

Figure 4.33 External oblique aponeurosis exposed.

- The upper and lower flaps of the external oblique are reflected and a self-retaining retractor inserted to expose the spermatic cord and inguinal canal.

- The spermatic cord is dissected out and separated from the posterior inguinal wall by sharp dissection in the region just lateral to the pubic tubercle. A soft tubing or a Stewart's hernial ring retractor is then placed around the spermatic cord so that it may be retracted upwards or downwards.

- The hernial sac is identified and with sharp dissection separated from the spermatic cord to its neck. The neck of an indirect sac will be traced to the internal ring (Figure 4.34). A direct sac should be inverted and the posterior inguinal wall flattened to facilitate placement of the mesh, by a running absorbable suture applied to the transversalis fascia (Figure 4.35).

- A patch of polypropylene mesh initially 8 cm by 16 cm is trimmed to the individual patient's requirements and the medial corner removed so that it will tuck between the external oblique and internal oblique muscles (Figure 4.36).

- The patch is laid on the posterior inguinal wall so that it lies parallel with the inguinal ligament, overlaps the pubic tubercle by 1–2 cm and tucks underneath the external oblique.

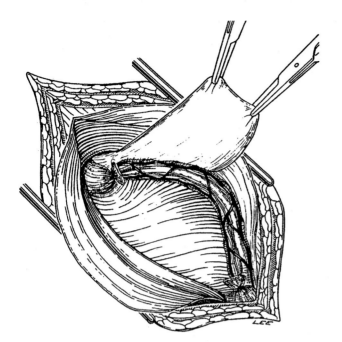

Figure 4.34 An indirect sac dissected to its neck.

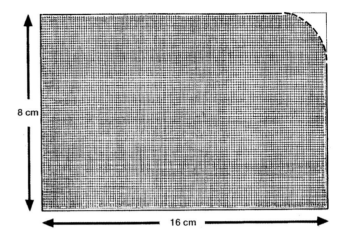

Figure 4.36 Shaping the mesh.

- A running suture is now begun at the upper medial rounded border of the mesh with a non-absorbable monofilament material and continued along the lower edge of the shelving margin of the inguinal ligament to a point lateral to the internal ring (Figure 4.37).

- Tacking sutures are then applied to the superior margin of the patch.

- The tails are overlapped and crossed and a single suture placed to create a new internal ring which is tested with an artery clip (Figure 4.38).

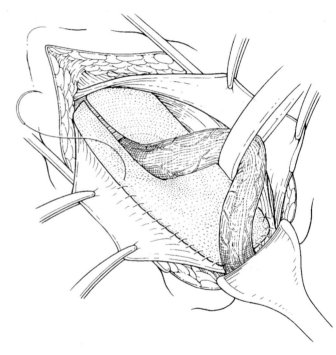

Figure 4.37 A continuous suture anchors the mesh to the inguinal ligament.

- The operation is completed by applying a running suture to close the external oblique over the spermatic cord and then the subcutaneous layers and skin are closed.

- The skin is closed with a subcuticular continuous absorbable polymer suture (Figure 4.39).

Hazards

- Haemorrhage may occur from accidental damage of the inferior epigastric vein or more seriously if a suture is placed in the femoral vein. Removal of the suture and firm pressure for a few minutes usually suffices to staunch the haemorrhage.

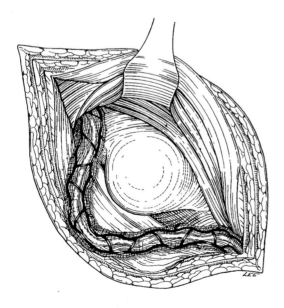

Figure 4.35 A direct sac such as this may be inverted with a running suture.

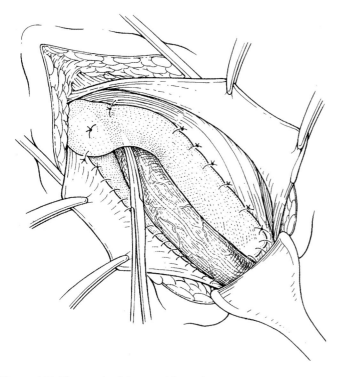

Figure 4.38 The completed fixation of the mesh.

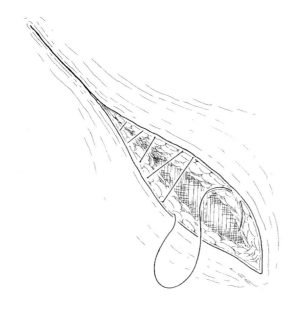

Figure 4.39 Skin closure.

- Sensory nerves should not be damaged or diathermised as this may lead to neuralgia. If sensory nerves get in the way, they should be cleanly divided and a small area of anaesthesia will result.

- Wound infection rate should be no higher than 2–3% for elective surgery. Minor infections can be dealt with by prescribing antibiotics but abscesses should be drained formally.

- 1–2% of patients will suffer ischaemic orchitis which results in fever, leucocytosis and testicular swelling for 4–5 days immediately following the operation, followed by testicular atrophy in one quarter of patients. The patient may sue for compensation.

- Urinary retention is more frequent after general anaesthesia in which it occurs in approximately 5% of patients and temporary catheterisation for 24 hours usually resolves the problem.

Postoperative management

- Early mobilisation is desirable; patients operated on under local anaesthesia are encouraged to ambulate within 1–2 hours of surgery and return home.

- Adequate analgesia is essential if patients are to return to early normal activity, but this is usually only required for the first 2–3 days after operation.

- Sedentary workers should be encouraged to return to normal activity and work 2 weeks after operation and those with more strenuous occupations may require up to 4 weeks of convalescence. Patients should be encouraged to exercise; physical activity does not increase the risk of recurrence.

FEMORAL HERNIA REPAIR

Approximately 40% of femoral hernias present as an emergency and many of these patients have been unaware of a lump in the groin prior to presentation with small bowel obstruction.

In elective cases, an irreducible lump may also be present but the sac does not usually contain bowel; extraperitoneal fat or omentum is more likely. There are a number of operative approaches to femoral hernia. The two most popular are:

- the modified McEvedy extraperitoneal operation, in which a transverse incision, two fingers breadth above the pubic symphysis extending from the midline laterally, is utilised to enter the extraperitoneal space to gain access to the hernia sac. This approach is optimal in acute emergencies

- the crural or low approach, which is favoured in elective femoral hernia repair and will be described here. Patient preparation and anaesthesia are similar to those used in inguinal hernia repair.

Procedure

- The skin incision is made over the fundus of the hernia sac and is approximately 5–6 cm long, parallel to and below the inguinal ligament.

- Incise the subcutaneous layers to expose the hernia sac, securing haemostasis.

67

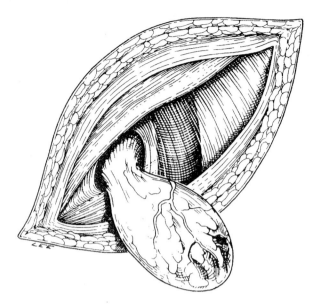

Figure 4.40 Sac mobilised.

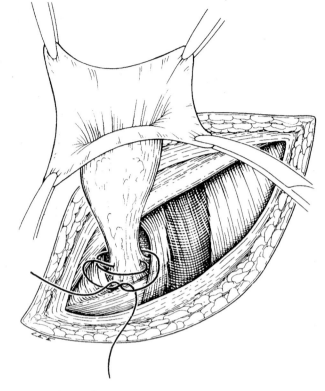

Figure 4.41 Closure of sac.

- The layers of the sac include fascia transversalis, extraperitoneal fat, cribriform fascia and the femoral fascial layer of the thigh which form 'onion skins'. These fascial layers are incised with a combination of blunt and sharp dissection and the sac is mobilised (Figure 4.40).

- The margins of the femoral opening are identified beginning at the medial margin, which is the lacunar ligament, and then opening up the plane anteriorly between the neck of the sac and the inguinal ligament and posteriorly between the neck of the sac and the pectineal fascia. Lateral to the neck of the sac lies the femoral vein where dissection should proceed with care.

- The fundus of the sac is grasped between haemostats, care being taken not to damage underlying bowel. The sac is opened and the contents inspected, adhesions divided and then omentum or bowel is returned to the general peritoneal cavity.

- The neck of the empty sac is closed with a transfixion suture (Figure 4.41).

- Repair of the femoral canal is then carried out with a figure-of-eight suture picking up the inguinal ligament, the iliopubic tract of fascia transversalis and the pectineal ligament as shown in Figure 4.42. Larger defects can be repaired with a Marlex mesh 'cigarette stub' as shown in Figure 4.43.

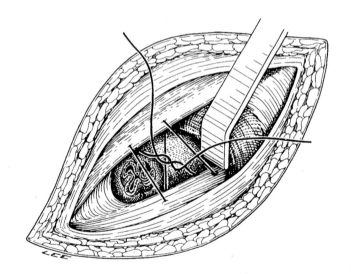

Figure 4.42 Figure-of-eight closure of femoral canal.

Hazards

- Haemorrhage from the femoral vein may occur from accidental damage or inadvertent placement of a suture in its wall. Removal of the suture and firm pressure will stop the bleeding unless damage is extensive.

- Wound infections are rather more common than in inguinal hernia because the incision is lower and nearer the groin crease. A single dose of prophylactic antibiotic is therefore advisable.

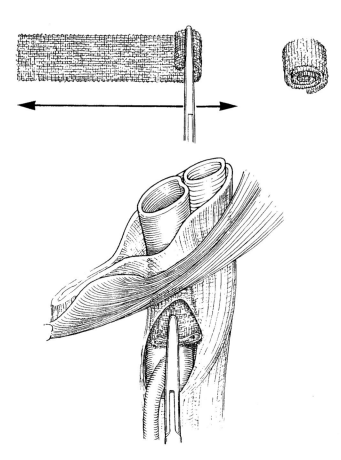

Figure 4.43 Cigarette stub placed in femoral canal.

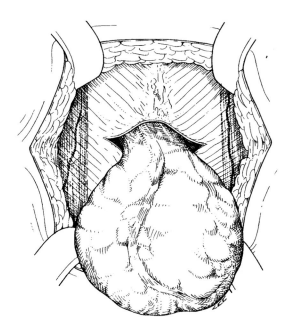

Figure 4.44 Neck of the sac is identified.

Postoperative management

As for inguinal hernia.

UMBILICAL HERNIA REPAIR

The operation in adults will be described. Recurrent umbilical hernias or those with a defect greater than 4 cm in diameter should be repaired with mesh placed in the preperitoneal retromuscular space. Smaller (less than 4 cm), primary umbilical hernias in adults are repaired by the Mayo operation which is described here.

Patient preparation

- General anaesthesia is required with full muscle relaxation and the patient is prepared accordingly.

- The skin is prepared and cleaned with particular attention to areas of intertrigo; umboliths should be removed.

- Carefully mark the palpable defect which may be umbilical, supra- or infraumbilical.

- Administer prophylactic antibiotics because of the higher than normal risk of postoperative wound infection.

- Thromboembolic prophylaxis will be required in many cases because of obesity.

Anaesthesia

- The patient lies supine on the operating table.

- A transverse incision is made over the defect extending laterally on each side to create an incision of approximately 4–5 cm. The incision does not include the umbilical cicatrix but skirts above it for supraumbilical and below it for infraumbilical hernias. An ellipse of redundant skin may be removed if it has become stretched over the hernia sac.

Procedure

- The incision is deepened to expose the fundus and subsequently the neck of the sac (Figure 4.44).

- Haemostats are applied carefully, avoiding damage to underlying bowel, and the fundus of the sac is opened and its contents inspected.

- Adhesions between the contents and the sac are divided and bowel or omentum returned to the general peritoneal cavity.

- The sac is excised carefully, coagulating blood vessels at the base of the neck before they retract into the extraperitoneal space.

- The margins of the defect are now picked up in haemostats (Figure 4.45).

- These margins are now repaired by an overlapping Mayo technique with interrupted non-absorbable suture material. Each suture is placed as follows: beginning 2–3 cm from the margin, the needle is passed from out to in, on the opposite side it is again passed from out to in and then in to out, and then finally back to the initial margin where the needle is passed from in to out (Figure 4.46).

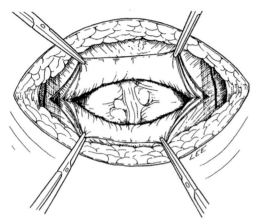

Figure 4.45 Margins of the defect are picked up in haemostats.

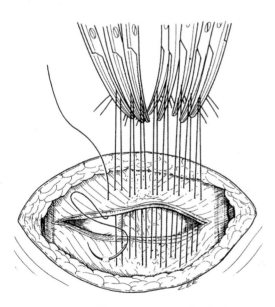

Figure 4.46 The first layer of deep sutures is now placed. The sutures enter the upper flap 3 cm from its margin. They go through both aponeurotic layers (anterior and posterior rectus sheaths) on eather side and through the full thickness of the linea alba in the midline. The sutures are then carried down to and then through the lower flap 1 cm from the margin. The sutures are left lax and held in haemostats.

- When the sutures are tied down the margins of the defect overlap and the free edge is then sutured down with a running suture (Figure 4.47).

- A small suction drain may be placed and the skin is closed with a subcuticular continuous absorbable suture.

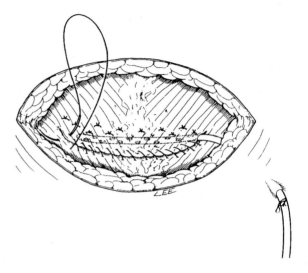

Figure 4.47 The upper flap is sutured to the anterior surface of the lower flap.

Hazards

- Beware adherent transverse colon within the sac.

- The deeply placed Mayo sutures should be placed under direct vision to ensure the needle does not damage underlying bowel.

- Careful haemostasis is required because postoperative haematoma is a precursor of wound infection.

Acknowledgements

Surgical drawings in this chapter are reproduced with permission from Chapman and Hall and Arnold publishers.

FURTHER READING

1   Devlin HB, Kingsnorth A. *Management of Abdominal Hernias*, 2nd edn. London: Chapman and Hall Medical

5

Anal and perianal diseases

Proctoscopy
Sigmoidoscopy
Haemorrhoids
  Outpatient treatment of haemorrhoids
  Haemorrhoidectomy

Anal fissure
  Outpatient treatment of fissure
  Subcutaneous lateral internal sphincterotomy
Anorectal abscess
  Incision and drainage
Anorectal fistula
  Operations

Richard Welbourn

Investigation of perianal and anal conditions begins with a clinical examination of the patient. General examination is carried out with particular reference to the alimentary tract and abdominal examination. Digital rectal examination is performed by turning the patient on the left side with the knees drawn up and the buttocks protruding over the edge of the couch. After careful examination of the perineum it is important to assess whether there is any contraindication to instrumentation such as spasm of the anal sphincters due to fissure. During digital examination, perineal contractivity of the sphincters is assessed and palpation undertaken for luminal and extraluminal masses, tracks or pockets of pus.

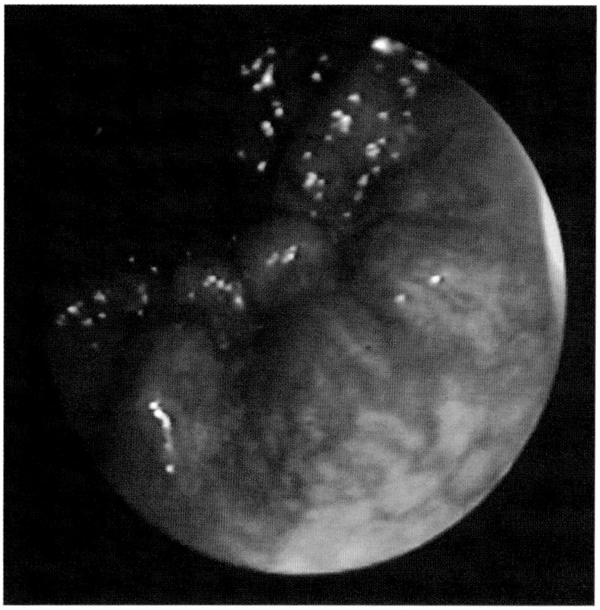

PROCTOSCOPY

The St Marks-type proctoscope has a light source and an obturator which is lubricated before passage into the anal canal. The instrument is then passed initially upwards and forwards and then upwards and backwards into the lower rectum. The obturator is now removed and as the instrument is withdrawn, the lower rectum, anorectal ring and anal canal can be inspected for pathology.

SIGMOIDOSCOPY

Bowel preparation is usually not required but if the lower rectum is loaded with stool, a phosphate enema will be sufficient to evacuate the rectum and allow clear visualisation of the mucosa. The patient lies in the left lateral position as for proctoscopy and the lubricated sigmoidoscope with obturator in place is gently passed by the same technique as for proctoscopy. Once the instrument has been passed 5–10 cm, the obturator is removed and a little air insufflated into the bowel lumen by pumping the bellows. The patient is warned that this may cause a little discomfort and the desire to pass flatus. At 15 cm the rectosigmoid junction is encountered and the instrument is manoeuvred backwards and then upwards to enter the distal sigmoid colon. Circumferential inspection is carried out as the instrument is withdrawn, gently applying insufflation to distend the bowel lumen. Mucosal and intraluminal masses are biopsied adequately and specimens sent for histological examination.

HAEMORRHOIDS

Clinical features

Haemorrhoids, or piles, are vascular anal cushions that produce symptoms (Figure 5.1). The most common symptoms are bright red bleeding, prolapse, itching or mucus discharge. Haemorrhoids are the most common cause of rectal bleeding but in all patients other causes must be sought. In a patient with simple rectal bleeding it is important to distinguish between 'outlet' bleeding and bleeding from further up the lower gastrointestinal tract that may

Figure 5.1 Haemorrhoids seen from inside the rectum on retroflexed view via colonoscope.

be mixed in with the faeces or associated with a change in bowel habit. Such symptoms may be the presenting features of colorectal cancer or inflammatory bowel disease.

Haemorrhoidal bleeding occurs during defaecation, is typically separate from stool and can drip from the anus (symptomatic, non-prolapsing haemorrhoids are sometimes called first degree). In women haemorrhoids commonly occur in pregnancy and may require treatment if symptoms do not resolve after the end of pregnancy.

Haemorrhoids may become larger and prolapse on defaecation (second degree). Persistent prolapse may develop and the haemorrhoids can only be pushed back digitally (third degree). Occasionally haemorrhoids may thrombose after prolapsing and cannot be pushed back (strangulation). Such haemorrhoids are very painful and may require immediate haemorrhoidectomy for pain relief. If left alone, strangulated haemorrhoids will resolve by themselves eventually and no further treatment may be required other than pain relief and antiinflammatory agents and measures to reduce oedema (e.g. a bag of frozen peas!).

In the outpatient clinic abdominal, rectal and sigmoidoscopic examination is mandatory. Rigid sigmoidoscopy (which examines the rectum) may be adequate for younger patients but flexible sigmoidoscopy allows views of the left colon as well and may be preferred for older patients. Biopsies should be taken if colitis or cancer is suspected. The flexible sigmoidoscope (or colonoscope) enables snare polypectomy to be performed if a polyp is found. If there are other lower gastrointestinal symptoms, such as a change in bowel habit, the whole colon should be examined by colonoscopy or barium enema. Rectal bleeding alone rarely arises proximal to the splenic flexure. Once other causes have been excluded rectal bleeding may be confidently ascribed to haemorrhoids.

Haemorrhoids are seen on proctoscopy (which examines the anal canal) as reddened or bluish mucosal bulges just above the dentate line on withdrawal of the instrument. Classically haemorrhoids are seen in the 3, 7 and 11 o'clock positions but often one pile mass in any position is predominant. There may be associated fleshy skin tags (below the dentate line) that may cause problems with cleanliness but do not usually cause symptoms.

It is important to reassure the patient that other, more serious, causes of bleeding have been excluded. Treatment of the haemorrhoids should be offered if they produce sufficient symptoms. Usually treatment can be given directly in the clinic.

Outpatient treatment of haemorrhoids

Several treatments for haemorrhoids are available. The two most frequently used for outpatients are:

- injection sclerotherapy
- rubber band ligation.

Injection sclerotherapy shrinks the haemorrhoidal tissue by inducing submucosal scarring with fibrosis. It has the advantage that it is quick to perform and side effects are minimal. Rubber band ligation works by causing ischaemic necrosis of the haemorrhoid. It requires a nurse assistant familiar with the technique and takes a little longer. It can cause pain afterwards and has an uncommon but important complication, secondary haemorrhage. Both techniques control symptoms.

Other treatments, such as anal stretch or cryotherapy, do not have any advantages, may cause local damage and should no longer be used. Regardless of the choice of treatment, bleeding can recur. To minimise the possibility of recurrent bleeding patients should be:

- encouraged to have bulky soft stools by increasing fibre intake or by using a bulk laxative
- told to avoid excessive straining at defaecation.

Injection sclerotherapy

Patient preparation

- Elicit any allergy to nut oil.
- Obtain verbal consent and ask a nurse chaperone to be present during the procedure.
- Consider giving the patient an enema if the rectum is loaded.

Position

Left lateral with back angled across couch, shoulders away from surgeon and buttocks towards edge of couch. Knees up and feet forward.

Procedure

- Always perform a rectal examination first, then sigmoidoscopy.
- Perform a proctoscopy and visualise the haemorrhoids.
- With the proctoscope in the left hand and the syringe in the right hand, insert the needle into the superior part of the haemorrhoid (Figure 5.2) just deep to the mucosa, above the dentate line.

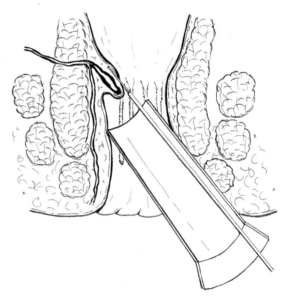

Figure 5.2 Injection of sclerosant into superior pole of haemorrhoid via proctoscope.

- Five percent phenol in nut oil, available in standard commercial preparation, is used for injection (Figure 5.3).
- Inject enough sclerosant to raise a bleb; usually about 5 ml is injected but in large haemorrhoids up to 10 ml of sclerosant may be needed.

Hazards

- Pain from injecting too near the dentate line.
- Too deep an injection in males may result in inadvertent injection of sclerosant into the prostate gland.

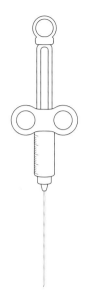

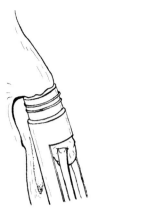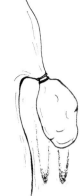

Figure 5.4 Rubber band ligation.

Figure 5.3 Disposable syringe and needle for injection sclerotherapy.

Postoperative management

- Warn the patient that there may be some postinjection bleeding.

- Advise the patient that injections may need repeating.

- Arrange to see the patient again in a few weeks if bleeding persists and consider further investigation.

Rubber band ligation

Patient preparation

- Discuss complications such as pain or secondary bleeding following banding.

- Obtain verbal consent and ask a nurse chaperone to be present during the procedure.

Position

As for injection sclerotherapy, viewing each haemorrhoid in turn.

Procedure

- The procedure is most easily performed with suction banding equipment but a handheld grasper is adequate.

- With the suction band applicator in the right hand, apply the suction part of the applicator onto the superior pole of the haemorrhoid. Apply suction by placing the thumb over the suction hole and wait for a few seconds.

- Pull the trigger and assess (Figure 5.4).

- Repeat the procedure for the other haemorrhoids.

Hazards

- Pain may occur from placing the band too near the dentate line. If pain persists reinsert the proctoscope and remove the band.

- Secondary haemorrhage may occur 1–2 weeks later from the ulcer produced by the band falling off. Bleeding can be severe enough to require blood transfusion.

Postoperative management

- Warn the patient that there may be some postbanding discomfort.

- Advise the patient that banding may need to be repeated.

- Arrange to see the patient again in a few weeks if bleeding persists and consider further investigation.

Haemorrhoidectomy

Haemorrhoidectomy is indicated if severe bleeding is not helped by outpatient treatment and especially if the patient is becoming anaemic due to chronic blood loss. The open technique (Milligan-Morgan) is the most commonly performed operation. The procedure may be performed as a day case provided the patient is given adequate instruction and analgesia.

Patient preparation

- Ensure that the patient is fit enough for a general anaesthetic.

- Obtain written consent for the procedure.

- Many surgeons prefer to give a rectal enema preoperatively.

Anaesthesia

General anaesthesia and topical local anaesthetic, e.g. 0.5% bupivacaine with adrenaline, to aid postoperative pain control and clarify the operative field via haemostasis.

Position

Lithotomy (patient supine with hips abducted and flexed).

Procedure

- Grasp each haemorrhoid and its external skin component with medium artery clips (Figure 5.5). As the assistant holds the other clips out of the way 2–3 ml of local anaesthetic is injected subcutaneously into each haemorrhoid.

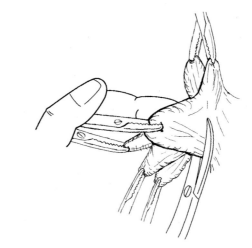

Figure 5.6 The skin incision is made first.

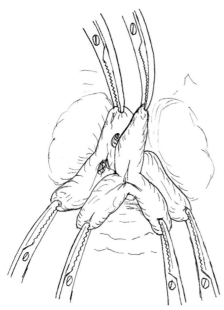

Figure 5.5 Each haemorrhoid and its external skin component are grasped by clips.

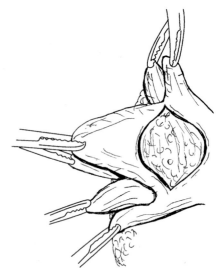

Figure 5.7 The incision is deepened to develop the plane between pedicle of haemorrhoid and internal sphincter.

- Using curved Mayo scissors, mark the circumferential extent of each excision margin.

- Insertion of a Parks retractor or Eisenhammer speculum into the anal canal may help to expose each haemorrhoid in turn.

- Place the index finger of the left hand inside the anal canal and gently stretch the tissues by tension on the artery clips.

- Join the incisions marking each haemorrhoid and deepen the incision to expose the internal sphincter. Diathermy dissection aids haemostasis (Figures 5.6, 5.7).

- Develop a plane to isolate the haemorrhoidal column on a pedicle away from the internal sphincter.

- Ligate the pedicle with a strong absorbable suture (e.g. 1/0 polyglactin) and excise the haemorrhoid, leaving the suture

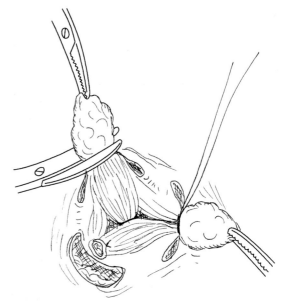

Figure 5.8 Each haemorrhoid is ligated and excised.

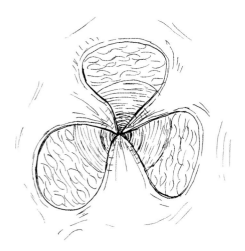

Figure 5.9 Skin bridges are left between each excised haemorrhoid.

long for retraction during excision of the other haemorrhoids (Figure 5.8).

- Leave adequate skin bridges of intact mucosa and anoderm (Figure 5.9).

- Excise the other haemorrhoids.

- Finally trim all the sutures.

- Inject local anaesthetic thoroughly.

- Apply a simple dressing, e.g. Vaseline gauze and pads.

Hazards

- Care must be taken not to divide mucocutaneous skin bridges as this may result in anal stenosis; repair any divided skin bridge with an absorbable suture (e.g. 3/0 polyglactin).

- Care with haemostasis avoids postoperative haemorrhage, which can be considerable.

Postoperative management

- Ensure that the patient is given adequate analgesia (preferably non-constipating).
- Give stool softeners or a bulk laxative postoperatively until bowel function returns.

Stapled haemorrhoidectomy

This is a newly described technique that excises the haemorrhoidal tissue as a circular cuff of mucosa via a stapling gun. Initial reports suggest it may be less painful than the Milligan–Morgan method.

ANAL FISSURE

Clinical features

The exact aetiology of anal fissure is unclear but it may be caused by the passage of a hard stool which tears the lining of the anal canal below the dentate line (Figure 5.10). Most fissures occur in the posterior midline but about 10% occur in the anterior midline. The skin below the dentate line, the anoderm, is exquisitely sensitive. Thus the classic symptom of a fissure in the anal canal is severe anal pain on defaecation. Pain usually subsides between times but many patients suffer pain from recurring fissures and the pain may be quite severe.

A fissure is associated with increased tone in the adjacent internal sphincter and although an acute tear may heal, the spasm often leads to further difficulty in defaecation and failure of healing, hence chronicity. A chronic fissure may lead to a characteristic skin tag of heaped up, hypertrophied anoderm (sometimes misleadingly called a 'sentinel pile') immediately inferior to the fissure. If a chronic fissure heals there may be scarring of the mucosa or submucosa that is easily palpated by the examining finger.

It is very important to differentiate an acute, simple fissure from inflammatory conditions (such as Crohn's disease) or malignancy (such as ulcerating rectal adenocarcinoma invading downwards or squamous carcinoma of the anal canal). Typically, in a younger patient with no other gastrointestinal symptoms or history to suggest otherwise, the finding of extreme tenderness posteriorly on digital rectal examination is sufficient. Usually the fissure can be seen but sometimes due to patient tenderness its presence must be inferred. If the clinical suspicion is of more than a simple fissure, and if pain allows, then sigmoidoscopy and proctoscopy with biopsy should be performed in the clinic. If this is not possible then examination should be performed under general anaesthetic.

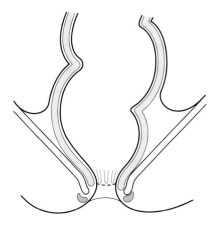

Figure 5.10 Diagram showing position of dentate line and sphincters.

Outpatient treatment of fissure

It seems logical that if internal sphincter spasm can be reduced by pharmacological means for a time sufficient for a chronic fissure to heal then an operation might be avoided. Internal sphincter tone appears to be nitric oxide dependent and enthusiasm for effecting a reversible chemical sympathectomy by applying topical glyceryl trinitrate (GTN, a nitric oxide donor) ointment is increasing. GTN 0.2% ointment applied 2–3 times daily for 2 months appears to work in about two-thirds of patients but there may be significant side effects such as headache due to systemic absorption. It is not known if GTN treatment prevents fissures recurring. Care should also be taken in treating patients with cardiovascular disease. At present it seems pragmatic to try the effect of topical GTN as first-line treatment for chronic fissure and to reserve operative treatment for those that do not heal. Other treatments such as topical botulinum toxin have also been suggested.

Subcutaneous lateral internal sphincterotomy

The mainstay of treatment is operative by performing a subcutaneous lateral internal sphincterotomy (SLIS). Forcible anal stretch (modified Lord's procedure) still has its advocates but should be applied with caution. Both operations aim to reduce the pressure in the anal canal so that evacuation can occur without pain and without causing more tearing stress on the anoderm. Forcible anal stretching may, however, result in uncontrolled tearing of the internal sphincter. It should be used with great care in any patient and especially women, whose pelvic floor following childbirth is already at risk of weakness in later life. The risk of varying degrees of incontinence after even a 'gentle' four-finger anal stretch is real, although small. SLIS can be carried out with more precision, the risk of postoperative problems with continence is low and it has therefore become the procedure of choice for most anorectal surgeons.

Indications

Operation is indicated if the fissure is not healed by non-operative means.

Patient preparation

- Ensure that the patient is fit for general anaesthesia.
- Obtain written consent for the procedure.
- Operation is performed as a day case procedure.

Anaesthesia

General anaesthesia and topical local anaesthetic, e.g. 0.5% bupivacaine with adrenaline, for postoperative pain control and haemostasis.

Position

Lithotomy (patient supine with hips abducted and flexed).

Procedure

- Examine the patient to ensure the diagnosis is correct.
- Insert a Parks retractor or Eisenhammer speculum into the anal canal.
- With the anal margin slightly stretched, feel the groove between the internal and external anal sphincters in the 3 o'clock position with the left index finger or with an instrument (Figure 5.11).
- Inject 1–2 ml local anaesthetic submucosally into the anoderm and between the sphincters for 1–2 cm or just above the dentate line (Figure 5.12).

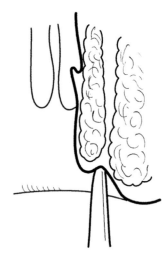

Figure 5.11 Fissure in posterior midline and instrument placed in intersphincteric groove.

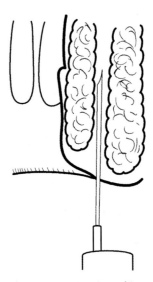

Figure 5.12 Local anaesthetic injection into intersphincteric groove.

- To reduce tissue bleeding allow sufficient time for the adrenaline to act.

- Make a radial incision about 1cm long in the groove (Figure 5.13).

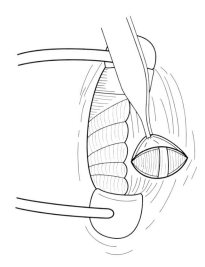

Figure 5.13 Radial incision in anoderm to expose internal sphincter.

- Insert McIndoe scissors and develop the plane between the sphincters up to the level of the dentate line (Figure 5.14).

- Divide the internal sphincter up to the dentate line, leaving a defect palpable through the mucosa.

- Apply a local dressing as for haemorrhoidectomy.

Hazards

- Ensure the correct sphincter is identified by palpation of the intersphincteric groove.

- Do not divide the internal sphincter above the dentate line.

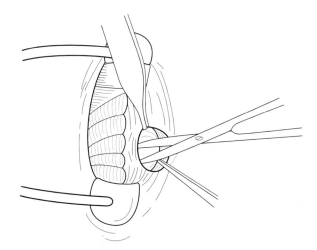

Figure 5.14 The internal sphincter is dissected away from anoderm and external sphincter and divided.

Postoperative management

Prescribe a stool softener or bulk laxative postoperatively to prevent the passage of hard stools.

ANORECTAL ABSCESS

Clinical features

Anorectal abscess is one of the most common surgical infections presenting to the trainee surgeon. The perineal skin may be involved with any of the skin conditions that present to the surgeon, e.g. infected sebaceous cyst, and therefore culture of the pus obtained for microscopy may be helpful in determining whether the cause is related to the gastrointestinal tract. Most anorectal abscesses arise from the deep part of an infected anal gland and therefore originate from the intersphincteric plane. The pus may point into any of the four surgical spaces identified (Figure 5.15).

- *Perianal abscess* (the most common anorectal abscess) points inferiorly via the intersphincteric space within 2–3 cm of the anal verge.

- *Ischiorectal abscess* points inferiorly lateral to the external sphincter.

- *Submucosal abscess* points between the anal canal mucosa and the internal sphincter.

- *Supralevator abscess* breaches the pelvic floor above the level of the anorectal ring (puborectalis muscle) and points into the rectum (rare).

An abscess presents with acute anal pain to one side of the anus and a reddened, raised, cellulitic area that may be pointing and is exquisitely tender. The patient adopts a characteristic position lying on the side and may have pyrexia, tachycardia and a raised white cell count.

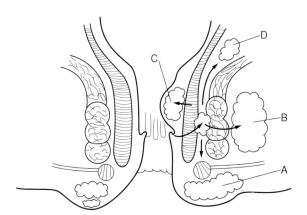

Figure 5.15 Classification of anorectal abscesses arising from intersphincteric abscess. **A.** Perianal. **B.** Ischiorectal. **C.** Submucosal. **D.** Supralevator.

Acute anal pain with pyrexia but no local signs must be taken to indicate anorectal infection and the patient should undergo examination under anaesthetic (EUA) the same day. Rectal examination and sigmoidoscopy should be carried out and a collection of pus carefully sought by digital examination and by using a retractor or speculum. If in doubt, a syringe with a 21 gauge needle may be helpful in localising pus.

Usually an abscess is unilateral but bilateral ischiorectal abscesses arise by pus tracking around posterior to the anus from one ischiorectal fossa to the other (horseshoe abscess). A submucosal abscess commonly drains spontaneously without operation but all others require incision and drainage. The object of treatment is to drain the abscess not only for pain relief but also to prevent the enlarging abscess breaching anatomic planes and giving rise to complications such as multiple fistulas.

At operation there are two important questions to answer. Can a fistula be found? If so, is it high or low (in relation to the anorectal ring/pelvic floor)? Because the anal glands open onto the skin at the dentate line, most fistula tracks open here also and are low fistulas. Many abscesses heal with simple incision and drainage but others recur unless the responsible epithelialised track is excised. Care should be taken to establish whether inflammatory bowel disease (e.g. Crohn's disease) is present.

Incision and drainage

Patient preparation

● Ensure that the patient is fit for general anaesthesia.

● Obtain written consent for the procedure.

Anaesthesia

General anaesthetic only. Local anaesthetic injection spreads infection and is not necessary (drainage of abscess provides immediate pain relief).

Position

Lithotomy (patient supine with hips abducted and flexed).

Procedure

● By rectal examination carefully delineate the anatomic site of the abscess.

● With a retractor or speculum in the anal canal, look for an internal opening of a fistula (Figure 5.16).

● Make a radial incision over the abscess, taking care to avoid underlying muscle. Incise the skin along the whole length of the abscess (Figures 5.17, 5.18).

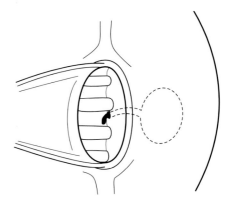

Figure 5.16 Pus pointing through the opening at the dentate line of an intersphincteric/perianal fistula.

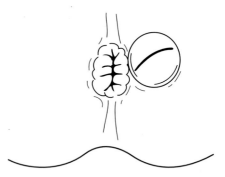

Figure 5.17 Radial incision over perianal abscess.

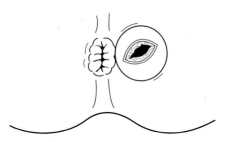

Figure 5.18 Abscess fully laid open.

● Evacuate all pus. A curette helps.

● With a finger make sure the cavity is fully opened.

● Take a pus swab for microscopy.

● Laying the abscess open adequately prevents skin closing over before it has healed.

● Perform a sigmoidoscopy and if there is suspicion of Crohn's disease take a rectal biopsy and send a piece of skin for histology.

● 'Packing' is a misnomer and should be avoided. A non-adhesive gauze dressing should be gently laid into the wound for ease of changing. A drain is unnecessary.

Large abscesses

● Require thorough laying open but try to preserve as much of a skin bridge as possible between horseshoe abscesses (Figure 5.19).

● Dressing may be too painful without anaesthetic and return visits to theatre may be necessary.

● Rarely, a horseshoe abscess may be so advanced that there is extensive gangrene of the tissues in the wall of the abscess and septicaemia. Extensive debridement and full supportive care (including antibiotics) together with defunctioning colostomy may be necessary.

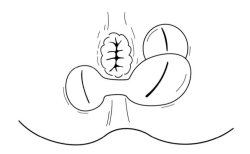

Figure 5.19 Horseshoe abscesses require incisions wherever pus points.

Hazards

● Do not attempt to lay open a fistula when draining an abscess if it cannot be established that the fistula is below the anorectal ring.

● Do not create a false passage by injudicious probing.

Postoperative management

● Change the dressings daily until healed.

● Encourage baths as soon as comfortable.

● Arrange an EUA if there is a suspicion of fistula or one is present.

ANORECTAL FISTULA

Clinical features

An anal fistula is an abnormal epithelialised communication between the mucosa of the anal canal and the perineal skin. Many anorectal abscesses heal primarily after adequate drainage but some fail to heal because of a persisting fistula. A patient with a recurrent anorectal abscess must be presumed to have a fistula and should have an EUA to see. Occasionally, a fistula will be seen to involve only the lower part of the internal sphincter and it may be easy to lay open at the same time as the abscess. Often a patient with a fistula presents *de novo* with a persistent discharge in the outpatient clinic. The aim of operation is to excise the epithelialised track while preserving continence.

Goodsall's rule states that: a fistula arising from any position anterior to the anus opens into the anal canal at a point radially inwards; and that a fistula arising from any position posterior to the anus tends to open into the posterior midline. Some patients have complex fistulas with multiple tracks extending superiorly, inferiorly, radially or circumferentially from the primary fistula. It is much easier to assess the anatomy of single or multiple fistulas at a separate EUA after the presenting abscess has been drained. An adjunct to clinical examination is magnetic resonance imaging which is an accurate non-invasive method of assessing complex fistulas.

Operations for fistula

The most important consideration in treatment is to preserve the integrity of the anorectal ring, without which complete incontinence is inevitable. In fact, division of even a small part of the internal or external sphincter may result in minor problems with continence. Rather than incise muscle, an alternative is firstly to mark the track by placement of a loose seton (from the French *seton* and the Latin *seta* = bristle). This can be placed at the time of initial abscess drainage if it appears that the internal opening is higher than the dentate line and the track thus crosses above a significant portion of internal or external sphincter. The suture is usually monofilament and non-absorbable. At a second procedure a loosely tied seton may be left *in situ* around muscle, after laying open or excising tracks up to their meeting with the sphincters. If healing proceeds the seton can be removed at a later date.

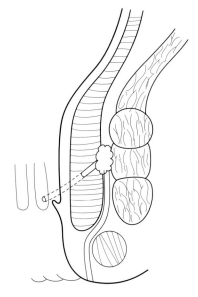

Figure 5.20 Intersphincteric/perianal fistula.

Sometimes it is preferable to place a tight seton around the fistula track and around the muscle. The principle is that a progressively tightened seton will cut through the external sphincter leaving an area of fibrosis in the muscle, rather than a defect. The muscle is still able to function as its circumferential integrity remains. In expert hands anal advancement flaps may have a place in the treatment of difficult fistulas that cannot be healed by other means.

Such complex sphincter surgery is needed for only a small minority of fistulas. Most patients in fact have a straightforward low fistula in which the amount of muscle involved is small and the risk of incontinence following laying open is low. Excision of a low fistula from an intersphincteric/perianal abscess is shown in Figure 5.20.

Patient preparation

Rectal enema is helpful.

Procedure

- Prepare the operative field by shaving the perianal skin with a surgical blade.

- Carefully feel the anal canal for the internal opening or track.

- Gently insert a curved fistula probe (e.g. Lockhart-Mummery) into the external opening.

- Using a retractor or speculum, visualise the internal opening and pass the probe through the fistula track from the external opening (Figure 5.21). Feel the position of the probe in relation to the anorectal ring.

- If the fistula is low make a radial incision over the track and lay open or core out the fistula with a blade or point diathermy (Figure 5.22), excising the lowest parts of the external and internal sphincters.

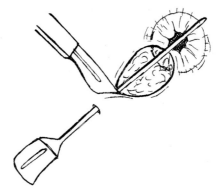

Figure 5.22 Laying open of low fistula.

- If the track appears to ascend above the anorectal ring, consider the placement of a seton.

- If the fistula appears more complex a diagram drawn in two or three planes should be placed in the records for future reference.

Hazards

- As for anorectal abscesses, do not create a false passage with a probe through the pelvic floor (Figure 5.23).

- Do not incise the anorectal ring. If in doubt, insert a seton.

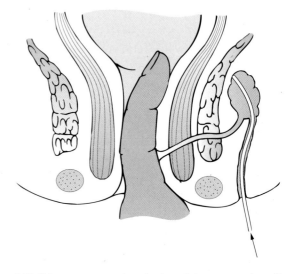

Figure 5.23 Take care not to push probe through levators, creating a false track.

Postoperative management

As for anorectal abscess. If a seton is placed a further EUA will be necessary before eventual removal.

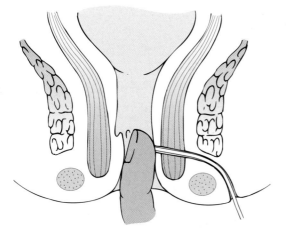

Figure 5.21 Careful delineation of the anatomy of the fistula.

FURTHER READING

1   Brisinda G. How to treat haemorrhoids. *BMJ* 2000; **7261**: 582–583

2   Grace R. Anorectal sepsis. In: Dudley HAF, Carter DC, Russell RCG, eds. *Atlas of General Surgery*, 2nd edn. London: Butterworths, 1986: 614-621

3   Kim DG, Wong WD. Anal fissure. In: Nicholls RJ, Dozois RR, eds. *Surgery of the Colon and Rectum*. Edinburgh: Churchill Livingstone, 1997: 233-244

4   Lund JN, Scholefield JH. A randomised, prospective, double-blind, placebo-controlled trial of glyceryl trinitrate ointment in treatment of anal fissure. *Lancet* 1997; **349**: 11–14

5   Mann CV. Open haemorrhoidectomy (St. Mark's ligation/excision method). In: Dudley HAF, Carter DC, Russell RCG, eds. *Atlas of General Surgery*, 2nd edn. London: Butterworths, 1986: 599-606

6   Mortensen N, Romanos J. Haemorrhoids. In: Nicholls RJ, Dozois RR, eds. *Surgery of the Colon and Rectum*. Edinburgh: Churchill Livingstone, 1997: 209-231

7   Notaras MJ. Lateral subcutaneous internal anal sphincterotomy for fissure-in-ano. In: Dudley HAF, Carter DC, Russell RCG, eds. *Atlas of General Surgery*, 2nd edn. London: Butterworths, 1986: 607-613

8   Phillips RKS, Lunniss PJ. Anorectal sepsis. In: Nicholls RJ, Dozois RR, eds. *Surgery of the Colon and Rectum*. Edinburgh: Churchill Livingstone, 1997: 255-284

9   Todd IP, Lockhart-Mummery H. Fistula-in-ano. In: Dudley HAF, Carter DC, Russell RCG, eds. *Atlas of General Surgery*, 2nd edn. London: Butterworths, 1986: 622-635

6

Common urological operations

Open surgery
  Surgery of the foreskin
  Scrotal surgery
  Groin surgery
Endoscopic surgery
  The instruments and equipment
  Cystoscopy
  Retrograde ureterography
  Placement of double J stent

Mark Fordham

OPEN SURGERY

The surgical trainee working on a urological unit will become involved in both open and endoscopic surgery. Most of the open surgery that the trainee will be taught will be on the male genitalia. These procedures may seem minor or trivial. Not, however to the patient, who will need careful counselling about possible fertility or potency problems that may be associated with the surgery, the likely level of postoperative pain and when normal sexual activity may be resumed. The endoscopic surgery that the trainee will learn is largely diagnostic in nature. The recognition of normal anatomy and differentiating it from pathological findings is an important first step in developing the skills needed for endoscopic resection.

Surgery of the foreskin

General points

Diathermy

Generally this is best avoided during surgery to the prepuce and penis. There is the danger of the current heating delicate penile vessels, causing thrombosis and ischaemic damage to the glans. Individual bleeding points should be clipped and tied with fine catgut. Most bleeding points will be controlled when the haemostatic skin sutures are placed.

Frenular artery

Bleeding can be troublesome and sometimes quite brisk. Active haemorrhage comes from the coronal end of the cut artery. When incising the frenulum, leave enough tissue to allow this area to be underrun with a catgut suture to control the bleeding.

Sutures

Absorbable catgut sutures and ties are ideal. A fine needle will traumatise the skin least. To allow the suture to run without snagging, lubricate the catgut. The lubricant that covers the wax paper which protects the Jellonet gauze can be used.

Dressing

Often no dressing is needed. Following a circumcision in an adult, a Jellonet gauze can be placed around the wound and held in place with a loosely wound 1 inch crepe bandage. The dressing usually protects the site until the patient is back in bed. In a child a gauze "sporran" will protect the penis for a short time (Figure 6.1).

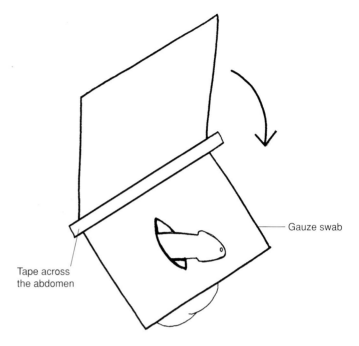

Tape across
the abdomen

Gauze swab

Figure 6.1 A gauze swab.

Reconstructive surgical use of the foreskin

Congenital abnormalities

If the distal urethra fails to develop and the glans has a blind pit at the tip the urethral opening will be on the ventral shaft of the penis. This is a hypospadias. The foreskin has a hooded appearance, incomplete ventrally with no true frenulum. Many surgical repairs of a hypospadias utilise the foreskin. A vascular pedicle flap is rolled into a tube to allow the urethra to be extended to the true meatus in the glans. In such cases the foreskin should not be excised.

Urethral stricture

In a similar manner a pedicled graft using the foreskin can be used to repair a urethral stricture. Preserve the foreskin in a man where this is a possibility.

Frenuloplasty

Indications

Tearing the frenulum during intercourse may cause troublesome bleeding. The injury heals by scarring, the frenulum becomes tighter and is more easily torn on subsequent occasions. Although circumcision is a more certain cure, the man may be reluctant to lose his foreskin. If there is no phimosis then a frenuloplasty will generally resolve the problem.

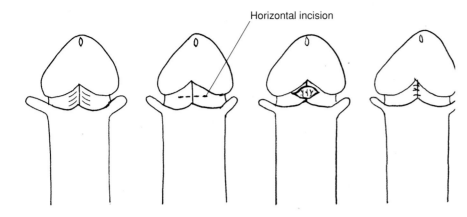

Horizontal incision

Figure 6.2

Anaesthesia

Although a local anaesthetic is perfectly adequate it is common for the patient to prefer a general anaesthetic.

Procedure

● The foreskin is retracted and the tight frenulum is demonstrated, causing the glans to be drawn ventrally.

● A short horizontal incision is made over the taut frenulum, allowing the tissues to retract under the tension (Figure 6.2).Continue to cut down to the vascular subcutaneous tissue which is freely mobile over the surface of the urethra.

● The horizontal cut is now closed vertically with haemostatic 4/0 catgut sutures.

● Replace the foreskin over the glans. This will act as an ideal dressing.

Hazards

Bleeding can be surprisingly brisk after the incision. Beware when taking deep sutures to control the bleeding as the urethra lies immediately deep to the tissues. If the vascular urethra is damaged more bleeding will occur and there is risk of causing a fistula.

Dorsal slit

Indications

The adult foreskin may be non-retractile due to scarring or thickening of the skin due to balanitis xerotica obliterans. Circumcision is the ideal treatment. However, sometimes a simple dorsal slit allows access to the glans either for catheterisation or occasionally to assess a possible lesion on the glans.

Anaesthesia

Local anaesthetic is adequate in most adults.

Procedure

● Blunt-nosed scissors should be used to avoid damaging the glans (Figure 6.3a). The lower blade is passed between the glans and prepuce and a cut made to enable the foreskin to be retracted easily (Figure 6.3b).

● The V incision is then sutured to control the bleeding (Figure 6.3c).

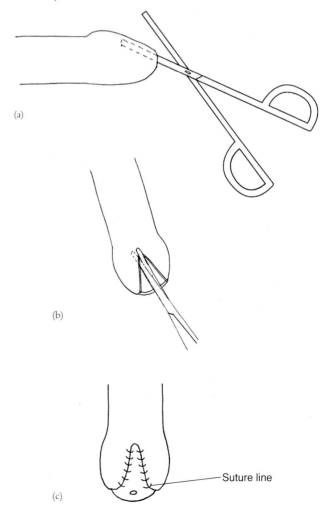

(a)

(b)

(c)

Suture line

Figure 6.3

Hazards

Take care not to pass the blades of the scissors down the meatus and so cut the glans.

Circumcision

Indications

After the age of two or three the normal prepuce is fully retractile. If it does not retract and the child suffers from recurrent balanitis despite careful hygiene, a circumcision may be appropriate.

In the adult a non-retractile foreskin (a phimosis) may require circumcision to allow proper hygiene or to assess a possible lesion of the glans.

Anaesthesia

Although it is possible to use local anaesthesia, general anaesthesia is usually preferred by the patient.

Procedure

Keep some of the sterile skin preparation fluid available to clean the glans when the foreskin has been retracted.

- Palpate the glans through the foreskin and mark the skin just distal to the corona. This can be done with marking ink or nipping the skin with an artery clip (Figure 6.4A).

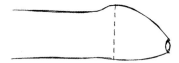

Figure 6.4A

- Pull the redundant foreskin proximally over the shaft of the penis and, holding the skin steady and on stretch, gently incise circumferentially with a blade down to the vascular subcutaneous tissue (Figure 6.4B).

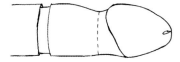

Figure 6.4B

- Now fully retract the foreskin to expose the glans, clean any remaining smegma that may be present and then incise 3 or 4 mm proximal to the corona around the penis. In this way the proximal and distal margins of the skin excision are defined. If the frenular artery causes troublesome bleeding this could be underrun with a catgut suture.

- Replace the foreskin over the glans and place artery clips on either side of the dorsal edge. Cut between the clips with scissors to the circumferential incisions (Figure 6.4C). Repeat this to the ventral surface. Divide the remaining subcutaneous tissue for each half of the foreskin. Clip the cut ends of the penile veins and tie with catgut. It is worth spending several minutes ensuring haemostasis at this stage (Figures 6.4D–F).

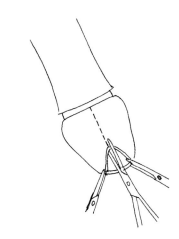

Figure 6.4C

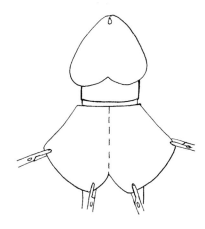

Figure 6.4D

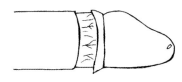

Figure 6.4E

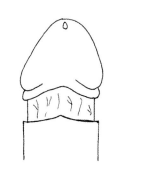

Figure 6.4F

● Start to oppose the cut ends by placing a suture at the dorsal and ventral points (12 o'clock and 6 o'clock) and use these sutures as anchors to hold the penis steady as the other sutures are placed.

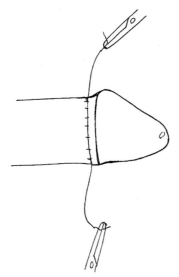

Figure 6.4G

Hazards

In an elderly male the foreskin may be very thickened and the inner aspect of the prepuce adherent to the corona and glans. To retract the foreskin an initial dorsal slit may be required. If the corona is obliterated, leave an adequate cuff of tissue so the closing sutures do not have to be placed in the glans.

Paraphimosis

If a foreskin retracts only with difficulty due to phimosis it may prove impossible to replace the foreskin back over the glans. This acute condition is termed paraphimosis. The inner layer of the prepuce is exposed and becomes oedematous (Figure 6.5A).

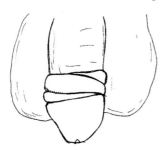

Figure 6.5A

To reduce the condition, the skin of the penis is stretched proximally over the shaft of the penis and direct pressure applied to the oedematous tissue in an attempt to reduce the swelling. The shaft skin can then be pushed distally to allow the tight band (XY in Figure 6.5B and C) to pass over the swollen tissue. A common mistake is to try and pull the oedematous inner layer of the prepuce (M and N) over the glans.

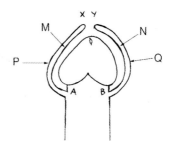

Figure 6.5B

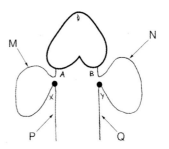

Figure 6.5C

This procedure can be attempted with a penile block or under general anaesthesia.

If the prepuce cannot be reduced the constricting ring must be incised. This will allow the foreskin to be replaced and will produce the appearance of a small cut at the edge of the foreskin. The tight band will lie beneath the oedematous skin.

If the procedure is performed under general anaesthesia, it is usual to proceed to circumcision as the healing is invariably satisfactory even though the foreskin may look swollen and bruised.

Scrotal surgery

Careful opening and closure of the scrotal sac together with complete haemostasis are the key steps to many scrotal procedures. A postoperative haematoma is a troublesome complication for both surgeon and patient which can take some weeks to resolve and has the potential to become infected.

For bilateral procedures a midline scrotal incision is ideal, otherwise a lateral incision of the testis is preferred. Generally, absorbable catgut or chromic catgut sutures are used for all scrotal surgery including skin closure.

Scrotal incision and closure

● Hold the scrotum firmly so the skin is taut and the subcutaneous vessels are demonstrated. For a midline incision cut along the median raphe and for a lateral incision select an area with few vessels.

- Coagulate vessels with diathermy as they appear and continue the incision down through the dartos muscle. In the midline incision a space will appear between the two sacs. Incise down to the tunica vaginalis on one side and then on the other. The tunica will bulge through the incision. Use some blunt dissection to create a space and the incision along the dartos can then be extended.

- Tissue-holding forceps can be applied to the dartos on each side and any remaining bleeding vessels coagulated with diathermy.

- The tunica vaginalis is incised and the testis delivered.

- Sutures for closure are haemostatic. The tunica vaginalis is closed with a continuous stitch using 4/0 chromic catgut and

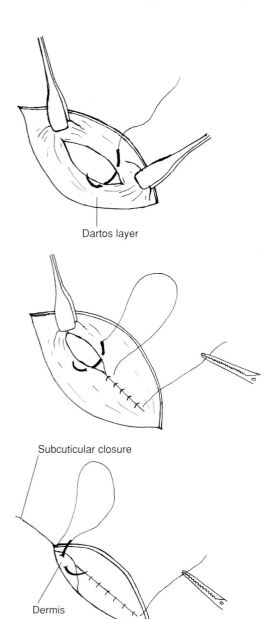

Dartos layer

Subcuticular closure

Dermis

Figure 6.6A

allowed to drop back into the scrotal sac. Clips are placed at either end of the incision to hold up the dartos layer (Figure 6.6A). Place an initial suture at one end, tie it and clip the free end. Run the suture continuously along the dartos layer and tether it at the end but do not cut it. In the midline incision close the opposite dartos layer by apposing it with another running suture to the suture line of the previous dartos closure, returning to the starting point. Now tie it to the clipped end. Close the skin with a subcuticular running suture and tie it to the dartos layer suture, thereby leaving no suture exposed.

- Plastic spray and a small gauze dressing are usually sufficient. A scrotal support is then fitted.

Excision of hydrocele

Indications

A large hydrocele may be a physical nuisance to a man. Simple aspiration will certainly remove the fluid but its recurrence is almost inevitable. Usually the clinical features can be demonstrated easily by transillumination. In a young man with a recently developed hydrocele, unless the testis can be palpated easily an ultrasound scan is wise to exclude a testicular tumour which would require urgent treatment. Occasionally, elderly men present with a long-standing scrotal swelling which transilluminates poorly or not at all. This may be a thick-walled chronic hydrocoele and an ultrasound scan will help establish the diagnosis.

Surgical options

The aim of the surgery is to obliterate the space between the parietal and testicular layers of the tunica vaginalis. In a thin-walled hydrocele the parietal layer can be opened, folded back and plicated with catgut sutures. In a thick-walled chronic hydrocele this layer is best excised. It is not uncommon to perform a combination of these two approaches so that the parietal layer is turned back on itself, without creating a very bulky remnant.

Procedure

- The scrotum is opened over the hydrocele and the incision extended down to the tunica vaginalis.

- Allis forceps can be placed on the dartos muscle and the layer around the tunica opened up for a centimetre or so. Incise the hydrocele and aspirate the fluid.

- Next plicate the tunica to create a concertina appearance around the testis. This may be done with minimal dissection of layers in a small hydrocele, but in a large hydrocele may require the whole testis to be delivered out of the wound. If the tunica is thickened and the plication will cause thick bunches of tissue, the tunica should be excised down to its reflection near to the epididymis.

- A 4/0 chromic catgut suture is then used as a haemostatic suture along the edge to plicate any excess remaining tunica (Figure 6.6B).

- The scrotum is closed routinely with careful haemostasis.

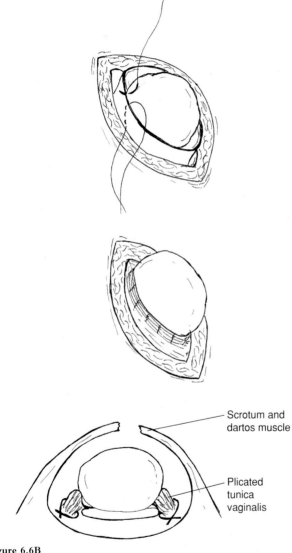

Scrotum and dartos muscle

Plicated tunica vaginalis

Figure 6.6B

Excision of epididymal cysts

Indications

Patients presenting with chronic or intermittent testicular pain may be found to have an epididymal cyst on clinical examination or on ultrasound scan. However, the majority of epididymal cysts are painless and discovered incidentally. Beware, therefore, of offering to excise an epididymal cyst in the hope that it will cure testicular pain; success is not guaranteed.

Dissection to remove these cysts may cause obstructive azoospermia on the operated side due to scarring around the tubules conveying sperms from the testis to the vas. In men hoping to father children, this operation is best avoided.

Procedure

- The scrotum is opened and the testis delivered through an incision in the tunica vaginalis.

- Each large cyst is dissected free using a combination of diathermy and fine scissors. Smaller cysts can be deroofed. If a large raw area of the epididymis has been exposed, this can be closed over with a 4/0 chromic catgut suture. In very large cysts, beware of damaging the cord and testicular artery adjacent to the upper pole.

- Routine closure, dressing and scrotal support.

Bilateral scrotal orchidectomy for hormone treatment of advanced prostate cancer

Indications

Pharmaceutical methods of suppressing the production of testosterone or blocking its action are now popular in the treatment of hormone-sensitive advanced prostate cancer. However, surgical castration remains a useful alternative to lifelong tablets or injections and is conveniently performed when a patient requires a general anaesthetic for endoscopic resection of an obstructive malignant prostate gland.

Complete excision of both testes and epididymis is performed easily by dividing the cord. However, excision of the seminiferous tubules alone (subcapsular orchidectomy) also results in reducing testosterone to castrate level but leaves reduced but cosmetically acceptable scrotal remnants.

Procedure

Via a midline scrotal incision, deliver each testis into the operating field.

SUBCAPSULAR ORCHIDECTOMY

- Incise the tunica albuginea from pole to pole. Compress the testis to squeeze out the yellow mass of seminiferous tubules. Hold the contents in a swab and free any attachments with scissors.

- At the base lies the hilum. Divide this with scissors. The brisk bleeding is then controlled with diathermy and oversewing with running catgut suture. Take some time to diathermy all the bleeding points within the testis. Pack a small swab into the empty tunica albuginea and then perform the procedure on the other testis.

- Return to the first testis, remove the swab and check for complete haemostasis. Close the tunica with a running 4/0 chromic catgut suture. Clip the free end of the suture and then return plicating the body of the testis to obliterate any potential space that may fill with haematoma (Figure 6.7).

- Repeat for the second testis and then return the testicular remnants within the tunica vaginalis and close with catgut.

- Close the scrotum routinely and fit a scrotal support.

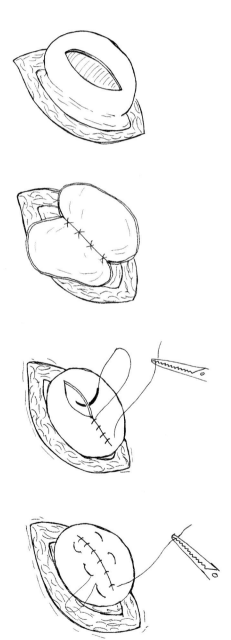

Figure 6.7

COMPLETE SCROTAL ORCHIDECTOMY

- Deliver the testis via the wound and identify the cord at the upper pole. It is convenient to open an avascular window within the cord, allowing two clamps to take a half thickness of the cord each.

- Divide, transfix and ligate with strong chromic catgut and repeat for the other testis.

- After careful haemostasis close routinely.

Postoperative care

A scrotal support or a crepe bandage dressing to minimise a scrotal haematoma is helpful.

Scrotal exploration for testicular torsion

Indications

The typical patient is an adolescent boy with a history of several hours lower abdominal pain and a painful tender testis. He may have woken with the pain, had resolving episodes in the past or suffered some mild scrotal trauma. However, similar symptoms due to torsion can be seen in young boys and adults. If at exploration the testes is not viable it must be excised. The patient or his parents must therefore have consented to this procedure before he is anaesthetised.

Procedure

- A scrotal incision is made over the affected testis. Bloodstained fluid in the tunica vaginalis may be released when the testis is exposed (Figure 6.8). Untwist the testis and place it between warm wet swabs to encourage vascular dilatation and watch to see if it pinks up. If the testis remains black incise the tunica albuginea to see if the testis bleeds. If there is no sign of viability excise the testis and epididymis by ligating and dividing the

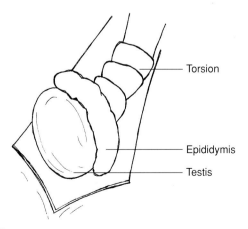

Figure 6.8

93

cord. However, if there is any doubt and areas are improving, be optimistic and preserve it.

- Fix the tunica albuginea to the dartos muscle with non-absorbable sutures to prevent a recurrence. Close the scrotal incision.

- The opposite testis is also at risk of torsion and this should be fixed at the same time. Use clean instruments to minimise any chance of infecting this side.

- Placing a prosthesis in the event of excising the testis is unwise at this stage. There is a potential for infection and a foreign body would compound this problem and result in delayed healing.

Vasectomy

Indications

This procedure is invariably carried out for social reasons at the patient's request. Any side effects, complications or postoperative pain are therefore particularly irksome to him as he had no symptoms beforehand. Vasectomy remains one of the most common reasons for medicolegal litigation. Careful preoperative explanation of the procedure and realistic expectations will pay dividends if any parts of the procedure do not run smoothly. Although it is common to obtain the partner's consent as well as the patient's, this is not a legal necessity.

Anaesthesia

The majority of cases are performed using local anaesthesia. This may involve infiltration of the cord as well as directly over the site of surgery. It is not uncommon for the patient to experience some discomfort and although further infiltration can be used this may be delayed while the vas is secured. Allow time for the local anaesthetic to work. A nervous or anxious patient, one with a bulky scrotum or one who has had previous surgery in this region would be best managed with a general anaesthetic.

Procedure

- The vas has to be identified, immobilised and an incision made through the scrotum directly over it so that a suitable grasper can be applied around it. With the non-dominant hand palpate the vas at the neck of the scrotum between index and middle fingers above and thumb beneath. Turn the hand so the fingers force the vas onto the thumb now in the upper position (Figure 6.9).

- An incision is made directly onto the vas and the vas grasped with tissue forceps. If the vas is very mobile it can be encircled through the scrotum with tissue forceps to steady it for the incision.

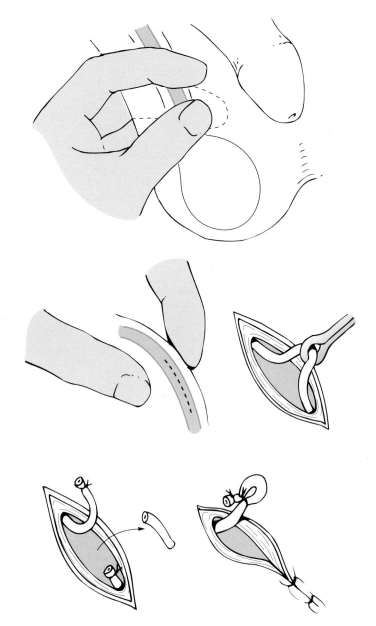

Figure 6.9

- Ensure the incision passes onto the vas so it can be lifted away from its sheath. A segment is excised and sent for histological examination. The cut ends are tied with Vicryl and the testicular end returned to the sheath which is then closed. The distal vas remains outside the sheath which, together with ligating a double-back loop on itself, is designed to minimise the chances of recanalisation.

- The scrotal incision is closed with one or two chromic catgut sutures. The procedure is repeated for the other side.

Postoperative care

If everything has gone well the patient may be tempted to be too active after the operation. However, he should avoid lifting or straining and preferably rest for 24 hours. Supportive underwear or scrotal support should be worn. The danger is of a scrotal haematoma developing which may take some weeks to resolve and require bedrest and antibiotics.

The patient is not sterile until all sperms distal to the vasectomy have been cleared. Two consecutive sperm counts must be clear of sperm and these are usually taken at eight and 12 weeks after surgery.

Groin surgery

Radical orchidectomy for testicular tumour

Indications

Orchidectomy for tumour is performed via a groin incision to avoid potential contamination by tumour cells of scrotal lymphatics which drain to the inguinal lymph glands, unlike the testicular lymphatics which drain to the paraaortic nodes.

Preparation

Take a sample of blood for tumour marker estimation (alphafetoprotein and beta HCG) and also a chest radiograph to assess for lung metastases preoperatively.

Some patients request a testicular prosthesis at the time of orchidectomy and consent for this should be obtained preoperatively. Prostheses of various sizes should be available in theatre.

As the scrotum may need to be handled during the operation, skin preparation and towelling up should include this area.

Procedure

- A routine inguinal incision is made exposing the external ring so that the inguinal canal can be opened.

- The cremasteric muscle is opened and the cord with its veins is picked up and clamped near the deep ring with a soft bowel clamp. This is to prevent tumour emboli passing along the veins while the testis is being mobilised from the scrotum.

- The cord is mobilised towards the scrotum and any small vessels cauterised. The testis can be delivered into the wound most easily by compressing the scrotum. Even for large tumours, with sufficient mobilisation the testis will pass through the neck of the scrotum.

- Attachments between the tunica vaginalis and the scrotum are divided by a combination of diathermy and clipping and cut-

ting. Careful haemostasis is essential. Take care not to button-hole the scrotum while dividing these attachments.

- Open the tunica vaginalis to confirm a testicular mass is present. If there had been any doubt about what may be found the patient will have been counselled preoperatively and a plan of action agreed upon.

- Double clamp the cord at the deep ring with Kocher's clamps. Excise the cord and testis, transfix and ligate the cord at each clamp with strong chromic catgut. Confirm haemostasis is satisfactory, especially in the scrotum, and close the incision routinely.

Postoperative care

Repeat tumour marker estimation the day after surgery and again a week later. Continue until it falls to the normal range or plateaus. This will show if any metastatic tumour remains after the primary has been removed.

Ligation of varicocele

Indications

Dilated pampiniform veins in the scrotum will swell with increasing intraabdominal pressure and present as a varicocele. Men involved in hot manual work may find this produces pain and discomfort in the varicocele and seek medical advice. Infertile men may be advised to undergo varicocele ligation in an attempt to reduce scrotal temperature with the aim of improving sperm production.

The patient should be warned that the veins are not going to be removed and so some residual mass may remain.

Procedure

- To ensure all tributaries to the pampiniform plexus are divided, those in the inguinal canal and those passing medially at the superficial inguinal ring must be divided.

- The inguinal canal is opened and the cremasteric muscle divided. The vas deferens and the testicular artery should be identified and preserved. All dilated veins are divided and tied. At the superficial inguinal ring the cord is mobilised and all small vessels divided and diathermied.

- Closure is routine.

ENDOSCOPIC SURGERY

The best way to learn how to handle urological endoscopic instruments is to begin by assisting the scrub nurse. Help prepare the trolley for endoscopic procedures, fit the telescope and cystoscopy sheath together and check all the taps and connections are functioning. Learn how to position the patient and to place the legs in stirrups (avoiding any pressure points or contact with metal), clean the genitals and drape the legs and perineum. On all appropriate occasions perform a pelvic examination of the anaesthetised patient to help learn the pelvic anatomy and to recognise pathological changes.

The instruments and equipment

To illuminate the bladder, modern instruments use fibreoptic light cables and commonly a microchip camera is attached to the telescope and the image is viewed on a TV screen. The bladder is distended with a clear fluid. Although sterile water is perfectly satisfactory any vascular absorption would cause haemolysis. If any electrosurgery is planned sterile isotonic glycine is used. This conducts the current without electrolysis and is less likely to cause problems if absorbed.

The flexible cystoscope

This fibreoptic instrument with a moveable tip allows cystoscopy to be performed under local anaesthetic for diagnostic examination. A small biopsy channel allows cup forceps to be passed down the scope to sample suspected tumours or to grasp and remove a ureteric stent.

The rigid cystoscope

This consists of:
1. cystoscopy sheath
2. obturator
3. bridge
4. rod lens telescope.

In the female the cystoscope sheath is passed along the urethra directly into the bladder with the obturator in place to avoid trauma to the tissues. The obturator is then removed and the telescope, fitted with the bridge, is then inserted along the cystoscope sheath.

In the male the cystoscope sheath, the bridge and the telescope are all assembled and under vision the scope is passed along the urethra through the external sphincter and prostatic urethra into the bladder. If urethral pathology is encountered a urethroscope is used.

The rod lens telescopes are not as manoeuvreable around the bladder as the flexible cystoscope and so to see around the bladder different angle objective lenses are used. The 30° is most generally used but a 70° and 120° are also available. The 0°, i.e. straight-ahead vision, is occasionally useful but more commonly used for urethroscopy.

The bridge has an operating channel which allows a diathermy wire to be passed down the channel to enable bladder lesions to be cauterised.

Biopsy forceps are available which are used instead of the bridge with the telescope passing down the centre, so the biopsy cups can be opened and closed under vision.

The Sachse optical urethrotome

This consists of
1. urethroscope sheath
2. obturator
3. blade
4. working element
5. 0° rod lens telescope
6. catheterisation attachment.

This instrument allows direct vision of the urethra together with a sharp blade that can be manipulated to cut an obstructing stricture.

The urethroscope sheath and obturator are passed into the urethra, the obturator is removed and the assembled working element, bladder and telescope connected.

An outer sheath, with a U-shaped cross-section, can be left in the urethra as the remaining scope is removed. A catheter can be passed down it into the bladder and the open section allows the sheath to be removed, leaving the catheter behind.

The Albarran catheter deflector

This substitutes for the bridge on a cystoscope. It passes to the end of the cystoscope sheath where a flat metal lever is positioned resting against the exit of the operating channel. When a ureteric catheter is passed down the cystoscope this metal lever can be deflected by a thumbscrew near the telescope eyepiece and enable direction of the catheter towards a ureteric orifice more accurately.

Ureteric catheters

These 60 cm long thin catheters are designed to pass down the cystoscope and up a ureter and are therefore much narrower than a urethral catheter. The slimmest, at 3 French gauge, will have a thin wire down the centre to keep the catheter rigid as it is passed down the cystoscope.Larger catheters, up to 10 or 12 French gauge, are sufficiently robust to be manipulated easily.

The catheter is marked with rings of 1 cm intervals, so the distance along the ureter can be measured.

Catheter tips vary. The round tipped have side openings. This allows the catheter to pass up to the renal pelvis without damaging the ureter. The bulb-ended Chevassu catheters have an open tip. This is designed to pass into the ureteric orifice and X-ray contrast can be injected directly up the ureter. The bulb prevents backflow out of the ureter.

Once in place a ureteric catheter can be used to collect urine from a single kidney for cytology or to inject X-ray contrast so the ureter and the renal pelvis can be demonstrated by X-ray screening.

Double J ureteric stent

This consists of:
1. ureteric stent
2. guidewire
3. pusher.

The ureteric stent is designed to allow urine to drain freely to the bladder in an otherwise obstructed ureter. The curled ends lie in the renal pelvis and bladder, preventing the stent from migrating up or down.

Antibiotics

For any urological endoscopic procedure where there may be urinary infection, antibiotics should be used prophylactically to minimise the risk of septicaemia.

Cystoscopy

Flexible cystoscopy

The same preparation is carried out as for passing a urethral catheter.

- In the male the cystoscope is advanced under direct vision. Examination of the bladder is similar to using a rigid cystoscope but as the tip is moveable, each segment of the bladder can be viewed this way.

- Advance the lens over the bladder neck a short distance to the trigone and the interureteric bar. At either end is a ureteric orifice. Rotate the instrument along its long axis, angling the end to examine each segment of the bladder.

- Finally advance the cystoscope directly towards the posterior wall of the bladder and allow it to loop back on itself so the bladder neck can be viewed with the cystoscope passing through it.

Rigid cystoscopy

The patient has the legs elevated in stirrups, the genitals cleaned and is then draped appropriately.

- In the female the cystoscope sheath with the obturator is introduced into the bladder via the urethra. The obturator is removed, the bladder drained and the telescope and bridge connected with the light lead and irrigation tubing attached.

- In the male the cystoscope is fully assembled and passed along the urethra under vision into the bladder. A 30° telescope gives adequate vision for this.

- To examine the bladder, begin at the bladder neck and advance to the trigone. This triangular patch at the bladder base has its apex pointing down the urethra and its base represented by the interureteric bar with a ureteric orifice at either end. Rotate the cystoscope about its long axis a few degrees from the midline to identify each orifice.

- Move the cystoscope back and forth as it is rotated so each segment of the bladder can be examined. Assess each lateral wall and then identify the air bubble at the dome of the bladder. To view the anterior wall of the bladder more easily, use your free hand to press suprapubically and bring down the bladder into view.

- If the bladder becomes too full it becomes more difficult to see the whole bladder and the ureteric orifices become flattened and more laterally placed. Empty some of the irrigating fluid out and reexamine.

- Look particularly for bladder stones, tumours and signs of bladder dysfunction such as trabeculation or diverticula. If the patient has had a catheter the mucosa will be oedematous and this can mimic a papillary tumour. Similarly if the bladder is underfilled the mucosal folds can look abnormal.

Biopsy can be performed with the endoscopic forceps. These can also be used to remove a ureteric stent by grasping it and pulling the whole instrument out. If areas require electrocautery a diathermy wire can be passed down the operating channel of the bridge.

Retrograde ureterography

This requires X-ray screening so put on a lead apron before scrubbing up.

- Assemble and pass the cystoscope and identify the ureteric orifices.

- Select a suitable ureteric catheter. Usually a 5 French gauge catheter is appropriate. Pass this down the operating channel, remove the guidewire and connect the syringe containing X-ray contrast. Inject contrast down the catheter to remove any air bubbles which could be misinterpreted if they appear in the ureter on X-ray screening.

- Pass the catheter into the ureteric orifice and screen the bladder and lower pelvis to confirm the orientation. Inject the contrast and screen the whole ureter and renal collecting system. Remove the catheter from the ureter and screen the contrast as it drains from the kidney to assess for any delay.

- If there are any difficulties in identifying the ureteric orifice, empty the bladder and reexamine with less fluid.

- If the catheter cannot be directed accurately, exchange the bridge for the Albarran catheter deflector.

Placement of a double J stent

Indications

Most commonly this is performed for an obstructed ureter, usually due to a stone. An initial retrograde ureterogram may have been performed.

Preparation

Wear a lead apron as X-ray screening will be needed. If there is any risk of urinary infection, postoperative antibiotics should be used. Ureteric stents are made in different sizes, both diameter and length. For the average adult a 6 French gauge stent of 26–30 cm length is appropriate.

Procedure

- Pass the cystoscope and identify the ureteric orifice. Select a ureteric stent and take hold of the guidewire. One end is stiff, the other end is floppy. Use the floppy end and pass it down the operating channel of the cystoscope until it is visible in the bladder.

- Place the objective of the telescope close to the ureteric orifice and now pass the guidewire up the ureter. Avoid any wire passing as a loop into the bladder as this will make it impossible to feed the wire up the ureter. Screen using X-rays to see that the wire is in the renal pelvis.

- Now slide the stent onto the guidewire and advance it down the operating channel. Still keep the cystoscope close to the ureteric orifice and advance the stent up the ureter under vision. If you encounter resistance, the guidewire may have advanced together with the stent and be jammed into the kidney. Screen the upper part and withdraw the wire so it lies just in the renal pelvis.

- The stent has to be pushed down the cystoscope's operating channel using the pusher (a simple hollow tube similar to a ureteric catheter). Continue to push the stent up the ureter until the pusher comes into view. Check the position by X-ray screening and then remove the guidewire while holding the stent in place with the pusher. The tip of the stent should then curl up into a J-shape in the bladder and also in the renal pelvis.

- Remove the pusher, empty the bladder and remove the cystoscope.

7

Head and neck

Thyroid lobectomy
    Indications
    Preparation
    Anaesthesia and positioning
    Procedure
    Hazards
    Postoperative management

Submandibular gland excision
    Indications
    Preparation
    Procedure
    Hazards
    Postoperative management

Denis Wilkins

THYROID LOBECTOMY

Thyroidectomy is an operation that requires considerable expertise if it is to be performed to a consistently high standard and with an acceptably low morbidity. It is important that the surgeon has decided on a clear strategy preoperatively, i.e. subtotal lobectomy, total lobectomy or near-total lobectomy.

Indications

The operation described will be a total or near-total lobectomy and a typical situation would be that of a substantial 'cold' nodule situated deep within the lobe.

Preparation

- Great care must be taken that thyrotoxicosis, if present, has been controlled (refer to Chapter 19). Drugs most commonly used include propranolol and carbimazole. Fewer surgeons now prepare patients with preoperative Lugol's iodine.

- The major source of morbidity in thyroidectomy is damage to the recurrent laryngeal nerve. For this reason it is important that the patient understands that there is a small (less than 1% in competent hands) risk of temporary or permanent damage to the recurrent laryngeal nerve during the procedure. Although the incidence is extremely low, many surgeons advocate inspection of the vocal cords preoperatively to exclude a preexisting palsy. Adequate counselling is important in those patients to whom the voice is particularly important, i.e. singers, switchboard operators, pilots, etc.

- The patient should also be made aware that there is a small incidence of permanent hypocalcaemia (refer to Chapter 19).

- The position and visibility of the scar will be of particular concern to young patients and should be discussed.

- DVT prophylaxis is contraindicated because of the risks of postoperative bleeding in head and neck surgery.

Anaesthesia and positioning

- The patient is placed supine on the operating table with the neck extended (Figure 7.1). Although this can be achieved using sandbags, an empty 1 litre, plastic fluid bag placed transversely underneath the shoulders and inflated using a sphygmomanometer bulb is ideal. This facilitates control over the degree of neck extension, which should not be excessive as the cervical spine can be strained.

- Most surgeons prefer the use of a fully supported endotracheal tube for the anaesthetic as laryngeal masks can easily become displaced if the larynx is manipulated.

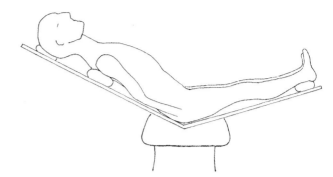

Figure 7.1 Positioning of the patient for thyroidectomy (note the headring supporting the head and the inflatable bag across the shoulders posteriorly).

- The surgeon generally stands on the side of the patient opposite to the diseased lobe, but some prefer to work from the same side.

Procedure

The general strategy is to mobilise the gland sufficiently to permit anterior dislocation. This will permit exposure of vital structures situated on the posteromedial aspect such as the recurrent laryngeal nerve and parathyroid glands.

- The shape and position of the incision is particularly important. There are a variety of techniques used, all of which aim to achieve symmetry and exact placement along Langer's lines. These include marking with a taut ligature, skin marking with pen and gentian violet or placement of the incision within a preexisting skin crease. Generally speaking, the incision should be placed approximately two fingers' width above the suprasternal notch and follows a fairly flat curve. Close proximity to the suprasternal notch will result in a more prominent scar. The lateral extent is a matter for judgement and will depend on the size of the gland (Figure 7.2).

- Following incision through skin and platysma, the knife is used to raise upper and lower flaps. These flaps, which comprise skin, subcutaneous tissue and platysma, will permit exposure of the strap muscles along their length. While dissecting

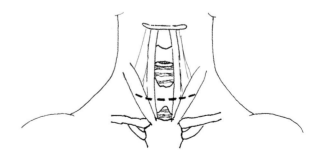

Figure 7.2 Position of incision for thyroidectomy (it is advisable to mark this out carefully before incising.

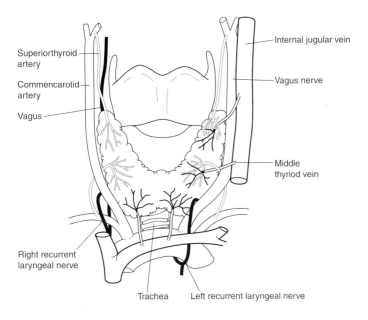

Superiorthyroid artery

Commencarotid artery

Vagus

Internal jugular vein

Vagus nerve

Middle thyriod vein

Right recurrent laryngeal nerve

Trachea

Left recurrent laryngeal nerve

Figure 7.3 Blood vessels and nerves related to the thyroid gland.

this layer it is better to angle the blade towards the surface rather than the deep structures.

● The upper extent of the dissection is the lower limit of the thyroid cartilage; the lower flap is mobilised to the level of the suprasternal notch.

● A Joll's retractor is then inserted after haemostasis has been achieved and opened so that it separates the flaps and exposes the deep fascia covering the outer layer of strap muscles.

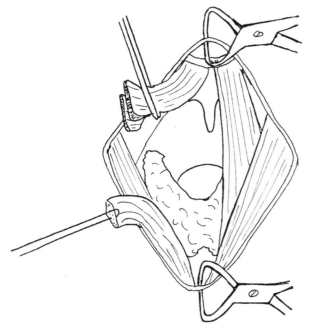

Figure 7.4 Muscles related to the thyroid gland. On the right side, the strap muscles have been divided to improve access. The medial edge of sternothyroid lies lateral and deep to sternohyoid.

● The deep fascia is then incised in the midline and the plane between the anterior surface of the thyroid gland and the strap muscles identified. This comprises a layer of filmy loose areolar tissue and it is important to look out for the attenuated medial edge of sternothyroid as the dissection proceeds laterally in order to stay in the correct, deep plane (Figure 7.4).

● The middle thyroid vein will usually be encountered as it enters the anterolateral aspect of the gland and here, as in the rest of the operation, haemostatic metal clips are helpful. Otherwise ligatures of fine absorbable material may be used throughout. Occasionally it will be necessary to divide the strap muscles to gain sufficient access to a very large lobe (Figure 7.4).

● When the anterior and lateral aspects of the gland have been thoroughly released, the upper pole is then mobilised. A well-defined plane will be found between the cricothyroid muscle and the upper pole of the thyroid gland close to the point at which the superior thyroid veins and arteries enter and leave the gland (Figure 7.5). Care must be taken here not to injure the external branch of the superior laryngeal nerve as it courses anteriorly on the inferior constrictor and for this reason it is advised that division of these vessels should be carried out in several stages rather than by mass ligation. The nerve contributes significantly to the tensioning of the vocal cords and although not easy to detect at laryngoscopy, patients thus affected will notice a deterioration in their voice. Once the superior pole has been mobilised by division of its vessels between the ligatures, it can be dislocated anteriorly by blunt but careful dissection of its posterior aspect.

● Identification of the recurrent laryngeal nerve and the parathyroid glands must then be carried out before vessels, veins or gland are divided (see Hazards). The recurrent laryn-

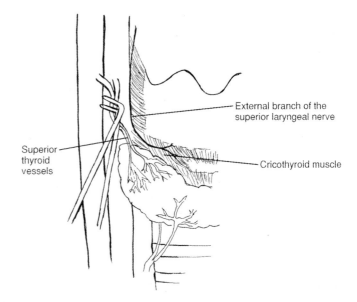

External branch of the superior laryngeal nerve

Superior thyroid vessels

Cricothyroid muscle

Figure 7.5 The structures related to the superior pole of the right lobe. The superior thyroid vessels should be clearly seen and taken cleanly to avoid damage to the external laryngeal nerve.

geal nerve is a branch of the vagus and generally arises in the superior mediastinum coursing on the right around the subclavian artery and on the left, the aortic arch. It usually ascends close to the oesophagus on the left side but slightly further away on the right, seeking the midline and tracking anteriorly as it proceeds towards the larynx. Here it penetrates the cricothyroid membrane. Posteriorly, therefore, it is very close, sometimes even tethered to the posteromedial aspect of the thyroid lobe (Figure 7.6).

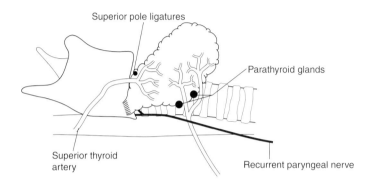

Figure 7.6 The right lobe of the thyroid viewed from the side. The right lobe has been turned anteriorly after ligation of the superior pole vessels. Note the close proximity of the recurrent laryngeal nerve to the attachment of the gland to the side of the larynx.

- Similarly the parathyroid glands identified as small, brownish-yellow structures, each rather the same size and shape as a lentil, should be identified where they lie on the posteromedial aspect of the thyroid gland usually at or about the level of the inferior thyroid artery (Figure 7.6).

- Once these vital structures have been identified, surgery may proceed. In the case of a total lobectomy most surgeons gently separate the parathyroid glands from the capsule of the thyroid itself, taking trouble to preserve as much of the blood supply as possible. In the case of a vascular thyroid gland, it is acceptable to ligate the main trunk of the inferior thyroid artery although this may jeopardise the blood supply to the parathyroid glands. If this is necessary, it should be carried out well lateral to the gland, taking care to ensure that the ligature is clear of the recurrent laryngeal nerve.

- There is little in the way of arterial blood supply to the inferior pole of the thyroid gland but there are many substantial veins which require ligation. This can be done with impunity once the recurrent laryngeal nerve has been identified.

- The next step depends upon the extent of the resection. It should be borne in mind that the thyroid is tethered tightly to the side of the larynx in the region of the posterior aspect of the cricothyroid membrane. Here tiny blood vessels run between the thyroid and the larynx in and around the point at which the recurrent laryngeal nerve pierces the cricothyroid membrane. Great care and patience is required here as the

gland is dissected free from these important structures, and the tiny vessels either clipped or ligated. When performing a subtotal lobectomy, a small portion of the gland should be left *in situ* at this point, so as to protect the nerve.

- The isthmus of the thyroid should be defined where it crosses the trachea in the midline and it is helpful if a plane between the trachea and the posterior aspect of the isthmus can be opened up by blunt dissection before the lobe is resected.

- If a remnant is to be left, the point of division of the capsule of the gland posteriorly is marked by attaching haemostats before incision. It is important that as the trachea is approached, the gland is divided anterior to the point at which the recurrent laryngeal nerve enters the larynx (Figure 7.7).

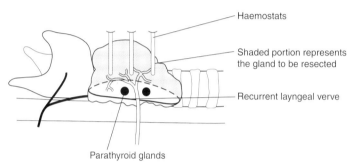

Figure 7.7 The line of resection of the thyroid in subtotal lobectomy. Note the line of haemostats attached to the capsule and marking the line of incision into the gland.

- The remnant of the gland, if present, is oversewn using a continuous absorbable stitch between the lateral capsule of the gland and the filmy fascia overlying the trachea at this point. Slight 'scalloping' of the cut surface of the gland will facilitate this step. A remnant equivalent in size to a level teaspoon or less is left (Figure 7.8).

- If total lobectomy is carried out, haemostasis of the very fine arteries in the region of the hilum of the gland should be achieved using fine ties or clips, clear of the nerve. The use of the diathermy in this position is contraindicated.

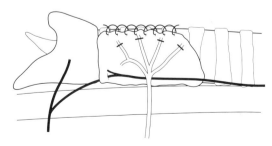

Figure 7.8 The remnant of the right lobe sutured to the anterolateral aspect of the trachea. A continuous absorbable suture is used between the capsule of the gland and the fibrous outer coating of the trachea.

- Thorough haemostasis is essential before the fascia and strap muscles are closed as a single layer in the midline.

- Most surgeons use a small vacuum drain placed in the bed of the resected gland.

- The flaps are closed using a fine (4/0) absorbable suture to platysma and the skin closed with clips, a continuous vertical mattress suture with 5/0 monofilament nylon or a subcuticular suture ensuring accurate skin apposition.

Hazards

Recurrent laryngeal nerve

The recurrent laryngeal nerve can be clearly identified as a white structure with a tiny surface blood vessel visible along its length.

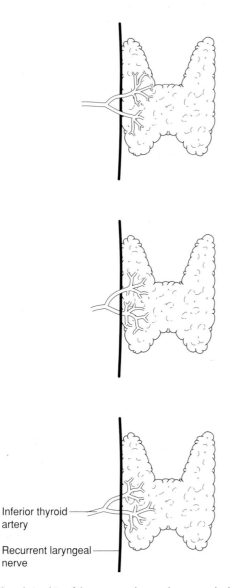

Inferior thyroid artery

Recurrent laryngeal nerve

Figure 7.9 The relationship of the recurrent laryngeal nerve to the branches of the inferior thyroid artery.

It can often be palpated against the side of the upper trachea as a thin 'cord'. It usually passes posterior to the inferior thyroid artery but may pass through the terminal branches or even anterior to them (Figure 7.9). In approximately 50% of cases the nerve divides into two branches as it approaches the larynx. An important landmark is the inferior cornu of the thyroid cartilage which can be palpated. It is just anterior to this that the nerve penetrates the cricothyroid membrane. Palpation of the cornu provides a very helpful landmark if location of the recurrent laryngeal nerve is proving difficult.

Damage to the recurrent laryngeal nerve is a significant injury which results in an inability to oppose the vocal cords. The services of a skilled throat surgeon will be required in this situation and laryngoplasty may well be required at a later date.

Parathyroid gland

Care should be taken to minimise the direct handling of these glands and to preserve their blood supply by dissecting close to the capsule of the thyroid gland in its posterolateral aspect. Fortunately, damage to one or two of these glands does not seem to cause significant problems but particular care needs to be taken when carrying out bilateral thyroidectomy. If persistent postoperative hypocalcaemia is encountered, treatment with a vitamin D analogue will be necessary. Careful monitoring of the blood calcium levels is required under these circumstances as hypercalcaemia may occur. In the case of acute hypocalcaemia, 10 ml of a 10% solution of calcium gluconate may be administered intravenously. It is important that this is given slowly to avoid cardiac dysrhythmia. Infusion over a period of 10 minutes is considered safe and may be repeated.

Postoperative haemorrhage

There is a small but significant incidence of haemorrhage into the deep tissues during the early postoperative period. It is important, therefore, to minimise the chances of haemorrhage by careful intraoperative haemostasis. Nursing the patient in a semirecumbent attitude and minimising neck movement for the first few hours following surgery is also important.

When haemorrhage occurs the patient may experience severe respiratory difficulties secondary to compression or collapse of the trachea.

Nursing staff should be instructed to be vigilant for the signs of respiratory difficulty. If there is clear evidence of a developing problem, prompt action must be taken. This may take the form of an immediate return to the operating suite if there is sufficient time. If not, then clips or sutures in the skin and deep fascia should be removed on the ward. Release of the haematoma usually results in immediate relief of the respiratory compromise after which the underlying haemorrhage can be treated appropriately.

In any situation where the airway may be compromised, skilled anaesthetic assistance should be summoned immediately.

Postoperative management

- Following extubation and as soon as the anaesthetist will permit, the patient should be nursed in a semirecumbent position at an angle of approximately 45° to minimise venous congestion. Respiratory difficulties at this stage may be caused by tracheal collapse or narrowing, as a result of oedema, vocal cord problems secondary to laryngeal nerve damage or even haemorrhage. Prompt corrective action must be taken and anaesthetic assistance is vital.

- Following return to the ward, the patient should be nursed propped up on pillows for the first few hours.

- Drains, if used, can be removed 24 hours postoperatively and the sutures removed on the fourth postoperative day. Traditionally, half the skin clips, if used, are removed at 24 hours and the remainder at 48 hours postoperatively.

- The serum calcium levels should be checked on the second postoperative day.

- Some units carry out routine postoperative vocal cord checks; others only if there are voice changes.

- Thyroxine replacement is at the discretion of the surgeon. Following a routine hemithyroidectomy for a solitary nodule the author places patients on 50 µg replacement thyroxine per day.

SUBMANDIBULAR GLAND EXCISION

Indications

- Sialoadenitis
- Sialolithiasis
- Suspicion of tumour (rare)

Preparation

The patient is warned about the scar and the small but finite risk of damage to the marginal mandibular branch of the facial nerve which supplies the lower lip on that side. Relaxant anaesthetic is usually employed. The patient is positioned on the table with a sandbag or inflatable cushion behind the shoulder blades, the neck slightly extended and with the chin pointing to the opposite side.

Procedure

- The incision should be placed at the lower border of the submandibular gland approximately on a level with the hyoid bone (Figure 7.10A).

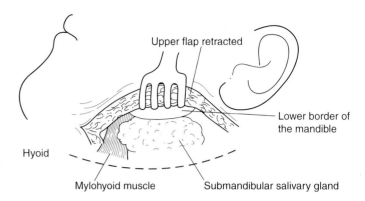

Figure 7.10A The line of the incision for an approach to the submandibular gland. The level of the hyoid bone is indicated. The submandibular gland relates to the free posterior margin of mylohyoid as if it is about to take a bite from it!

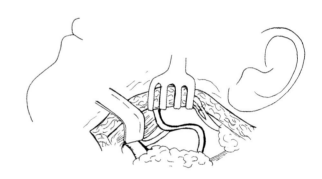

Figure 7.10B The submandibular gland attached only by its duct which passes deep to the mylohyoid muscle.

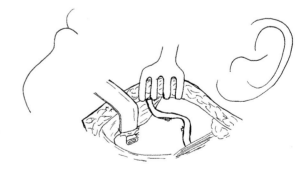

Figure 7.10C The bed of the submandibular gland after removal. The ligated branches of the facial artery and the ligated duct deep to the mylohyoid.

- The skin, subcutaneous fat and platysma are dissected superiorly in a plane immediately adjacent to the gland which can be recognised by its pink and slightly lobulated appearance. It is during this dissection or the subsequent retraction of the upper skin flap that damage to the mandibular branch of the facial nerve occurs and this can be avoided by dissecting strictly in a

105

plane adjacent to the gland itself. For this reason some surgeons advocate intracapsular dissection for benign disease. During the elevation of the upper skin flap either the main trunk or small branches of the facial artery will be encountered and these may require ligation just below the horizontal ramus of the mandible.

- The gland itself is wrapped around the free posterior margin of the mylohyoid muscle dividing the gland into superficial and deep components. The submandibular duct arises anteriorly from the deep portion.

- Once the anterior and superior portions of the gland have been dissected attention can be turned to its deep surface where it can usually be elevated without difficulty although the facial artery may again require ligation. The hypoglossal nerve is an immediate deep relation of the submandibular gland but it is not at risk if the dissection is kept strictly close to the gland (Figure 7.10B).

- When the gland has been dissected free, downward traction will reveal the flat band of the lingual nerve in the floor of the mouth behind the horizontal ramus of the mandible. Tiny secretomotor fibres to the gland will need to be divided allowing the gland to be separated from the nerve which disappears from view behind the mandible.

- The gland is now only attached by the duct which can be clipped, ligated with an absorbable suture and divided. It is not necessary to follow the duct anteriorly where it comes into close relationship to the lingual nerve (Figure 7.10C).

- The wound is closed with a fine subcuticular suture. If accurate haemostasis has been obtained a suction drain is not required.

- When gross infection is present the surgeon may choose to leave the wound open.

Hazards

- *The marginal mandibular branch of the facial nerve.* The best way to avoid damage to the nerve is to make the incision low enough in the neck (about two fingers' breadth below the mandible) and to avoid superficial dissection and retraction in the subplatysmal plane.

- *The facial artery and associated veins* frequently come into the operative field. Their anatomical relationship to the gland is consistent and predictable and they may require ligation.

- *The lingual nerve* is usually seen in the floor of the mouth just inside the horizontal ramus of the mandible where it appears as a flat white band. Great care may be needed in cases of chronic infection where the tissue planes are obliterated and difficult to identify.

- *Haemorrhage.* As with any operation in the head and neck, careful haemostasis should be observed throughout and a point made of checking for bleeding points at the end of the operation. Anticoagulant DVT prophylaxis is not necessary for this type of operation and is relatively contraindicated because of the vascularity of the area.

Postoperative management

In most instances the patient will be ready for discharge either on the same day (a day case) or on the following morning. The sutures are removed on the fourth postoperative day.

8

Vascular surgery

Introduction
Outpatient treatment of varicose veins
   Sclerotherapy
Surgical treatment of long saphenous varicosities
   Preoperative preparation
   Procedure
   Hazards
   Postoperative management
Control of venous bleeding

Vascular suture/vascular anastomosis
   Common faults and complications
   Postoperative care
Fasciotomy
   Indications
   Preparation
   Procedure
   Hazards
   Postoperative care
Further reading

D. Wilkins

INTRODUCTION

All trainee surgeons should be familiar with the basic techniques of vascular surgery as they apply to both arteries and veins. The commonest procedures to which the young surgeon will be exposed are those carried out for varicose veins associated with straightforward superficial long saphenous incompetence. This surgery provides excellent training opportunities but it must be emphasised that adequate supervision by more senior colleagues is essential. The trainee must ensure that he or she is familiar with the patient, the theoretical aspects of the techniques and how to deal with potential problems. Stripped deep femoral veins, divided femoral arteries and damaged deep femoral veins figure prominently in the claims encountered by the medical defence societies.

Surgery to peripheral arteries is demanding of proper technique, enjoyable and rewarding. All surgeons should be able to carry out simple arterial suture. The descriptions of basic techniques in venous and arterial surgery which follow concern the procedures most likely to be encountered by young surgeons in the early parts of their careers.

OUTPATIENT TREATMENT OF VARICOSE VEINS

The successful treatment of varicose veins is crucially dependent upon correct assessment. This is a skill which is developed over a period of years by practitioners in the field and has been much assisted by the widespread availability of ultrasound equipment and expertise. For an introductory account of the clinical assessment and investigation of varicose veins the reader is referred to *Fundamentals of Surgical Practice*, pages 322–325.

Sclerotherapy

Indications

Whereas several decades ago, injection techniques (sclerotherapy) were the norm, the pendulum has now swung very much in favour of surgical treatment. Nonetheless, there are occasions when injection sclerotherapy is appropriate. These include trivial varicosities not obviously associated with major superficial venous incompetence, patient preference and for the treatment of some residual or recurrent varicosities.

Obese or immobile patients, those on the oral contraceptive pill and others with a history of previous deep vein thrombosis should be considered unsuitable for sclerotherapy because of the risk of deep venous thrombosis.

Preparation

The procedure is usually carried out in the outpatient department. It is important that in obtaining informed consent, the patient is given a realistic expectation of the outcome, including cosmetic effects and the likelihood of recurrence. Possible complications which should be mentioned, although not unduly emphasised, include:

- skin staining at the injection site

- scarring

- deep vein thrombosis.

It is important that the patient realises that the likelihood of inducing a deep vein thrombosis is minimised by a regime of vigorous exercise and effective compression following injections. Sclerotherapy is contraindicated in those patients who are unable to comply with a vigorous exercise regime or who are too obese for the application of effective leg compression (see below). An information sheet reinforcing the above points and giving clear instructions is extremely helpful.

Procedure

With the patient standing, injection points are marked. A series of small (1 or 2 ml) syringes with 30 gauge needles mounted may be introduced into the individual varices and taped into position once a flashback of blood into the syringe confirms correct intraluminal placement.

The patient is then assisted to sit and then lies supine on a strategically placed couch. During this manoeuvre the leg is held straight, supported by an assistant and elevated as the patient lies back.

Injection of the sclerosant (usually a solution of sodium tetradecyl sulphate ([STD] 0.2–3%) is made into each site. It is important that the injection is made only into the empty varix. The maximum dosage to be injected at each site and the maximum overall dosage is stipulated in the manufacturer's instructions which must be carefully adhered to. For example, no more than 1 ml and usually half this amount of 3% STD may be injected at any one site and no more than four sites injected at one sitting. It is vital that extreme vigilance is maintained when injecting and if there is the slightest sign of extravasation, such as local pain, the appearance or palpation of a 'bleb' or blanching of the skin, injection is discontinued immediately and the needle withdrawn.

With the leg elevated and the needles and syringes withdrawn, it is the author's practice to place small lengths of soft rubber foam over the injection sites and in the line of the varicosities before applying compression. This ensures that the individual veins are compressed satisfactorily. A full-length elastic stocking (class 2) of the correct size or elastic bandaging is then applied and the patient instructed to walk for the next 20 minutes.

Hazards

Injection outside the vein

Careful attention to placement of the needles and the subsequent manoeuvring of the leg during elevation will help to avoid dislodgement of the needle. Careful observation and palpation of the injection site at the commencement of injection will detect the earliest signs of extravasation. If there is the slightest suspicion of extravasation injection at that site should be terminated.

Injection into an artery

This is a catastrophe and little can be done to rectify the situation when it has occurred. The smaller calibre arteries around the ankle and on the foot are vulnerable (particularly behind the medial malleolus) and it is inadvisable, therefore, for the inexperienced practitioner to attempt sclerotherapy in these areas.

Deep vein thrombosis

The incidence of this complication should be negligible if the correct procedure is followed. It is to guard against this that injection should be made only into an empty vein, that effective compression is applied immediately following injection and that a vigorous exercise regime is followed postinjection. Injection into varicosities above the knee should be carried out only by experienced practitioners and with extreme caution lest a propagating thrombus be induced in the upper reaches of the long saphenous vein.

Postprocedure care

The patient should be instructed to keep the ankle joint as active as possible during the following weeks. He or she should avoid standing still or sitting with the knee bent. Daytime should be spent keeping the leg active; sitting with the legs up and toes moving or lying down.

At the end of two weeks the stockings may be removed by the patient. The leg may be inspected in outpatients at one or two months following this and further injections carried out as necessary.

SURGICAL TREATMENT OF LONG SAPHENOUS VARICOSITIES

Preoperative preparation

The patient should be informed of the significant possibility of residual or recurrent varicosities, the small but definite risk of minor sensory nerve damage and the importance of early postoperative activity in minimising the risk of a deep vein thrombosis. The advisability of offering varicose vein surgery to a patient unable to achieve full mobility immediately following surgery should be carefully considered.

Patients should have stopped taking the oral contraceptive pill for two months and some surgeons also cover the operation with subcutaneous heparin or one of its analogues.

The patient is positioned supine on the table and a side extension board for the lower limb is helpful to give a degree of abduction, particularly in the case of bilateral operations. A degree of head-down tilt is helpful in achieving haemostasis. If short saphenous vein surgery is being carried out under the same anaesthetic it is usual for the patient to be placed first in the prone position and then to be turned into the supine position and redraped after the wounds have been closed.

The long saphenous vein, together with any perforating branches, should be carefully marked as should any superficial varicosities which are to be removed by phlebectomy. Perforating branches may be marked using duplex ultrasound (Figure 8.1).

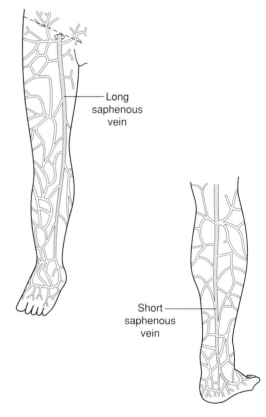

Figure 8.1 Showing the typical course of the long and short saphenous veins. The short saphenous vein usually penetrates the deep fascia at the junction of upper and middle thirds of the calf. Both of these veins are closely approximated to major cutaneous nerves in the distal part of their courses.

Procedure

A skin crease incision measuring between 2.5 and 5 cm in length is made over the saphenofemoral junction. This is located approximately 4 cm below and lateral to the pubic tubercle (Figure 8.2).

The incision is carried down through the deep fascia and once this has been incised, the long saphenous vein may be exposed by sweeping the tissues aside in the direction of the vein using a finger covered by a gauze swab.

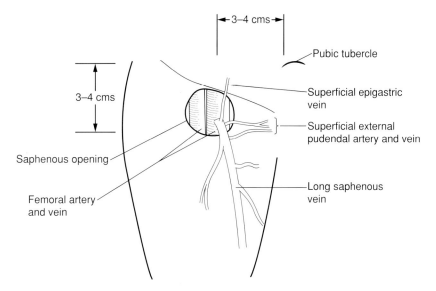

Figure 8.2 Saphenous opening showing the surface marking and major structures.

The dissection of the saphenofemoral junction and its branches is then completed using scissors and atraumatic forceps (DeBakey's or similar). It should be appreciated that dissection in a plane which is very close to the surface of the vein is both easier and less hazardous than dissection in a plane that leaves an overlying film of connective tissue. Dissection along the length of the long saphenous vein is a good starting point.

The long saphenous vein is traced to the saphenofemoral junction, dissecting out and ligating tributaries as they are isolated. There are two clues which are helpful as the saphenofemoral junction is approached. The superficial external pudendal artery usually, but not always, follows a course which results in it crossing transversely the caudal aspect of the saphenofemoral junction. Secondly, the cribriform fascia, a filmy, almost cobweb-like lattice of connective tissue, becomes apparent and surrounds the vein as it turns deep to join the femoral vein.

The saphenofemoral junction is then identified and in order to do so, the surgeon must visualise the femoral vein, a massive venous structure immediately adjacent to the femoral pulse and with the long saphenous vein clearly entering it as a separate structure. The importance of being certain that the junction has been correctly identified cannot be overemphasised. The saphenofemoral junction is then ligated between haemostats (Figure 8.3).

The majority of surgeons strip the long saphenous vein only to the upper third of the calf so as to avoid damage to the long saphenous nerve. Removal may be achieved in the majority of cases by passing a proprietary intraluminal stripping device (such as a wire or rod) retrogradely from the groin. If using a wire, the tip is brought through the vein wall and skin by way of a small stab incision in the calf (Figure 8.4).

Turning once more to the groin, the surgeon then ties a ligature of sufficient strength and length around the vein and its contained

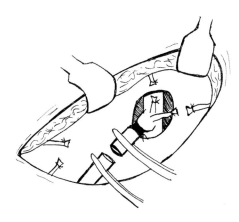

Figure 8.3 Showing the sapheno-femoral junction exposed and the long saphenous vein divided between haemostats.

stripper. Stripping the vein from groin to calf then takes place by pulling on the exposed distal end of the stripper. Once this has been done, an important step is to deliver the end of the vein, still impaled on the stripper, through the stab wound in order that it may be divided at its distal point.

Traction on the groin end of the thread may then be used to deliver the vein and stripper into the wound where it can be removed. Pressure over the track of the stripped long saphenous vein may be applied for a few minutes so as to achieve haemostasis and minimise bruising (Figure 8.5).

Phlebectomies are usually carried out as an adjunct to saphenofemoral ligation and stripping. A fine, sharp-pointed blade (Beaver™ or similar) is used to make stab incisions over the varicosities. It is important that the incisions are orientated along Langer's lines, which for the most part run longitudinally in the lower limb. If carried out correctly, an almost invisible scar results, whereas a transverse incision in the leg invariably results in an ugly mark (Figures 8.6–8.8).

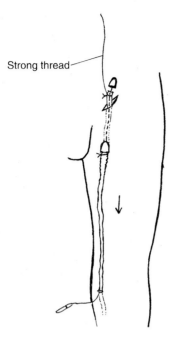

Strong thread

Figure 8.4 The vein stripper has been passed down the long saphenous vein and out to the surface in the lower leg via a small stab incision. Stripping has been started.

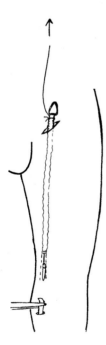

Figure 8.5 The distal long saphenous vein has been divided and is being removed through the groin incision together with the vein stripper.

Through the stab incision, a fine purpose-designed hook, of which there are several varieties available, is used to deliver the varicosity to the surface. A haemostat may then be applied and the varicosity teased out by traction until it fractures. Pressure over

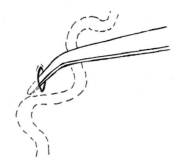

Figure 8.6 Stab avulsions. A small stab incision has been made and a pair of mosquito forceps (or vein hook) introduced.

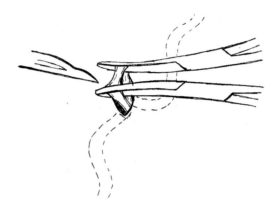

Figure 8.7 The superficial varix has been delivered and is about to be divided between forceps.

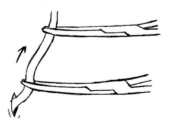

Figure 8.8 Using gentle, persistent traction, it is possible to deliver sizeable lengths of superficial varices through the stab wounds before they fracture.

the track for a few minutes will minimise haematoma formation and haemorrhage before moving to the next site.

After haemostasis, the stab wounds are closed using skin tapes. The groin wound should be closed using an absorbable suture to approximate the deep tissues and either an absorbable or removable subcuticular suture for closing the skin.

At completion the limb is elevated and either a suitable compression stocking is applied or the limb bandaged using one of a variety of elasticated bandages.

Hazards

Venous haemorrhage during surgery

This is covered in a subsequent section (see below). It is important that senior help is summoned immediately by the trainee should there be a problem.

Venous haemorrhage can almost invariably be controlled in the first instance by direct pressure over the damaged vein using a swab, together with elevation of the limb.

Nerve damage

There is a small incidence of damage to cutaneous nerves arising from the phlebectomy incisions. Care should be taken to identify that the structure being avulsed is indeed a vein and not a superficial nerve. This is particularly important when avulsing varicosities at the ankle or on the dorsum of the foot.

If stripping the entire long saphenous vein, great care needs to be taken at the ankle to separate the long saphenous vein and nerve where they are very closely applied one to the other.

The femoral nerves in the groin are lateral to the femoral artery and should not be significantly at risk. If local anaesthetic is injected into the groin wound before closure, temporary femoral nerve paralysis may occur and can result in the patient falling on initial mobilization due to weakness of the hip flexors.

If short saphenous vein surgery is being carried out the sural nerve is at risk in the popliteal fossa and great care needs to be taken with this dissection.

Hazards associated with excessive compression of the limb

Care needs to be taken that, whilst the compression applied to the limb is sufficient to minimise swelling and bruising, it does not compromise the arterial blood supply or deep venous return from the leg or damage major nerve trunks. In this respect, full-length elastic stockings, especially those with a waist loop for support, are ideal since the pressure is distributed evenly over the limb. If using bandages, a layer of wool may help to distribute the pressure. The lateral popliteal nerve where it courses over the neck of the fibula is particularly vulnerable to localised pressure at this point.

Nursing aftercare includes a routine check on the circulation of the foot. Any indication of circulatory compromise, such as excessive (ischaemic) pain in the limb, alterations of sensation or colouration of the toes, should be dealt with by urgent release of compression and rebandaging.

Deep vein thrombosis

Deep vein thrombosis in this situation is at best a nuisance and at worst life threatening. The risks of this occurring may be minimised by ensuring full mobilisation up to and immediately following surgery, DVT prophylaxis using heparin or its analogues if there is deemed to be an increased risk and careful instructions to the patients on their postoperative activity. Lack of mobility through conditions such as arthritis and obesity is a relative contraindication to varicose vein surgery.

Postoperative management

It is important that the patient achieves full mobility as rapidly as possible after surgery. Patients are mobilised as soon as they have recovered from the anaesthetic and will usually be discharged on the same day as surgery. They should be advised that exercise of the calf and ankle muscles is imperative during the next 10 days and that this may be achieved by walking and by simulating 'piano playing with the toes' when the limb is at rest. Elevation of the limb when the patient sits and the avoidance of substantial periods with the knee flexed, as in driving, is important during this period. Patient information sheets emphasising these points are very helpful.

Most surgeons advise the removal of stockings at between one and two weeks following surgery together with tapes and sutures. The patient is warned to expect a degree of bruising and an inspection to gauge the final result at approximately two months is helpful.

CONTROL OF VENOUS BLEEDING

Unexpected venous haemorrhage from a major vein can be a very frightening experience for the young surgeon. Inexpert attempts to control venous haemorrhage can also be extremely dangerous for the patient. A situation can rapidly deteriorate until it is out of control, with a raggedly torn vein bleeding copiously. However, with the knowledge of appropriate steps to be taken in the initial stages to avoid such a situation, the haemorrhage can be quite easily rectified.

The young surgeon is most likely to encounter serious venous bleeding during the groin dissection for varicose vein surgery. Whereas the jet of blood makes the source of arterial bleeding relatively easy to identify and control, venous bleeding manifests as a 'welling up' of blood which quickly fills the whole of the wound, making the origin difficult to identify. The blind insertion of clamps into this pool of blood in misguided attempts to control matters will often result in serious damage to a major vessel.

Remember PAMS.

● *Pressure and position.* First, control bleeding by pressure with a gauze swab or swabs. Can the venous pressure be reduced by tilting the table head up (head and neck surgery) or feet up (lower limb surgery)? On its own, this manoeuvre can make a dramatic difference to the bleeding but beware of the risks of air embolus should too much negative pressure be induced.

- *Access.* If necessary, increase the size of the wound.

- *Manpower.* Call for assistance. The trainee surgeon will undoubtedly call for senior help and, indeed, this is probably the only step that needs to be taken apart from pressure to control the bleeding.

- *Suction.* A large end-suction device is the most important tool for a vascular surgeon. Properly used by an assistant, this will clear the wound of blood and usually is all that is required to give the operating surgeon a view of the tear in the vein, while one or two judiciously placed vascular sutures are inserted.

The control of serious venous haemorrhage from major vessels secondary to trauma is clearly beyond the scope of the trainee surgeon. Proper attention to less serious, iatrogenic venous haemorrhage, however, using the principles outlined above will save the young surgeon (and patient) much misery!

VASCULAR SUTURE/VASCULAR ANASTOMOSIS

The basic technique of vascular anastomosis is one that should be mastered by all surgical trainees from an early stage; suitable workshops are now available on this subject. Fine, non-absorbable monofilament vascular sutures mounted on round-bodied needles are freely available and for most work on major peripheral arteries 4/0 or 5/0 will be ideal. Certain principles apply, as follows.

- Before clamping any vessel it is vital that the surgeon addresses the question of heparinisation. On most occasions systemic heparinisation using an intravenous injection of a standard dose (5000 units) of heparin or a dose which is titrated against weight will be appropriate. Occasionally regional heparinisation using a heparin/saline mixture flush into the artery will be deemed sufficient.

- Use atraumatic vascular forceps and handle the internal, endothelial surfaces of veins and arteries as little as possible.

- Insofar as the arteries are concerned, always try to suture from inside to outside so as to minimise the chances of raising an intimal flap.

- Apposition of vascular surfaces should be such that the join is everted.

- In general terms, the surgeon will produce the best work if operating from a position of comfort.

- Avoid handling the tip of the needle with any instrument and in particular the needle holder. Needle points are highly polished and once scratched, their performance degrades considerably.

- At the 'heel' and 'toe' of an end-to-side anastomosis or patch, place the sutures close together so as to avoid constricting donor or recipient vessels.

- Always ensure excellent exposure, lighting and vision. Increasingly, vascular surgeons are using low-powered magnification spectacles as well as headlights to improve suturing accuracy.

- An end-suction device should be used to keep the operating field clear of blood and tissue fluid.

An illustration of the general principles of vascular suturing is provided in the performance of an end-to-side anastomosis suture for a femoropopliteal vein bypass. This is an excellent training procedure, as is the application of a vein patch for closing a longitudinal arteriotomy. The steps are illustrated in Figures 8.9–8.11).

Common faults and complications

- *Suturing a diseased artery from 'outside to inside' results in the raising of an intimal flap.* Avoid this by reversing the needle at a convenient point on the suture line so as to maintain 'inside-to-outside' suturing on the artery if possible.

- *Following clamp release, there is doubt about the patency of the anastomosis.* This may be due to a number of technical problems.

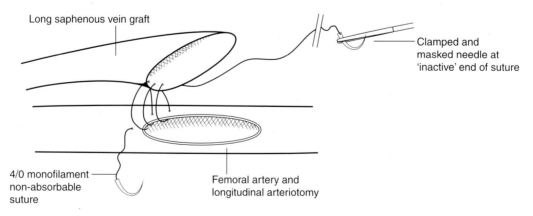

Figure 8.9 Vein parachuted down by tightening the suture after 4–6 passes at the heel. 'Inactive' needle brought into play and reversed to continue inside/outside sequence on the artery.

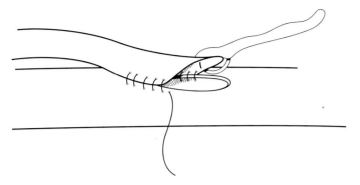

Figure 8.10 Vein parachuted down by tightening the suture after 4–6 passes at the heel. 'Inactive' needle on the far side of the arteriotomy is brought into play and reversed, to continue inside/outside sequence on the artery.

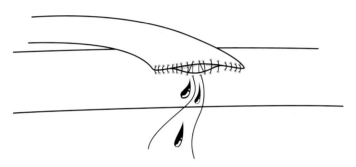

Figure 8.11 The suture line is almost completed and after one or two more passes the needles will be cut off and the suture tied using at least six throws. Before tightening, the vessels will be flushed clear of any blood clot or debris by momentary release of the clamps. Note that the knot is at the centre of the suture line.

The first priority is to establish whether in fact there is flow and in most vascular units one of a variety of techniques will be used as a routine at the completion of an anastomosis to confirm this. These techniques include Doppler ultrasound, on-table angiography and magnetic flow meter measurement. The presence of pulsation at the anastomosis site is, on its own, an unreliable indicator.

- *Lack of flow.* If there is doubt or it is proven on testing that there is no flow, action must be taken at that time rather than adopting a 'wait and see' approach. It may be necessary to refashion the anastomosis or merely remove stray blood clot by flushing or by the passage of a balloon catheter.

- *The suture line is not haemostatic.* A few minutes' pressure following clamp release is usually all that is required for the average suture line to become dry. Any obvious large defects will require the placement of a further suture. It is important that the arterial inflow is briefly interrupted while this is carried out and that *two* passes through the vessels are made to close the defect.

- *Defects of suture handling.* During suturing it is very important that the assistant who is 'following' by holding on to the run-

ning suture keeps a proper tension in place. The assistant should be vigilant for the development of tangles and knots which can usually be forestalled. If a running knot forms in the suture it should be either undone, pulled tight so that it does not snag on the tissues as it is pulled through or dealt with by cutting out and recommencing with a new suture tied in at that point. A careful check for looseness of the suture line should be made before the final knot is tied.

- *Narrowing of the anastomosis or contributing vessels.* Usually this is due to poor shaping of the vessel ends or the incorporation of excessive amounts of vessel wall. It must be dealt with by refashioning the anastomosis.

Postoperative care

Certain principles apply to most types of vascular surgical procedures.

Anticoagulation

Many surgeons continue anticoagulation either temporarily or permanently following a vascular procedure. There are no agreed guidelines and it is a matter of individual practice. It is important, therefore, to specify a protocol to be followed at the completion of surgery so that nursing and medical staff responsible for the postoperative care have a clear indication of the management plan.

Nursing care

It is undoubtedly an advantage if such patients are cared for by nurses experienced in the management of vascular patients. The circulation in the limb should be monitored using the capillary refill time, any palpable pulses and/or handheld Doppler devices. Wound care is particularly important, as is attention to the relief of pressure on vulnerable areas of skin such as heels and buttocks.

Antibiotics

Again, practice is extremely variable except to say that if prosthetic graft material has been used, perioperative and postoperative antibiotic cover will invariably be needed. Prosthetic graft infection at a later stage is an extremely serious complication which will usually not be resolved until the graft is removed.

Postoperative haemorrhage

In the early postoperative period, this may manifest as an expanding haematoma in a wound. The usual principles of control of the haemorrhage and resuscitation of the patient apply. An early return to the operating theatre for surgical correction is advisable.

FASCIOTOMY

Indications

Fasciotomy can be a limb-salvaging procedure. It has an application in many emergency and urgent situations where oedema of the deep tissues can increase compartment pressures to the extent that the circulation is compromised. A typical example would be the revascularisation of a leg which had been severely ischaemic for more than 12–24 hours. Another situation would be that of a severely contused limb with or without an associated fracture. Failure to recognise and deal with these 'compartment' syndromes can result in severe permanent damage, such as a Volkmann's contracture in the arm or a useless lower leg.

The most frequent situation encountered will involve the lower leg. This is therefore described in more detail, but the same principles apply to the arm.

Preparation

The procedure is carried out under general anaesthetic but in an emergency may be carried out under local anaesthetic.

The surgeon must decide which of the three deep compartments should be decompressed. In the case of general injury, all three must be dealt with (Figure 8.12). It is the author's preference to deal only with the major posterior compartment in less severe cases. Tension may be judged in the anterior compartment by palpation of the deep fascia through the skin. In general terms, 'if in doubt, open it' is the maxim. In some centres the equipment and expertise are available for direct measurement of intracompartment pressures using fine-bore cannulas but the performance of such a test should not be allowed to introduce unnecessary delay. A pressure that is less than 30–40 mm below the systolic pressure should be taken as an indication for decompression.

A further decision needs to be made regarding the necessity to open the skin as well as the deep fascia. It is the author's preference to release the deep fascia using a 'closed' method (see below) initially and if the skin then seems to be limiting the decompression, to release this in addition. An extensive incision of this nature may be necessary but inevitably leads to a much more prolonged period of recovery involving delayed healing, skin grafting, etc. It is important to realise, however, that damaged muscle and nerves are much more susceptible to ischaemia than normal tissues and if there remains any doubt about the adequacy of decompression the safest course is to lay the whole compartment open.

Procedure

The patient is placed on the table in the supine position and the whole limb is prepared and draped. The incision necessary to gain access to the main posterior compartment is as shown (Figure 8.13). The incisions for the anterior and lateral compartments are shown in Figure 8.14.

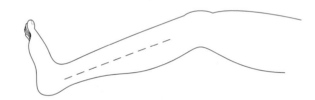

Figure 8.13 Incision for fasciotomy. The medial side of the right leg is shown.

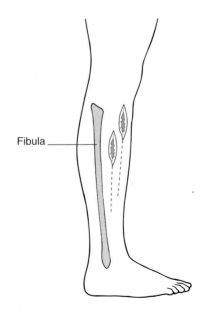

Figure 8.14 Incisions necessary for decompression of the anterior and lateral compartments of the leg.

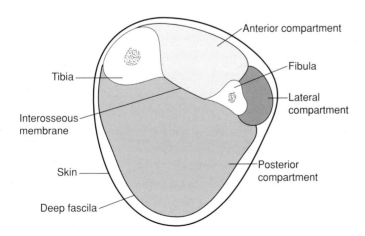

Figure 8.12 A cross section of the lower limb showing the major compartments.

116

A longitudinal incision may then be made in the deep fascia at this level and a long pair of scissors with the tips open used to extend this incision along the length of the lower limb. If using this closed technique, several points need to be borne in mind. First, the scissors can be pushed along the desired line with the tips slightly open and engaging the fascia. This will be sufficient to split the fascia along its length. A scissoring action is not usually necessary, except perhaps at the distal end. It is important that the fasciotomy is continued to the ankle. If resistance is encountered here or elsewhere, it is wise to make another incision (Figure 8.15).

Once released, the tension of the skin can be gauged and, if still relatively loose, the remainder of the skin may be left intact.

The wounds are left open and packed with gauze soaked in a weak solution of iodine and the limb is wrapped with wool and a loose crepe bandage. A back slab may be helpful.

Hazards

The major hazard using the closed procedure, and indeed the open one, is haemorrhage. Careful interoperative haemostasis is important and if excessive haemorrhage using the 'blind' technique is encountered, then a conversion through the skin may be necessary.

There is usually marked loss of serosanguinous fluid and sometimes frank haemorrhage on the ward which may need countering by transfusion and indeed firm bandaging to obtain control.

Damage to cutaneous nerves is another potential hazard which is largely unavoidable using either closed or open techniques.

Postoperative care

The limb should be kept well elevated and it is reasonable to give perioperative antibiotics for 24 hours. Subcutaneous DVT prophylaxis should be given in the form of heparin or its low molecular weight analogues and consideration may be given to systemic anticoagulation, bearing in mind the considerable risks of haemorrhage associated with such extensive wounds.

At a time which is variable and commensurate with the damage to the limb, the wounds may be closed or grafted. Physiotherapy in the early stages to preserve limb mobility is essential. It must be emphasised that close observation of the limb in the early perioperative phase is essential and that if there is any doubt regarding the adequacy of the fasciotomy, further exploration is indicated.

FURTHER READING

Bell PRF, Jamieson CW, Ruckley CV. *Surgical Management of Vascular Disease*. London: Saunders, 1992

Ruckley CV. *A Colour Atlas of Surgical Management of Venous Disease*. London: Wolfe Medical, 1998

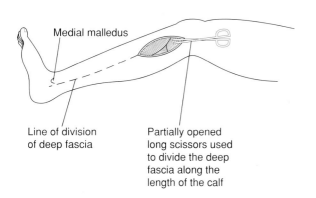

Figure 8.15 Partially opened long scissors used to divide the deep fascia along the length of the calf. The skin along the whole length of the leg should be opened if there is the slightest doubt regarding the adequacy of decompression.

9

Thoracic surgery

Endotracheal intubation
   Indications
   Technique
   Procedure
   Difficult intubation
   Hazards and complications
   Special situations and techniques
   Double-lumen tubes
Cricothyroidotomy
   Indications
   Contraindications
   Technique
   Complications
Tracheostomy
   Indications
   Types of tracheostomy tubes
   Technique of insertion
   Care and complications
   Tracheostomy weaning and removal
Foreign bodies in the airways
   Pathophysiology
   Diagnosis
   Removal

Investigation
   Late complications
Bronchoscopy
   Indications
   Types of bronchoscopy
   Technique
   Complications
CVP line insertion
   Indications
   Catheters
   Technique
   Complications
Opening and closing the chest
   Thoracotomy
   Median sternotomy
Chest drain insertion
   Indications
   Types of chest drains
   Technique for relief of pneumothorax
   Complications
Harvesting the long saphenous vein
   Indications
   Technique
   Complications

Aljafri Majid

ENDOTRACHEAL INTUBATION

Indications

1. Emergency, e.g. during cardiopulmonary resuscitation.

2. Elective:
   - general anaesthesia for surgical procedures.
   - elective ventilation for respiratory failure or chest wall trauma, especially flail chest.
   - airway protection in CNS disorders, e.g. CVA, trauma
   - neuromuscular disorders – polio, myesthenia gravis, Guillain–Barré.

Technique

The patient

- Have you got the correct patient?

- What are the indications for intubation?

- What associated medical conditions are there?

Equipment (Figure 9.1)

- Laryngoscope (make sure the light is working) and a selection of blades.

- Intubation forceps, e.g. Magill forceps.

- Bag (e.g. Ambu) masks, tubing, angle pieces, connectors, oxygen supply, suction pump, suction catheters.

Endotracheal tubes

Cuffed tubes are either low pressure, high volume (usually made of PVC) (Figure 9.2) or high pressure, low volume (usually made of red rubber).

The cuff is connected via a fine tube to a balloon, which indicates the degree of inflation of the cuff. On the other end of the balloon is a Luer connection for inflation whilst deflation of the balloon is prevented by a one-way valve or a cap. These should be checked to ensure that they are not leaky. Uncuffed tubes are used for neonates, infants and small children. Cuffed tubes may cause injury to the tracheal wall resulting in tracheal stenosis.

For adults, tubes with a 9 mm internal diameter (ID) are generally suitable for men and tubes with an 8 mm ID are suitable for women. For children, a number of formulas based on the age of the child are used to calculate the most appropriate tube size. Bear in mind that these formulas are only estimates; once inserted, if the tube is found to be too loose and causing too large an air leak, or too tight fitting such that it may cause damage to the cords or tracheal mucosa, it should be changed to a more suitable size.

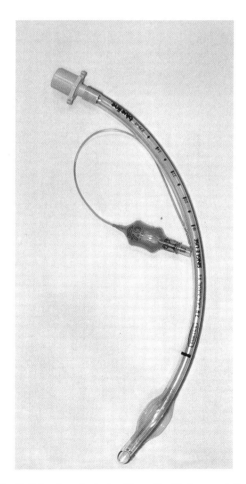

Figure 9.2 Cuffed endotracheal tube. The cuff and balloon are inflated.

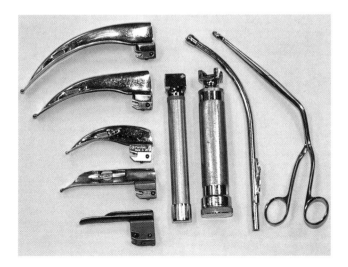

Figure 9.1 Some items of equipment used for endotracheal intubation. (From left) a selection of laryngoscope blades, two laryngoscope handles, sucker and Magill forceps.

Drugs

The appropriate dosages should be calculated, the drugs drawn up and the syringes properly labelled.

- Induction – thiopentone, propofol, etomidate.
- Muscle relaxation – suxamethonium, pancuronium, vecuronium, etc.
- Analgesia – morphine, fentanyl.
- Anaesthesia – halothane, nitrous oxide, isoflurane.

Support

- Nursing support – the nurses assisting should preferably have had some experience with intubation of patients.
- Senior medical support (preferably an anaesthetist) should be available.

Procedure

Position the patient supine, with a headrest.

Preoxygenation

A tight-fitting mask is placed over the nose and mouth and 100% oxygen administered. An anaesthetic bag is attached to the circuit and the patient asked to breathe normally. If available, a pulse oximeter is useful to monitor the procedure.

Induction and muscle relaxation

The usual sequence is induction first followed by muscle relaxants after intubation, if needed. For rapid sequence induction, the induction agent is administered and quickly followed by the muscle relaxant before intubation.

Intubation

- Introduce the laryngoscope blade through the mouth and position the tip in the vallecula fossa.
- Lift the laryngoscope to bring the tongue and epiglottis forwards; external pressure on the cricoid helps to displace the larynx posteriorly and allows the laryngeal inlet to be more easily seen.
- Visualise the cords and introduce the lubricated endotracheal tube; the Magill forceps and a stylet are useful. Aim to position the tip of the tube midway down the length of the trachea.
- Connect the tube to the oxygen supply and begin ventilation.

Ventilation

Observe the movement of the chest and auscultate both sides for breath sounds which should be heard clearly on both sides. If only the right side appears to be being ventilated, this may be because the endotracheal tube has been inserted too deeply and has intubated the right main bronchus. The tube should be withdrawn 1–2 cm and both lungs reauscultated for normal breath sounds. The epigastrium should also be auscultated to exclude the possibility of oesophageal intubation.

Once the tube is properly in position, mark or note down the position of the incisors or lips (22 cm for males, 20 cm for females) on the tube and secure it in place with tapes. Any excess length of the endotracheal tube may be cut off to reduce the volume of dead space.

The maintenance of anaesthesia, analgesia, sedation, etc. will depend on the indications for intubation and the procedure that is to be used.

Extubation

Prior to extubation, assess the:

- level of consciousness – the patient should be awake and responsive.
- depth and rate of spontaneous ventilation.

After extubation, infants and small children are particularly vulnerable to airways obstruction from laryngeal oedema. Thus it is important to ensure that the air or oxygen administered is well humidified since drying of secretions can lead to obstruction of air flow. This risk is increased if there has been any difficulty with intubation or if the patient has been intubated for some time (a day or more) or if the tube is too tight fitting. Besides humidifying the oxygen, regular use of a saline nebuliser and even corticosteroids may be needed to reduce the oedema.

Difficult intubation

This can be caused by:

- increased weight
- decreased flexion/extension at the head and neck
- decreased ability to open the mouth as measured by the inter-incisor gap
- receding chin
- large incisors
- an oropharyngeal aperture in which the faucial pillars, soft palate and uvula are not easily seen on opening the mouth.

After three unsuccessful attempts at intubation, ventilate with a tight-fitting mask and call for more experienced assistance.

Hazards and complications

- Hypoxia – during attempts at intubation, monitor the oxygen saturation with a pulse oximeter.

- Oesophageal intubation.

- Intubation of the right main bronchus.

- Tracheal stenosis.

- Trauma to the lips, tongue and larynx in the case of orotracheal tubes.

- Tube dislodgement.

- Cuff deflation – air leak and hypoventilation.

- Self-extubation.

- Laryngeal oedema – especially in neonates, infants and small children particularly if the endotracheal tube is too tight and can result in airway obstruction after extubation. This is managed with intravenous steroids prior to extubation and humidification via a nebuliser to keep the secretions moist until the oedema settles.

Special situations and techniques

Alternatives to direct laryngoscopy to visualise the larynx during intubation include:

- a fibreoptic bronchoscope or laryngoscope used to visualise the larynx and guide the ETT into the trachea

- blind intubation – skilled anaesthetists may opt to use this technique under special conditions, e.g. cervical spine injury, ankylosing spondylitis

- lighted stylet – this can improve the success rate and speed of blind intubation. Intubation needs to be performed in a darkened room. The stylet is introduced directly through the orotracheal or nasotracheal routes or via a port in a laryngeal mask. The light at the tip of the stylet is transilluminated through the neck and indicates its position as it passes through the larynx into the trachea. A brilliant glow indicates its position in the trachea whilst a diffuse glow indicates that it has entered the oesophagus.

- Retrograde intubation – under very special (difficult) circumstances, a guidewire may be inserted through a needle into the trachea and passed retrogradely through the vocal cords into the pharynx and out through the mouth. The guidewire can then be used to guide the endotracheal tube into the trachea.

Double-lumen tubes

Double-lumen tubes (Carlens, Robertshaw) are used for:

- single lung ventilation during thoracotomy

- independent lung ventilation

- bronchoalveolar lavage.

Double-lumen tubes consist of two tubes bound or fused together. They are moulded into a shape which will allow them to be positioned within the airways without becoming kinked. The tubes are of different lengths and the longer of the two is positioned to open into the bronchus (the bronchial tube) whilst the shorter of the two opens into the trachea (the tracheal tube). There are two cuffs, one for the bronchial tube and the other for the trachea. It is possible to ventilate just one lung, both lungs simultaneously or both lungs independently. For example, to ventilate one lung both the tracheal and bronchial cuffs are inflated, the proximal end of the tracheal tube clamped and ventilation performed through the bronchial tube.

CRICOTHYROIDOTOMY

Indications

- Access to the airway for ventilation under special circumstances where endotracheal intubation through the orotracheal or nasotracheal route is not possible, e.g. facial, especially oropharyngeal trauma.

- Access to the airway under circumstances where intubation is not easily performed, e.g. in a road traffic accident where a patient is trapped in a vehicle.

- As a temporising manoeuvre after failed oro- or nasotracheal intubation.

- For removal of secretions or blood causing life-threatening airway obstruction.

- As an elective procedure for aspiration of secretions although some controversy exists regarding whether tracheostomy or cricothyroidotomy is the preferred procedure.

- Suspected or proven cervical spine injury.

- To improve oxygenation (needle cricothyroidotomy – see below). This is a temporising manoeuvre to provide supplemental oxygen to a patient in whom there are difficulties in providing a good airway.

Contraindications

- Laryngeal trauma.

- Infants – the space between the cricoid and thyroid cartilage is too narrow for an airway to be inserted.

Technique

At least three techniques are available:

1. open technique
2. percutaneous technique
3. needle cricothyroidotomy.

Open technique (minitracheostomy, 'mini-trach')

- Incise the skin transversely over the cricothyroid membrane, i.e. between the lower border of the thyroid cartilage and the upper border of the cricoid cartilage.
- Incise the cricothyroid membrane.
- Dilate the wound and hold the edges open with the dilator/ artery forceps.
- Insert a (paediatric) endotracheal or tracheostomy tube with an internal diameter of about 4 mm.

Percutaneous technique

- Insert a needle into the trachea through the cricothyroid membrane.
- Insert the guidewire through the needle into the trachea and withdraw the needle.
- Pass the dilator over the guidewire to dilate the puncture site and repeat with increasing sizes of dilators to dilate the stoma as in the Seldinger technique.
- The tube can then be inserted and the dilator and guidewire removed.

Needle cricothyroidotomy

This is used as a temporising manoeuvre which aims to provide supplemental oxygen in cases where endotracheal intubation through the nasal or orotracheal route is not possible, e.g. oropharyngeal trauma.

A 5 inch 12 or 14 needle-cannula is connected to a small (5 ml) syringe. Whilst aspirating on the syringe, the needle is inserted through the cricothyroid membrane in the midline. Aspiration of air indicates entry into the tracheal lumen and the needle and syringe are then removed. The cannula is then advanced into the trachea pointing in the direction of the tracheal bifurcation. The cannula hub is joined directly to tubing connected to the oxygen supply and oxygen at 15 l/min is then administered. By intermittently connecting and disconnecting the cannula hub to the oxygen tubing, inspiration and expiration are made possible. It must be emphasised that resistance to airflow through such a small cannula greatly increases the work of breathing. In addition, since ventilation is reduced CO_2 retention occurs and, even in the absence of lung pathology, limits the usefulness of this procedure to a maximum time of half an hour.

Once the cricothyroidotomy tube is no longer required it can be removed and the wound sealed with a dressing.

Complications

Early

- Haemorrhage, from damage to:
  - veins – there is usually a fine venous plexus over the cricothyroid membrane and sometimes larger veins (>2 mm diameter) traverse this area
  - small arteries
  - uncinate lobe of the thyroid.
- Subcutaneous and/or mediastinal emphysema from leakage of air from around the stoma which may enter the subcutaneous tissue or track down to the mediastinum.

Intermediate

- Risk of aspiration from abnormalities of swallowing.

Late

- Subglottic stenosis.
- Dysphonia.

TRACHEOSTOMY

Indications

- Removal of secretions, particularly from patients who are unable to clear their own airway because of neurological problems, e.g. after a CVA, head injury or neurosurgery.
- Relief of upper airway obstruction.
- Postlaryngectomy.
- Patients expected to require long-term ventilation.
- Diphtheria.
- As an emergency in patients in whom there has been a failed intubation.

Types of tracheostomy tubes

Metal tubes made of silver, German silver or stainless steel are usually indicated for long-term use (months or years). There are a number of designs, the common ones consisting of a removable inner tube (which can be removed for cleaning) and an outer tube that has a flange for anchoring it to tapes to keep the tube in place (Figure 9.3).

Plastic tubes are usually indicated for shorter term use and are made of various plastics such as polyvinyl chloride. They may be cuffed or uncuffed and are usually kept in place by tapes attached to a special flange (Figure 9.4).

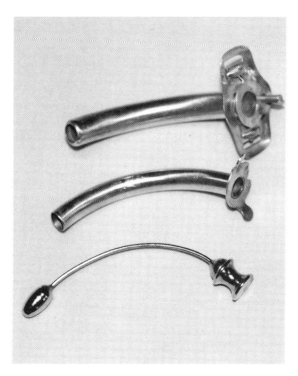

Figure 9.3 Silver tracheostomy tube showing the outer tube (top), inner tube (middle) and obturator (bottom).

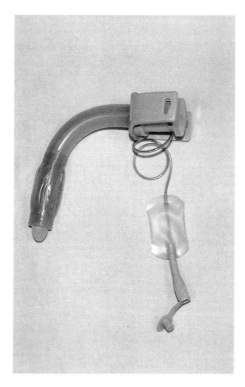

Figure 9.4 Cuffed tracheostomy tube with obturator inserted.

Technique of insertion

Open technique

Tracheostomy is best performed in an operating theatre under optimum conditions. Good lighting and proper instruments, including diathermy (turned down low), decrease the hazards of this procedure. Occasionally tracheostomy has to be performed as an emergency at the bedside but this does increase the risk of the procedure.

- General anaesthesia, sedation or local anaesthetic.
- Nasal or orotracheal tube in place (usually but this may not always be possible).
- The patient should be lying supine, with the head supported by an O-ring.
- Skin preparation and square drape or head drape.
- Skin incision over 2nd tracheal cartilage.
- Separate the strap muscles.
- Divide the thyroid isthmus.
- Identify the trachea.
- Incise the trachea through the 2nd–4th tracheal rings; vertical incision is quickest, no proven advantage to any other incisions – transverse, flap or excision of disc.
- Ask the anaesthetist to deflate the cuff and withdraw the endotracheal tube – at this time the secretions which have collected around the endotracheal tube are released and may even obstruct the trachea so they should be immediately removed by suction.
- Using the tracheal hooks to hold open the edges of the incision, insert the tracheostomy tube through the stoma and inflate the cuff.
- Connect the tracheostomy tube to the ventilator tubing and hand ventilate.
- Auscultate the lungs and ensure that there is equal air entry on both sides.

Percutaneous technique

Tracheostomy is often required for critically ill patients in the ICU, who are often already ventilated via an endotracheal tube and require continuous monitoring and infusions of drugs. For such patients, even transfer to the operating room may constitute a considerable additional hazard. Such patients are often operated on in the ICU itself where the conditions are often suboptimal. The percutaneous technique introduced relatively recently is becoming more popular for such patients. It is usually performed by an experienced intensivist and is briefly described here.

- A needle and cannula are inserted into the trachea at about the 2nd or 3rd tracheal ring. The needle is withdrawn and a guidewire is inserted through the cannula into the trachea.

- The tracheal stoma is then dilated. There are two methods of dilatation with special dilating forceps or by dilators. The dilators are available in two forms: either in a set of graduated sizes or as a single tapered dilator.

- Once the stoma has been dilated to a sufficient size, the guidewire is threaded through a perforation in the tracheostomy obturator. The obturator and tracheostomy tube are then inserted into the trachea through the tracheostomy stoma after which the obturator and guidewire are removed.

Care and complications

All tracheostomy tubes require specialised nursing and medical care in order to reduce the incidence of complications.

- Dislodgement – occurs easily if the tracheostomy tube is not secured properly.

- Blockage from accumulated secretions, blood or blood clot.

- Kinking.

- Vessel erosion.

- Tracheal stenosis.

- Pulmonary aspiration – often silent, due to abnormalities in swallowing, and often in older patients and may defeat the original purpose of keeping the airway clear.

- Fracture of the tracheostomy tube (rarely).

Tracheostomy weaning and removal

Once the patient's general condition has improved and when he/she no longer requires a tracheostomy (e.g. minimal secretions), he/she can be weaned off the tracheostomy. In general the patient should be alert, cooperative and self-ventilating.

FOREIGN BODIES IN THE AIRWAYS

Pathophysiology

Common foreign bodies in children include balloons, coins and small toys. Toys made of material which can conform to the shape of the airways (balloons, soft plastics) are particularly dangerous since they can obstruct airflow and result in asphyxiation. Silent aspiration may occur in patients with neurological disorders, e.g. head injury or stroke patients.

The effects depend on:

- the level of obstruction – the upper airways, lower airways

- the degree of obstruction – complete or partial airway obstruction

- whether there is a ball valve effect.

Airway obstruction occurs:

- immediately if the foreign body is large enough to obstruct but not pass through the airway

- momentarily if it is small enough to pass through the upper airways before being lodged in the lower airways (bronchi)

- intermittently if it alters its position, e.g. moves from the trachea to the bronchus and back again, or if it swivels or rotates to obstruct the airway.

Diagnosis

A child may have been seen to place an object in its mouth prior to a bout of choking and coughing, with inability to speak and cyanosis.

An adult may have been eating and suddenly appears distressed. The patient may point to the throat. There may be coughing, noisy breathing and wheezing.

Removal

If the patient appears to be in distress and unable to breathe emergency measures must be taken immediately. The Heimlich manoeuvre is performed for adults and children over one year of age. To do this manoeuvre first stand behind the patient and place the fist of one hand on the abdomen midway between the xiphoid and umbilicus. Cover the fist with the other hand and then compress the abdomen suddenly several times to raise the intraabdominal and hence intrathoracic pressure to expel the foreign body.

For children less than one year of age the head-down position and back slaps are recommended. There is some controversy regarding blind finger sweeps. They may push the object further into the larynx although in some cases this manoeuvre may be life saving. If the object is suspected to be in the larynx, laryngoscopy is performed under local or general anaesthesia using a laryngoscope and Magill forceps to extract the foreign body.

Bronchoscopy is performed for removal of foreign bodies in the trachea and larger bronchi (see 'Bronchoscopy' below).

Investigation

If the condition of the patient is relatively stable various investigations may be performed with a view to identifying the foreign body and establishing the level at which it is located within the airways. Radiographs may be useful in the case of radioopaque foreign bodies.

When the foreign body is suspected to be in the pharynx or larynx, AP and lateral radiographs of the neck may be useful. If the foreign body is suspected to be lower down in the respiratory tree, AP chest radiographs taken on inspiration and expiration as well as lateral views are taken in the emergency department to detect the foreign body and to determine if there is any air trapping.

If the patient is not too distressed, he may be transferred to the radiology department for PA views as well as fluoroscopy.

Early radiographic features include hyperinflation of one lung with mediastinal shift and a depressed hemidiaphragm with reduced excursion on inspiration seen on screening. Later features include collapse, consolidation, pneumonic changes and lung abscess.

Late complications

Bronchiectasis may occur years later.

BRONCHOSCOPY

Indications

Diagnostic

- To visualise pathology, e.g. endobronchial lesions:
  - primary tumours, benign or malignant
  - secondary spread of tumours, e.g. from oesophageal carcinoma
  - mediastinal lymph node enlargement – blunting of the carina.
- To obtain brushings and washings for cytology or biopsy.
- Fluorescence for early diagnosis of carcinoma.

Therapeutic

- Removal of foreign bodies, blood or secretions.
- Dilatation of tracheal stenosis
- Insertion of tracheal stents.
- To assist in endotracheal intubation of difficult airways.

Types of bronchoscopy

Fibreoptic bronchoscopy

Fibreoptic bronchoscopes are available in various sizes for paediatric and adult work (Figure 9.5). The larger adult ones are just over 5 mm external diameter and usually include biopsy and aspiration channels and are storeable. They utilise a fibreoptic

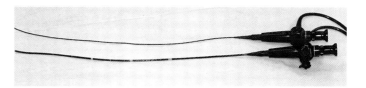

Figure 9.5 Paediatric (above) and adult (below) fibreoptic bronchoscopes.

light source and cable to provide illumination. Accessories such as brushes and biopsy forceps and alligator forceps enable brushings and biopsies to be taken as well as removal of some small foreign bodies.

Briefly, the technique involves sedation or a general anaesthetic, local anaesthetic to the vocal cords as well as transtracheal injection of local anaesthetic to anaesthetise the tracheal luminal surface. The bronchoscope may be inserted through the nasal route (use plenty of lubricant), oral route (use a bite guard) or through an endotracheal tube if the patient is intubated (a good way to gain initial experience). If the patient is not anaesthetised the cords should be observed for movement with respiration (unilateral vocal cord palsy may indicate sinister pathology) and the tracheal bifurcation should be sharp (blunting of the tracheal bifurcation suggests subcarinal lymph node enlargement).

Rigid bronchoscopy

Rigid bronchoscopes are of two types:

- open tube – the patient must be anaesthetised using a self-ventilating technique or ventilated through a Sanders jet ventilation system which uses a Venturi effect to entrain air into the bronchoscope
- ventilating bronchoscope – the bronchoscope is connected to a ventilator circuit (Figure 9.6).

Parts of the rigid bronchoscope include the beak (which is shaped to enable it to pass through the cords with minimal trauma), the shaft, connections to ventilatory system, light source and eyepiece. Accessories include the Hopkins lens, 0°, 30° and 60°-angled lenses to view the major bronchi, suction tubes, biopsy forceps and alligator/crocodile grasping forceps (Figures 9.7 and 9.8).

Indications

Biopsy of endotracheal and endobronchial lesions as well as removal of foreign bodies but because of its rigid shape, its use is somewhat limited to the larger bronchi.

Technique

Position of patient and operators

- Patient lies supine on an operating table which has an adjustable headrest with the head on an O-ring.

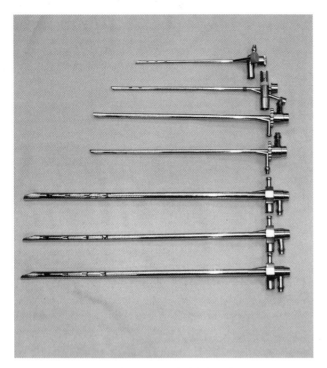

Figure 9.6 A selection of infant, child and adult bronchoscopes.

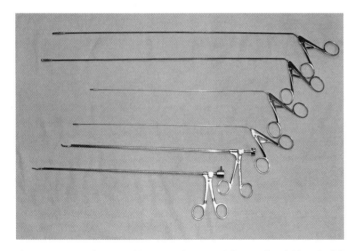

Figure 9.7 A selection of biopsy and grasping forceps for child and adult bronchoscopes.

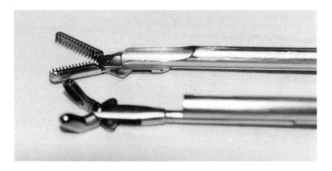

Figure 9.8 The tips of the alligator (above) and biopsy (below) forceps.

- The head should be facing slightly superior, i.e. slight flexion of the lower cervical and extension of the upper cervical, vertebral and atlantooccipital joints ('sniffing the morning air').

In this procedure, anaesthetist and surgeon 'share the airway' and it is important that both have access to it without interference and can hand over the airway to each other smoothly. Positioning of the surgeon, anaesthetist and their nursing assistants around the patient is therefore important. One arrangement is for the surgeon to stand (kneel) at the head end of the patient with the anaesthetist on the surgeon's right. The theatre nurse may be on the surgeon's left and the trolley with the bronchoscope and other equipment should be readily to hand.

Anaesthesia

Preoxygenation with a tight-fitting mask and ventilation through a bag and 100% oxygen.

Local anaesthesia and sedation are now rarely used for rigid bronchoscopy except in emergency circumstances. General anaesthesia and sedation include topical analgesia to the pharynx and larynx with 4% lignocaine. There are variations in the technique of anaesthesia which are beyond the scope of this chapter. However, in general terms they are to do with whether the patient should be self-ventilating, partially self-ventilating or completely paralysed and fully ventilated by positive pressure ventilation. For foreign body removal it is preferable for the patient to be self-ventilating, at least initially, to avoid forcing the foreign body further into the bronchial tree by positive pressure ventilation.

Methods of ventilation

- Sanders jet ventilation (open tube bronchoscope).
- Self-ventilation (open tube or ventilating bronchoscope).
- Positive pressure ventilation (ventilating bronchoscope).

Monitoring

It is essential to monitor:

- the status of oxygenation via a pulse oximeter to detect the oxygen saturation.
- the rate and rhythm of the heart with an electrocardiographic monitor; bradyarrhythmias and ectopics may occur as a result of vagal stimulation or hypoxia.

Procedure

- Once the patient is anaesthetised, insert the bronchoscope into the patient's mouth and, whilst looking through it, advance the bronchoscope into the oropharynx.

- Hyperextend the neck by dropping the headrest posteriorly and advance the bronchoscope to the laryngopharynx; elevate the epiglottis and visualise the vocal cords.

- If a self-ventilating technique of anaesthesia is used, observe the movement of both vocal cords with respiration.

- Rotate the bronchoscope 90° along its axis so that its beak is aligned with the axis of the vocal cords and then pass the bronchoscope through the cords.

- Rotate the bronchoscope back to the normal position (i.e. turn the point of the beak anteriorly and view the trachea; the tracheal rings should be visible anteriorly).

- Advance the bronchoscope down the trachea until the carina is seen, taking note of any abnormalities within the lumen. The normal carina is sharp, a blunt carina is suggestive of enlarged mediastinal nodes.

- Advance the bronchoscope down the right main bronchus and identify the orifices of the lobar bronchi. It will be necessary to use the angled telescopes to visualise the upper lobe bronchi.

- If an endobronchial lesion is seen, a biopsy is taken. If a foreign body is seen, it should be removed (the details of foreign body removal are beyond the scope of this chapter).

Complications

- Hypoxia may occur if there is difficulty with intubation causing significant periods of apnoea during insertion of the bronchoscope. This can be avoided by paying particular attention to the pulse oximeter.

- Foreign bodies or secretions can obstruct the airway.

- During inspection (and ventilation) of a main bronchus, underventilation of the opposite lung may occur.

- Bleeding may result from traumatic insertion of the bronchoscope.

- Trauma to the teeth and lips from the shaft of the bronchoscope.

- Nosocomial infection – proper care and cleaning of the bronchoscope are needed to prevent transmission of micro-organisms such as the tubercle bacillus.

CVP LINE INSERTION

Indications

- Monitoring of central venous pressure.

- Short-term infusion of drugs which cannot be administered through the peripheral veins, such as dopamine or potassium chloride.

- Long-term administration of chemotherapeutic agents, parenteral nutrition, antibiotics and blood products.

Catheters

- Single-lumen tubes have a larger bore and hence can be used for rapid infusion of fluids, blood or blood products. They should not be used to infuse more than one drug at a time (e.g. an inotrope and a vasodilator), as a change in infusion rate of either drug (accidentally or deliberately) is likely to create profound confusion and possibly catastrophe.

- Triple-lumen tubes – these allow multiple functions to be performed through each of the lumens, e.g. pressure monitoring, infusion of maintenance fluids as well as infusion of drugs, particularly inotropes.

- Broviac, Hickman, Cook's catheters are inserted into a large (subclavian) vein and tunnelled and are usually indicated for long-term use.

- Long lines are designed to end in the right atrium whilst short lines are designed to end in a large vein, e.g. internal jugular.

Technique

- Basilic vein – the basilic vein is punctured in the antecubital fossa and a long line is passed into the vein, aiming to end in one of the larger veins such as the superior vena cava.

- Jugular vein – there are two approaches, the 'high' and the 'low', but they both aim to puncture the internal jugular vein prior to its junction with the subclavian.

- Subclavian vein – the subclavian vein is punctured just before it enters the thoracic inlet, the surface marking being just below the junction of the middle and medial thirds of the clavicle.

- Femoral vein – the femoral vein is punctured in the femoral triangle located just medial to the femoral pulse.

Complications

- Haemorrhage.

- Pneumothorax at the time of insertion (subclavian route).

- Malposition – long lines inserted into the basilic vein from the arm may pass into the neck rather than into the superior vena cava and down into the right atrium.

- Thrombosis – this is a problem associated with long-term central venous catheters and may cause:
  - venous access failure due to catheter-tip thrombosis
  - asymptomatic venous thrombosis
  - symptomatic thrombosis of large veins such as the axillary, subclavian and internal jugular.

- Infection catheter colonisation occurs in about 25% of ICU patients whilst the incidence of catheter-related infection is in the region of 5%. Methods of preventing catheter-related infection include:
  - tunnelling
  - polyester Dacron cuff, to create a vigorous fibrotic reaction around the catheter to prevent microorganisms from reaching it
  - regular catheter changes. It has been the practice of many ICUs to change the catheters weekly but this approach is not universally shared. How often catheters should be changed (if at all) is currently being debated. There is a morbidity (and mortality) associated with central venous catheter changes and if the infection rate in a particular ICU is low the risks of changing the catheter must be seriously weighed. There is as yet no consensus on regular catheter changes.

  Recently it has been shown that new catheters impregnated with antibiotics (minocycline and rifampicin) or antiseptic agents (chlorhexidine-silver sulphadiazine) are associated with greatly reduced rates of catheter-related infection. It is now becoming apparent that in the pathogenesis of catheter-related infections, both the intravascular and extravascular routes are important. Thus it may be important to coat both the inside and outside of the catheters with an antimicrobial agent (be it an antibiotic or an antiseptic) to reduce the infection rate.

- Arteriovenous fistulas.

OPENING AND CLOSING THE CHEST

Entry into the thoracic cavity may be achieved through a number of approaches including:

- median sternotomy
- mediastinotomy
- thoracotomy
- mini-thoracotomy
- thoracoscopy.

Thoracotomy

Indications

Operations on the lungs, pleura (and contents), chest wall, mediastinal structures, pericardium and heart.

Approaches

- Anterolateral – this is not used much nowadays but was previously used to approach the heart to perform a closed lateral valvotomy.

- Posterolateral thoracotomy.

The 3rd, 4th or 5th intercostal spaces are often used to perform closed heart operations, such as modified Blalock shunts, co-arctation of the aorta, or for operations on the lungs such as upper lobotomy.

Lower approaches such as through the 5th, 6th or 7th intercostal space may be used to perform pneumonectomy, lower lobectomy or lower oesophageal work.

Anaesthesia and positioning

Single- or double-lumen endotracheal tubes are needed for thoracotomy. A single-lumen tube is used in paediatric patients since no double-lumen tubes are available for children. It may be used in adult patients if the procedure does not involve major surgery on the lungs or occasionally if there are difficulties involved in inserting the double-lumen tube.

The patient is placed in the lateral position (check the notes and radiographs to make sure that the patient is lying with the side to be operated on uppermost, i.e. 'correct side up'). The arm is abducted and protracted forward so that the intercostal space to be approached is not covered by the scapula.

Procedure

- The incision starts just posterior to the angle of the scapula and is continued forwards along the line of the ribs to the anterior axillary/midclavicular line or further if needed.

- The latissimus dorsi and the serratus anterior muscles are divided along the line of the incision.

- The intercostal muscles are divided along the upper border of the rib, taking care to avoid puncturing the lung and pleura.

- Ventilation is withheld momentarily to allow the lung to collapse and the pleura is then incised to enter the pleural cavity.

- Insert an intercostal rib spreader (e.g. Finochetto) and gradually retract the ribs.

Closure

- Marcaine is infiltrated into the intercostal spaces to block the intercostal nerves.

- Alternatively the nerves can be blocked with an extrapleural infusion of marcaine.

- Intercostal drains are inserted.

- Pericostal sutures (3 or 4) made of absorbable material (polydioxanone or chromic catgut) are inserted and the ribs approximated. Absorbable sutures are used since they will not be long lasting and hence decrease the likelihood of intercostal neuralgia occurring from entrapment of a nerve with the suture.

- The deeper muscle/aponeurotic layer (serratus anterior) and the more superficial layer of muscle (latissimus dorsi) are closed in layers.

- Subcutaneous suture.

- Subcuticular absorbable sutures are used for the skin.

Median sternotomy

Elective

A midline skin incision is made, extending from just below the suprasternal notch to the xiphisternum. The subcutaneous tissue and periosteum are diathermied along the line of the incision. The xiphisternum is divided with a pair of heavy (Mayo) scissors.

The sternum is then divided with an oscillating saw and after application of wax to the cut sternal edges, the sternum can be retracted open with a sternal spreader.

Emergency

After open heart surgery, the sternal wound may need to be reopened:

- to relieve cardiac tamponade – cardiac tamponade causing a low cardiac output may occur if the mediastinal and pericardial drainage tubes become blocked

- to control pericardial or mediastinal bleeding – as a rough guide, in an adult, if the rate of bleeding exceeds 300 ml of blood in the first postoperative hour, 200 ml in the second and 100 ml in the third in the presence of normal coagulation, these are indications for exploration.

The decision to reopen the sternum is usually made after consultation with senior staff. It is preferable to transfer the patient back to the operating theatre for the procedure but in critical situations the patient may need to have the sternum reopened on the cardiac ICU.

Technique

Under general anaesthetic and preferably with blood and good venous access available, the technique is as follows:

- Open the skin wound and divide the presternal sutures.

- Divide the sternal wires with wire cutters; if no wire cutters are available untwist the wires and remove them with a firm tug.

- Insert a sternal retractor and evacuate blood and blood clot from the anterior mediastinum.

- If the pericardium has been closed, divide the pericardial sutures and open the pericardium.

- Scoop out any large blood clots.

- Common bleeding sites include the periosteal and pericardial edges, suture lines on heart or great vessels and ties on vein grafts which may have become loose. Pressure on the bleeding site may be performed until more senior help arrives.

- Once the problem has been controlled, flushing with saline should unblock the chest drains.

- The sternum is then closed using stainless steel wires to approximate the skin.

CHEST DRAIN INSERTION

Indications

In general chest drains are inserted to remove gas or fluid (blood, pus) or both from the chest cavity. The presence of a significant amount of gas in the chest cavity may compress the lungs and if under tension, may also cause shift of the mediastinum and compromise venous return.

- Post thoracotomy for drainage of air and blood or after any procedure within the chest such as lung resection, oesophagectomy, resection of a mediastinal mass or a closed heart procedure.

- Pneumothorax – spontaneous + tension pneumothorax, posttraumatic + tension pneumothorax.

- Haemothorax – posttraumatic.

- Malignant – may be haemorrhagic.

- Pleural effusion.

- Empyema thoracis.

Types of chest drains

Intercostal drains are usually made of plastic, e.g. clear PVC or thromboresistant silicone. There are a number of designs which usually have an open tip and side eyes, a radioopaque sentinel line with a sentinel eye and a flared or bevelled proximal end to facilitate connection to tubing connectors. They may be straight or angled and be supplied with or without a trocar.

Sizes range from 8 to 32 French. Larger tubes have a lower chance of being obstructed by blood clot although the size of the patient's intercostal space is an obvious limitation. Larger intercostal drains can be uncomfortable and the size of tube should be tailored to suit the size of the patient.

Technique for relief of pneumothorax

● Review the patient and chest radiograph.
  – How breathless is the patient and are there obvious causes for the pneumothorax?
  – Is the pneumothorax apical/loculated?
  – Is there any sign of adherence of lung to the chest wall, e.g. fibrotic areas?
  – Consider also the differential diagnosis of a large emphysematous apical bulla; this can easily mimic an apical pneumothorax on a chest radiograph.

● Plan the most appropriate site for insertion of the chest drain. The 2nd intercostal space in the mid-clavicular line or the 5th intercostal space in the mid-axillary line is commonly used.

● Explain the procedure to the patient.

● Select instruments and material and inform the nursing staff of the plan. You will need the following.
  – Local anaesthetic.
  – Needles, 20 ml syringe, three-way tap.
  – Chest drain – appropriate size, type of material.
  – Suction pump which should be capable of aspirating high volumes at relatively low pressure, e.g. Tubbs. High vacuum regulators attached to 'wall' suction, although useful, have a tendency to drift at low suction pressures of −10 to −20 cm H_2O.

● Position the patient in a semirecumbent position of about 45°.

● Infiltrate local anaesthetic and allow sufficient time for it to work.

● However, if the patient is obviously distressed, the pneumothorax will need to be relieved immediately. Under such circumstances attach the 16 or 18 G needle to the three-way tap and connect it to the 20 ml syringe. Withdraw the plunger to the 10 ml mark and insert the needle into the intercostal space and watch how the plunger moves; if it moves outwards, it suggests there is air under tension. Use the three-way tap to alternately evacuate air from the chest and empty the syringe.

● Make an incision about ½ inch long over the intercostal space and deepen the incision through the intercostal muscles (staying close to the upper border of the rib of the intercostal space).

● Insert a finger or blunt instrument such as an artery forceps into the intercostal space; remember that if the lung is adherent to the chest wall it is still at risk of being punctured, even with this technique. If the patient is being ventilated by positive pressure ventilation, aim to deflate the lung by either temporarily disconnecting the patient from the ventilator or pausing ventilation during the expiratory phase.

● Insert the intercostal drain and ensure that all side holes are within the chest.

● Secure the intercostal drain with sutures and insert an additional purse-string suture around the drain site but leave it untied; this is to be used for closure of the drain site when the drain is subsequently removed.

● Connect the drain to an underwater seal drainage system. This is usually connected to suction of between −10 and −20 cm H_2O.

For removal of fluid

Besides the chest radiograph, ultrasound may also be used to plan the siting of the chest drain, especially when the effusion is loculated. It should be noted that after a pneumonectomy, suction is not applied to the postpneumonectomy space and that the chest drains are clamped and the clamps released periodically (half hourly or hourly) to monitor blood loss.

Complications

● The lung may be punctured during chest tube insertion and this can result in a large air leak as well as considerable haemorrhage, especially when a large pulmonary vessel is punctured. It may occur because of:
  – adhesions between lung and parietal pleura
  – insertion of the intercostal drain into a bulla which has been misdiagnosed as a pneumothorax.

● Punctured abdominal viscera (liver, spleen, stomach, colon) because the drain is inadvertently inserted too low. This may occur:
  – because the depth of inspiration may be considerably limited by pain caused by trauma to the chest or abdomen so that the position of the diaphragm is much higher than usual
  – in short obese patients where the position of the diaphragm may be quite high within the chest.

HARVESTING THE LONG SAPHENOUS VEIN

Indications

● Coronary artery bypass grafting.

● Femoropopliteal bypass.

● Carotid artery surgery.

● Spiral (for SVC bypass grafting).

Technique

● A 3–4 cm long incision is made over the medial aspect of the leg just above and anterior to the medial malleolus.

- The long saphenous vein is identified and a tunnel superficial to the vein is created. The incision is then extended in the cephalic direction by cutting down onto the tunnel with either a knife or a curved Mayo scissors.

- The vein is then dissected free from the surrounding tissue. In the lower third of the leg the saphenous nerve crosses the vein to run anterior to it towards the foot. Care should be taken to avoid handling or dividing this nerve as it can result in anaesthesia over the medial malleolus.

- Great care must be taken to avoid handling and applying traction (tension) to the vein during the dissection as this results in intimal disruption. One technique to minimise handling is to pick the vein up by the adventitia with forceps. Alternatively a tape (preferably elastic) around the vein may be used to retract the vein during dissection.

- Side branches are ligated flush with the wall of the vein, taking care to avoid any narrowing of the vein.

- Once sufficient length of vein has been obtained (Figure 9.9) it is divided between artery forceps and doubly ligated.

- A Redivac drain may be inserted if the vein has been harvested to a level above the knee.

- Wound closure is undertaken with subcutaneous and subcuticular sutures.

- A compression bandage with crepe over rolled wool is applied whilst the leg is elevated.

Complications

- Mild leg oedema, particularly around the ankle, may occur in the first few months after harvesting the vein due to a degree of venous insufficiency from the removal of the long saphenous vein. This oedema subsides over the following months with the development of other venous collaterals. Elastic stockings may be useful.

- Transient or permanent hypoaesthesia near the ankle may also occur if the saphenous nerve has been damaged or divided.

FURTHER READING

1   Johnson DS, Condon VR. Foreign bodies in the paediatric patient. *Curr Prob Surg* 1998; **35**(4):279–332

2   O'Leary M, Bihari D. Central venous catheters – time for a change? *BMJ* 1998; **316**:1918–1919

3   Pescovitz MD. A history of surgical suction from Delafoy to Gomco. *Surg Gynecol Obstet* 1989; **169**:266–274

4   Veenstra DL, Saint S, Saha S, Lumley T, Sullivan SD. Efficacy of antiseptic-impregnated central venous catheters in preventing catheter-related blood stream infection. *JAMA* 1999; **281**:261–267

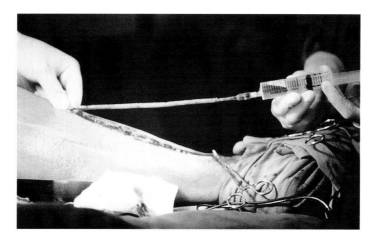

Figure 9.9   A segment of vein sufficient for a single coronary or sequential bypass graft.

10

Orthopaedic surgery

Aspiration and injection of joints
    Indications
    Patient preparation and anaesthetic
    Hazards
Application of splints and plaster casts
    Patient preparation
    Procedure
    Hazards
    Postoperative management
Colles' fracture
    Anaesthesia
    Procedure
    Hazards

Postoperative management
Ganglia
    Patient preparation
    Procedure
    Hazards
Closed reduction of an anterior dislocated shoulder
    Anaesthesia
    Procedure
    Hazards
    Postinjury management

Godfrey Charnley

ASPIRATION AND INJECTION OF JOINTS

Indications

In orthopaedic practice aspiration of joints is performed to reduce the pain associated with swelling caused by a joint effusion or a haemarthrosis. Aspiration is also useful in the diagnosis of evolving septic arthritis or inflammatory conditions including gout or pseudogout. In these cases the aspirated fluid is sent for urgent microscopy and culture and to see whether any urate or calcium pyrophosphate crystals are present.

Joint infiltration is useful to reduce pain in the early stages of degenerative or inflammatory arthritis. A combination of local anaesthetic such as bupivacaine with a corticosteroid such as hydrocortisone acetate, methylprednisolone acetate or triamcinolone hexacetonide is commonly used.

The knee, shoulder, ankle and joints of the hand may be injected or aspirated in the ambulant patient but deeper joints such as the hip require general anaesthetic rather than local anaesthetic.

Patient preparation and anaesthetic

- Strict aseptic technique must be utilised to avoid introducing an infection. The skin is therefore meticulously cleaned with chlorhexidine or iodine in a clean environment, preferably an operating theatre.

- After draping the area, a small amount (1 ml) of 0.5% plain bupivacaine may be initially infiltrated into the skin and subcutaneous tissue using a 25 gauge needle.

- Once the local anaesthetic is acting, a large 19 or 21 gauge needle attached to a syringe is inserted into the joint cavity.

- For example, the knee joint is usually approached laterally between the femur and tibia or beneath the retropatellar surface and the femoral condyles.

- If there is joint space narrowing or the patient has a large build, the use of image intensification with traction applied to

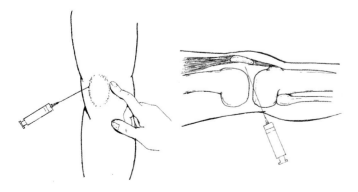

Figure 10.1 Aspiration and injection of joints.

the limb distally will increase the joint space and confirm the needle's position.

- Depending on the size of the effusion or haemarthrosis, a 10, 20 or 50 ml syringe is attached to the needle and the joint aspirated. The presence of fat in the blood of a haemarthrosis raises the possibility of an intra-articular fracture. Similarly, an effusion that is turbid or cloudy might alert the surgeon to the possibility of a joint infection.

- For joint infiltration the procedure is identical except that a combination of anaesthetic and steroid is inserted into the affected joint.

Hazards

If in the near future the patient is likely to require a joint replacement then infiltration of the joint with local anaesthetic alone is recommended rather than corticosteroids because of the risk of introducing infection.

APPLICATION OF SPLINTS AND PLASTER CASTS

Despite advances in orthopaedic technology and implants to treat fractures, plaster casts and splints are still the most common mode of treatment for fractures of the upper and lower limbs. Immobilisation of an injured limb provides pain relief and, if carefully applied, can hold the reduced fracture over several weeks until bony union.

Plaster of Paris is widely used for acute injuries but other materials, including synthetic casting materials and thermoplastics, may be used subsequently. The former has the benefit that it is cheap and easy to mould whilst the others tend to be lighter in weight, stronger and more water resistant.

Patient preparation

- The key to successful cast and splint application is to have a comfortably positioned patient and assistance from colleagues to hold the injured limb whilst the surgeon applies and moulds the cast to immobilise the fracture. Adequate analgesia is necessary prior to and during the manipulation of the displaced fracture and application of the splint.

- To save time and minimise discomfort, the plaster bandages and dressings should be prepared in advance. The size and number of plaster bandages necessary will depend on the age of the patient and size of the limb and whether an above-knee or elbow plaster is required. As a general guide, for the upper limb three to four bandages of 5–7.5 cm width are necessary whilst for the lower limb the same number of 15–20 cm bandages are required.

- If the injured limb is very swollen then back slabs or three-quarter slabs are utilised. These are made from several layers of

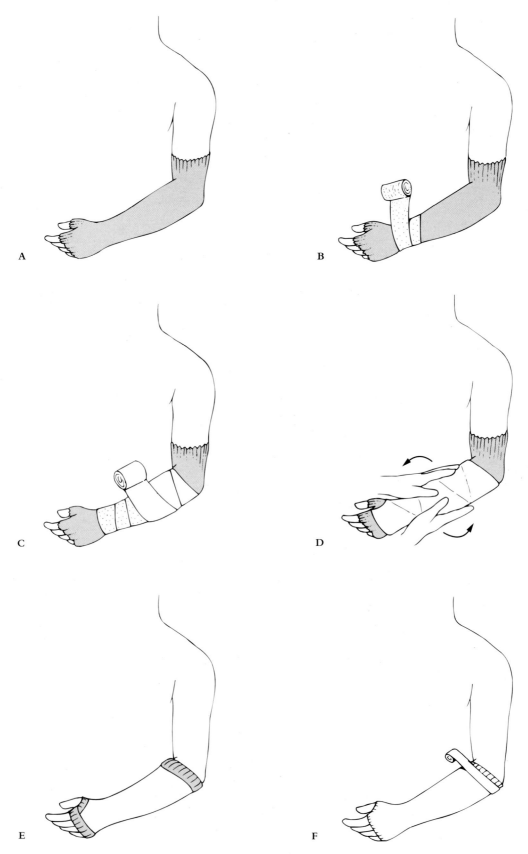

Figure 10.2 Application of splints and plastic casts. **A.** Layer of stockingette. **B.** Layer of orthopaedic wool e.g. Softban is then applied with extra padding over bony prominences. **C.** Apply plaster of Paris half overlapping the previous layer with half of the roll. **D.** Mould the plaster to hold the fracture position. **E.** Fold back the stockingette. **F.** Complete the cast.

plaster bandage cut and shaped to give support whilst at the same time allowing any swelling to escape. Usually 10 layers of plaster are necessary.

- The back slabs can be 'templated' and measured against the uninjured limb.

Procedure

- To protect the skin a non-elasticated bandage is applied such as stockinette.

- Over this and without excessive tension, synthetic wool is rolled with each layer covering 50% of the previous layer. Slightly more wool may be required over bony prominences.

- A plaster of an appropriate width is then applied over the fracture. The author's preference is that the plaster is thoroughly soaked in cold water as this will allow more time to mould and contour the plaster.

- The plaster is continued to just short of the ends of the stockinette bandage which is then turned back to avoid rough plaster edges causing skin abrasion. These overturned edges can then be secured with one or two final turns of the plaster.

- As the plaster dries, it can be 'worked' to strengthen it, whilst at the same time moulding the cast over the fracture to prevent subsequent displacement of the reduced bony fragments.

- If back slabs are used they can be held in position by a thin crepe bandage secured with a thin strip of plaster.

Hazards

- If the limb is swollen and a complete cast applied, particularly if it is synthetic, pressure damage may occur to the underlying neurovascular structures.

- Too much wool will prevent adequate moulding. Conversely, too little padding may cause pressure sores under the plaster.

- Avoid overlong plasters which may impede the function of the elbow or knee or small joints of the hand and foot.

- Hot water or too little water will result in a poor bandage that can delaminate and cannot be moulded.

- Excessive moulding pressure with the fingers or thumbs rather than the palms of the hand can cause ridges which may create a potential for pressure sores.

- If synthetic materials are used they need to be applied with gloves to avoid abrasion of the surgeon's hands.

Postoperative management

- All patients should be checked before discharge to ensure that their cast is comfortable and that they can use those joints that do not need to be immobilised.

- Patients should be discharged with adequate analgesia and usually a sling in the case of upper limb fractures.

- Elevation of the injured limb for 1–2 days is advisable to reduce postfracture swelling.

- Each and every patient should be given a list of instructions on how to care for their cast and contact telephone numbers in case they develop problems with their splint.

- If a back slab or three-quarter slab has been applied, this can be completed by simply wrapping further rolls of plaster over the slab once the swelling has reduced.

- At the first fracture clinic review, radiographs are normally taken to confirm that the reduced fracture position has been maintained.

COLLES' FRACTURE

First described by Abraham Colles in 1814, this distal radial fracture remains the most common upper limb fracture seen in orthopaedic practice today. Although many distal radial fractures are called Colles' fractures, the original injury described is an extraarticular fracture with dorsal angulation of the distal radius, creating a 'dinner fork' deformity following a fall on the outstretched hand. It is particularly common amongst elderly patients with osteoporotic bone.

As for any fracture, the key steps are: reducing the deformity, holding the reduced fracture in a satisfactory position to allow bone healing and, in due course, rehabilitation of the local soft tissues.

Anaesthesia

Haematoma infiltration, regional anaesthetic or general anaesthetic can all be used to facilitate reduction of the displaced fracture and to allow for a satisfactory immobilisation in a plaster cast. The most important factor is that the patient is comfortable and relaxed during the manipulation and that there is adequate time for the application of a moulded plaster splint and imaging of the reduced fracture position. The choice of anaesthesia depends on the anaesthetic facilities available, the experience of the surgeon and the patient's general medical history and health.

Procedure

- Preparation (in advance) of the plaster, wool and bandages or back slab required saves time.

- The classic deformity comprises shortening with dorsal angulation and radial deviation of the distal radial fragment. This is corrected by applying traction in the opposite palmar and ulnar directions. If the fracture ends are impacted, increasing dorsal angulation, initial disimpaction will aid the subsequent manipulation of the fracture fragments.

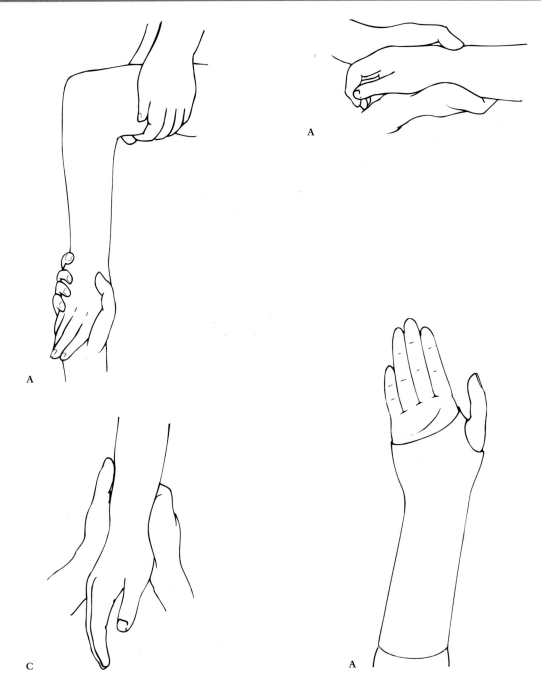

Figure 10.3 Colles' fracture. **A.** Apply traction. **B.** Palpage the distal radius and apply volar pressure. **C.** Add additional ulna deviation. **D.** Hold the reduction in a moulded plaster allowing finger and thumb movements.

- To achieve the reduction, countertraction at the elbow applied by a colleague is necessary.

- The fracture is reduced by the 'operating' surgeon with the use of the thumbs to restore the alignment of the distal radius by local pressure on the distal radial fragment. A non-elasticised stockinette bandage can then be applied gently over the wrist and forearm with subsequent application of plaster wool. Particular attention should be paid to protecting bony promi-

nences including the ulnar and radial styloid processes (see Application of plasters).

- As the injury may be complicated by further swelling, an incomplete plaster is applied, preferably a three-quarter back slab.

- Whilst the plaster splint dries it should be moulded to maintain the position of the reduced fracture with pressure around

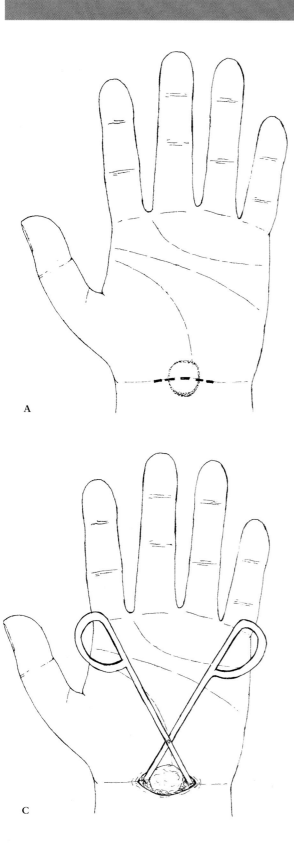

A

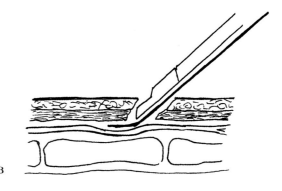

B

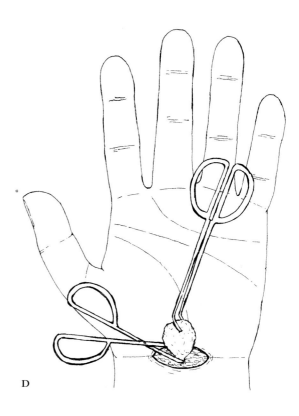

D

C

Figure 10.4 Ganglion incision. **A.** Skin crease incision. **B.** Splitting the retinaculum. **C.** Use blunt dissection to define the boundary of the ganglion. **D.** Excise at the base.

the fracture site being applied by the thumbs or palm of the hand. The splint must permit flexion of the fingers at the metatarsophalangeal joint level and should not prevent full flexion or extension of the elbow nor limit movements of the thumb.

- At the end of the manipulation and once the plaster has dried, post-reduction radiographs in AP and lateral projections should be obtained.

Hazards

- Acute swelling may be contained in a full plaster, leading to pressure on the median nerve and radial artery.

- Avoid excessive flexion of the wrist as this may also cause abnormal pressure over the median nerve.

- The most important deformity to be corrected is radial shortening with an abnormal relationship between the radial and ulnar articular surfaces and the carpus. Persistent radial shortening or incongruity of the radial articular surface will lead to permanent pain and disability.

- Inadequate trimming of the plaster or poor padding can cause complications, including pressure sores or restricted movements of the fingers and elbow during immobilisation.

Postoperative management

Most patients, especially those with unstable fractures, must be reviewed with new radiographs one week later. If these later radiographs confirm that the reduced fracture position has been maintained then application of further plaster over the back slab can be undertaken to reinforce and complete the plaster, providing there is no persistent swelling. Most patients require 5–6 weeks of plaster immobilisation with review and further radiographs at the end of this period.

On further review at five or six weeks postinjury, if there is adequate new bone on the follow-up radiographs then the plaster can be removed and gentle supervised movement of the wrist and physiotherapy management will restore function of the wrist joint.

GANGLIA

Ganglia are commonly found around the wrist and ankle joints and are caused by mucoid degeneration. They have a fibrous 'capsular' wall and contain clear gelatinous material. Occasionally they can be dispersed by multiple puncture with a large-bore needle under local anaesthetic. However, they are often multilobulated with extensions reaching into the joints and will thus recur. They also sometimes overlie bony prominences and a radiograph is useful in excluding any abnormal bony pathology prior to definitive surgical excision.

Patient preparation

- Because wrist ganglia can overlie important structures, general or regional anaesthetic with exsanguination and tourniquet control is recommended (refer to Chapter 1 for method of Bier's block).
- For ganglia around the wrist joint, the upper limb can be placed on a separate arm table.

Procedure

- A transverse, skin crease incision over the apex of the lesion usually provides adequate access.

- After the incision, it may be necessary to divide the extensor retinaculum if the ganglion is on the dorsal surface of the wrist. Gentle soft tissue dissection of the ganglion away from local tendons can be performed by blunt dissection using either McIndoe's scissors or a small curved haemostat.

- It is helpful to use small Langenbeck type retractors to identify one side of the ganglion initially and work around the ganglion until its 'neck' is defined.

- Once the capsular sac has been exposed a small self-retaining retractor can be positioned to fully expose the sac, its neck, its base and the surrounding tissues. It may then be excised at the neck with a scalpel or sharp scissors.

- Sometimes ganglia will burst but by placing a haemostat on the 'deflated capsule', traction can be applied to allow the dissection and excision to be completed.

- The ganglion should be sent for histology.

- After the ganglion has been excised the tourniquet can be released and with bipolar or coagulative diathermy, haemostasis is achieved.

- Deep structures may be approximated using 3/0 polyglactin and the skin closed either with subcuticular untied sutures of a similar material or using 3/0 nylon interrupted sutures.

- For postoperative pain relief it is worth infiltrating 5–10 ml of 0.5% plain bupivacaine. A wool and crepe bandage also helps to reduce the postoperative swelling.

Hazards

Dorsal wrist ganglia may be located around branches of the superficial radial nerve. Volar wrist ganglia may be located close to the median nerve or its terminal branches or radial artery. In this situation it is essential to define the boundaries of the ganglion and protect these important neurovascular structures prior to its excision.

CLOSED REDUCTION OF AN ANTERIOR DISLOCATED SHOULDER

The shallow glenoid cavity does not easily contain the humeral head. Because of this and despite the rotator cuff musculature, anterior dislocation and, much less frequently, posterior disloca-

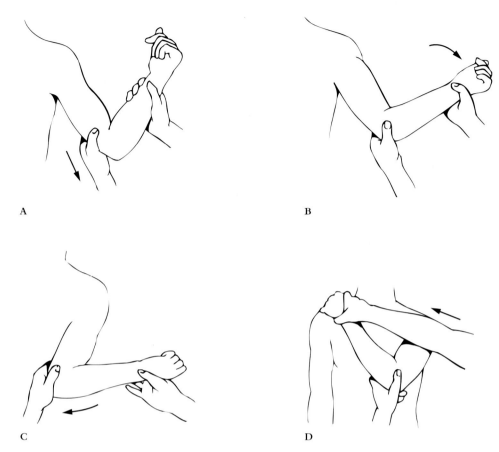

Figure 10.5 Shoulder reduction. **A.** Apply traction. **B.** Add additional upper arm external rotation. **C.** Continue with some abduction.. **D.** Once the shoulder reduces adduct and internally rotate the arm.

tion of the glenohumoral joint can occur. This injury was described as far back as 3000 BC!

The most common (over 90%) dislocations are anterior following trauma or sporting activities such as skiing and rugby. The clinical presentation is of loss of function of the injured arm with pain. The rounded deltoid contour is lost and the shoulder appears 'squared off'.

The injury requires traction and manipulation to restore the relationship between the articular surface of the humerus and the glenoid surface of the scapula.

Before any attempts at reduction, it is essential to obtain adequate X-rays and perform a neurovascular examination of the shoulder and affected upper limb (see Hazards below).

Anaesthesia

General anaesthesia or sedation can be used. With the latter, a variety of agents including valium and midazolam can be used but if the patient feels *any* pain this will provoke spasm and prevent a successful reduction.

Procedure

- Ideally the 'operating' surgeon should have an assistant to help in the reduction. However, it can be achieved single-handedly providing the patient is fully relaxed and without pain.

- For the common anterior dislocation gentle traction is applied with one hand whilst the other hand feels the displaced humeral head in the pectoral region or the axilla.

- Increasing the traction is then followed by abduction and external rotation of the humerus with the fingers in the axilla gently helping to push the displaced head back into the glenoid.

- Once a click or clunk is palpated or heard (as the humeral head reduces), the arm is adducted across the shoulder and the arm internally rotated with the elbow flexed.

- The arm is then held in this position in some form of sling or support whilst X-rays of the shoulder are obtained.

143

Hazards

- Before any attempt at reduction it is essential that the local neurological supply is examined. The brachial plexus, axillary and musculocutaneous nerves may all be damaged in fractures and dislocations around the shoulder girdle. If such injuries are documented initially then you cannot be blamed for creating them during the reduction! Less commonly, damage to the axillary artery and vein can be caused by dislocations and fractures of the shoulder and once again, early recognition is required.

- Dislocations of the shoulder can occur with fractures of the great tuberosity and the humeral neck. Whilst a great tuberosity fracture may reduce as the dislocation itself is reduced, beware more distal fractures which may require internal fixation.

- It is imperative to obtain X-rays in two planes. The anterior view of the shoulder is necessary plus a lateral scapula view to confirm that the humeral head has displaced in an anterior direction to the glenoid. Rarely, posterior dislocations occur, particularly in epileptic patients or following electrocution.

- After the reduction it is mandatory to obtain repeat antero-posterior and lateral scapula X-rays to confirm the reduction.

Postinjury management

The patient should rest the shoulder for 2–4 weeks in a double-loop collar and cuff as this provides more comfort than a simple sling.

Supervised outpatient physiotherapy will minimise a potential risk of recurrent anterior dislocation approaching 50%.

FURTHER READING

1   Surgery Apley's system of orthopaedics and fractures.

11

Head injury and the surgeon

Coma
Raised intracranial pressure
Intracranial clots
  Extradural haematoma
  Acute subdural haematoma
  Chronic subdural haematoma

Acute intracerebral haematoma
Open (compound) depressed skull fracture
  Surgery for open depressed skull fractures
Spinal fracture complicating head injury

Terry Hope

Each year thousands of patients are seen in the accident and emergency departments of Britain. A large number are capable of being discharged after examination, according to head injury guidelines (see *Fundamentals of Surgical Practice*, Chapter 19, pages 464–468). Only a small percentage of those admitted for observation will require surgical intervention, usually but not always in the neurosurgical unit. The purpose of this chapter is to give the general surgeon in training a basic knowledge of emergency head injury in neurosurgery.

COMA

The unconscious head-injured patient is managed according to ATLS guidelines. It is important to realise that prompt resuscitation is essential in preventing so-called secondary insults. These secondary insults are essentially abnormal physiological variables, which lead to increased brain damage following the initial insult. An impaired airway leads to hypercarbia and hypoxia, both of which can cause increased intracranial pressure from cerebral vasodilatation. A set of blood gases is essential in managing the comatose patient.

Head injuries are often complicated by other injuries and hypotension is a potent factor in secondary insult. All patients who are hypotensive must be energetically resuscitated before transfer to the neurosurgical unit. There is a good ground rule: hypotension is not usually due to head injury alone; there is either an obvious or occult source of bleeding present.

RAISED INTRACRANIAL PRESSURE

In a simplistic sense, comatose patients can be divided into those with rapidly evolving cerebral oedema caused by an acceleration-deceleration shearing injury to the brain and those who harbour an increasing space-occupying blood clot. In the latter group there are usually signs of rapidly rising intracranial pressure. This results in:

- deterioration in the level of consciousness as seen on the Glasgow Coma Chart (Figure 11.1)

- a dilated pupil with a sluggish reaction to light on the side of the expanding clot

- possibly an increasing blood pressure with bradycardia (the Cushing reflex caused by progressive compression of the medulla)

- an increasing, contralateral hemiparesis.

A patient showing rapidly rising intracranial pressure needs urgent treatment, probably with intubation (to lower the PCO_2), possibly mannitol, a group and crossmatch of blood and an urgent CT.

INTRACRANIAL CLOTS

It is important to realise that patients may have severe brain injury and die without marked changes on the CT. Most will show cerebral oedema with slit-like ventricles and subtle signs of brain coning which are difficult to see on CT.

Intracranial clots may be extradural, subdural or within the parenchyma of the brain itself (intracerebral haematomas). These space-occupying clots are acute lesions, which develop within minutes or hours after impact. A combination of these may occur.

Extradural haematoma

This is not the most common sequel from head injury but an extradural haemorrhage, if recognised early, has a good prognosis after surgical evacuation. The kinetic injury from the impact is enough to cause skull fracture, yet there may not be more than a brief period of loss of consciousness and then recovery to be followed by deterioration (lucid interval). In the history of the accident, sporting injuries to the side of the head and assaults are more common than road traffic accidents. Often the fracture is

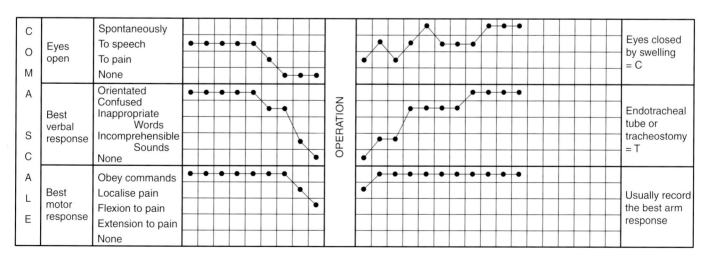

Figure 11.1 The Glasgow Coma Scale.

along the line of the middle meningeal artery or its branches (Figures 11.2 and 11.3). Sometimes it is the accompanying vein that bleeds, which may result in a slower accumulation of clot.

In extradural haematoma the volume of the clot is small (Figure 11.4) but there is not room for expansion within the intracranial space. As a consequence there is rapid neurological deterioration with a dilating pupil being the rule. This is from compression of the ocular motor or third cranial nerve on the side of the lesion. Initially, the pupil becomes sluggish in its response to light and then fixed and dilated.

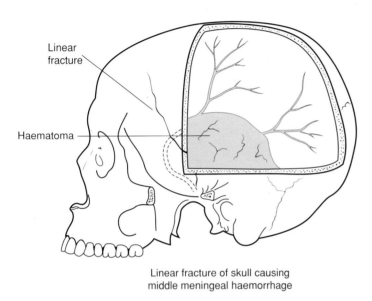

Linear fracture of skull causing
middle meningeal haemorrhage

Figure 11.2 Linear fracture of skull causing middle meningeal bleeding.

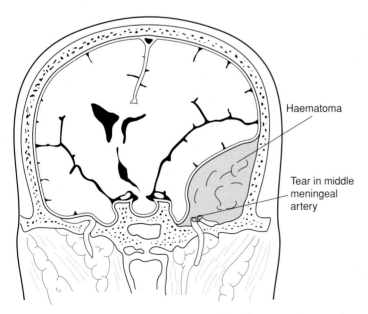

Figure 11.3 Extradural haematoma due to tear of middle meningeal artery at the foramen spinosum by fracture of the base of the skull.

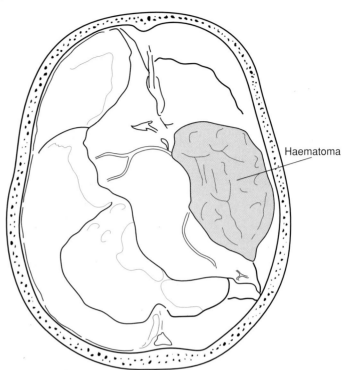

Figure 11.4 Clot exposed on skull base by reflection of dura.

CT diagnosis

It is important to consider whether the airway needs protection prior to CT scanning (intubation). The benefit of hyperventilation is not only protection of the airway but also induced hypocapnia, which temporarily lowers intracranial pressure (Figure 11.5). Intravenous mannitol acts as an osmotic diuretic, crossing the blood–brain barrier but promoting a rapid diuresis.

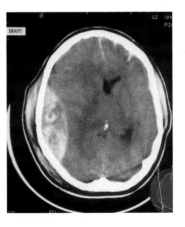

Figure 11.5 Acute extradural haematoma. Note extracranial subgaleal blood.

Surgery for extradural haemorrhage

- Urgent crossmatch of blood necessary.

- In infants it may be important to transfuse prior to surgery itself.

- Speed is life saving.

- Morbidity and mortality result from delay and those who talk after head injury should not die. Burr hole for diagnosis and evacuation of extradural haematomas has become outmoded in the CT age.

- CT scanning allows the placement of a suitable (often temporal) craniotomy. A craniotomy is a series of burr holes connected by a saw cut. The craniotomy bone flap hinges on the temporalis muscle (osteoplastic flap) or may be free (Figures 11.6–11.8).

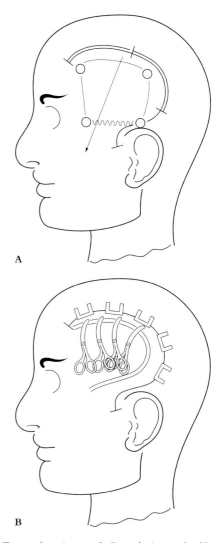

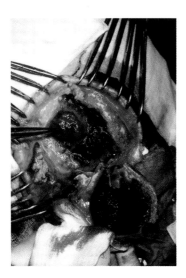

Figure 11.6 Craniotomy. Bone flap turned and acute extradural haematoma.

Figure 11.8 Temporal craniotomy. **A**. For a classic extradural haematoma. Scalp incision pulled down in direction of arrow, burr holes as shown joined by Gigli saw or cutting powered craniotome. **B**. Note technique to ensure scalp homeostasis. Raney spring clips to outer edge of incision. Curved haemostatic forceps to inner edge. 20 ml of 1% lignocaine with 1:200 000 adrenaline is injected subcutaneously prior to incision.

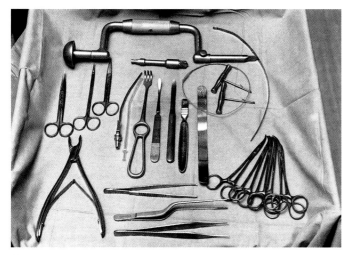

Figure 11.7 Basic craniotomy set of instruments. Note that the instruments are simple.

Acute subdural haematoma

This neurosurgical complication, in contrast to an extradural haemorrhage, results from high-speed kinetic energy in part to the brain (Figure 11.9). There is often clearing of the brain parenchyma and a tear in the cortical vessels and therefore the outcome, even with prompt evacuation of the clot, is variable. Here the patient is unconscious from the moment of impact. The haematoma beneath the dura, is from a torn cerebral artery or vein. Frequently brain contusions occur. As the patient arrives in the casualty department the pupil is already enlarged from the side clot and the coma score is progressively deteriorating.

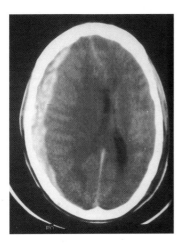

Figure 11.9 CT scan of acute subdural haematoma. Note shift of brain and concave lens appearance of the clot.

Surgery for acute subdural haematoma

As with an extradural haematoma, the best operation is a suitably placed craniotomy guided by the CT scan. On turning the bone flap the dura will be found to be tense and blue. The dura is then opened widely and the clot is sucked away from the cortical surface (Figure 11.10) and the bleeding point on the cortex may be found and coagulated by bipolar diathermy. There is then a tendency in some cases for a rapid and devastating swelling of the brain requiring hyperventilation, intravenous mannitol and removal of the bone flap.

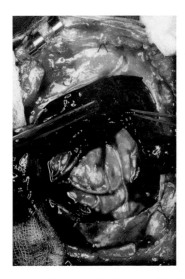

Figure 11.10 Craniotomy. Dura turned and acute subdural haematoma being sucked off.

Postoperative management

Following craniotomy for acute subdural haematoma, most patients are transferred to the intensive care unit where intracranial pressure monitoring is recorded. There is a tendency for further cerebral oedema, even with the best medical management, which may include several days of sedation, moderate hypothermia and maintenance of good cerebral perfusion pressure. The mortality and morbidity is high similarly.

Chronic subdural haematoma

With an ageing population this is becoming an increasingly common neurosurgical event. With ageing of the brain, cortical atrophy occurs. With cortical atrophy there is a 'bow string' effect on the parasagittal veins. The head injury is often mild and might have occurred weeks ago and thus been forgotten. Anticoagulants (warfarin), alcohol abuse and non-accidental injury in paediatric practice are well-known factors.

History

The clinical picture is not acute. There is a slow deterioration in neurological function over days or weeks; confusion, headache and mild motor weakness are typical features in an elderly person who might mistakenly be diagnosed as having had a stroke.

In paediatric practice the infant fails to thrive, vomits feeds and is lethargic with tense fontanelle when at rest. These children are usually victims of non-accidental injury. Here a cranial ultrasound is often diagnostic.

Surgery for subdural haematoma

Burr-hole drainage is appropriate (Figures 11.11A and B). Often both frontal and parietal burr holes are necessary. The dura is coagulated and divided with a cruciate incision, allowing the release of the subdural collection (often under pressure). Local anaesthesia may be quite appropriate for what is a simple and quick procedure. The prognosis here is often good. Continuing drainage of the subdural space with a catheter into a collection bag is useful.

Acute intracerebral haematoma

Within the confines of the skull the brain is supported by its dural attachments, with cerebrospinal fluid acting as a buffer. These, however, afford modest protection during cranial impact. A contracoup injury occurs when a force is applied to one side of the skull, leading to the brain striking the opposite bony inner table. These contusions commonly occur in the frontal, temporal and occipital poles of the brain, where the convexities strike against the cranial fossa. Contracoup contusions can increase with

The most important question, that can only be answered by surgical exploration of the wound, is 'Has the dura been breached? CT scanning with so-called bone window settings (Figure 11.12) enables the extent of the compression to be gauged and whether intracranial air (torn dura) is present.

Many depressed skull fractures gives rise to localised inflammation of the skull where kinetic energy is absorbed and therefore serious neurological deterioration may not result.

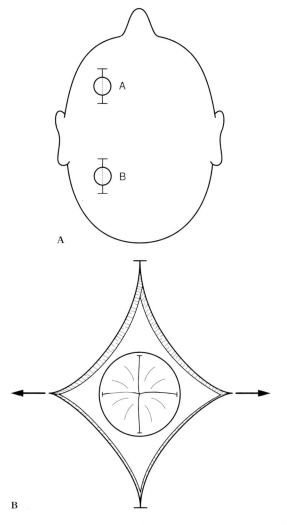

A

B

Figure 11.11 A. Burr-hole positions for chronic subdural haematoma (often under local anaesthesia). Burr hole A approximately 2 inches from midline at coronal suture. Burr hole B at or near parietal eminence. **B**. Burr-hole technique for chronic subdural haematoma. (i) 1.5 inch scalp incision (infiltrate with lignocaine adrenaline). (ii) Retraction in line of arrows with self-retraining retractor. (iii) A Hudson drill with perforator and then a burr is used. (iv) Dura is coagulated in the line of the cruciform fossa. (v) Dura incised with pointed scalpel and subdura released then washed out and drained.

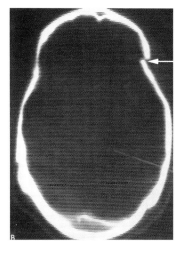

Figure 11.12 CT scan. 'Bone-window' setting showing depressed skull fracture (arrow).

size in time (within the first 24–48 hours), leading to delayed neurological deterioration from rising intracranial pressure. In the case of non-dominant intracerebral haematoma in the temporal lobe, lobectomy may be helpful in controlling intracranial pressure.

OPEN (COMPOUND) DEPRESSED SKULL FRACTURE

Historically these lesions have always been taken seriously because of the potential for intracranial invasion of bacteria leading to meningitis, cerebral abscess and ventriculitis.

Surgery for open depressed skull fractures

- Debridement (contused devitalised skin breeds bacteria).

- The incision is extended in an appropriate direction.

- A burr hole is made on the intact bone at the fracture edge so as not to angle bone inwards.

- A small craniectomy is made around the depression.

- The bone fragments are removed by sliding them outwards.

- A dural inspection and repair may be necessary.

- Antibiotics and anticonvulsants are used when the dura is torn and with cortical injury present.

SPINAL FRACTURE COMPLICATING HEAD INJURY

Cervical spine fractures, in particular, are common in head-injured patients (Figures 11.13 and 11.14). A useful aphorism is: if

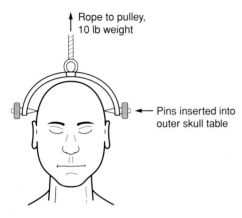

Rope to pulley,
10 lb weight

Pins inserted into
outer skull table

Figure 11.13 Skeletal (skull tongs) traction in cervical spine fracture, Scoville pattern.

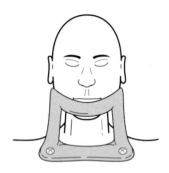

Figure 11.14 Cervical spine immobilisation. 'Bivalved' rigid brace – applied from scene of accident in suspected neck fracture (all unconscious head injuries).

a force is imparted to the skull sufficient to render the patient unconscious it is sufficient to cause a spinal fracture.

- All unconscious patients should be managed with log rolling and spinal fixation from the scene of the accident to the casualty department and thereafter.

- A full series of cervical spine X-rays are necessary including, if possible, an open mouth odontoid view.

- CT scanning of the whole of the body spine is often necessary to exclude an occult fracture.

12

Plastic surgery

Methods of wound closure
    Basic principles
    Direct closure
    Serial excision
    Tissue expansion
    Skin grafts
Skin flaps
Abnormal scars (hypertrophic and keloid)
    Clinical features
    Aetiology

Treatment
Breast reconstruction
    Introduction
    Techniques
    Contraindications
    Subcutaneous mastectomy
    Nipple-areola reconstruction
    Partial mastectomy defects
    The silicone controversy
    Soya bean oil implants

Loshan Kangesu

Plastic and reconstructive surgery aims for the restoration of appearance and function. Although initial emphasis was on skin, most surgery involves manipulation of underlying tissue, fascia, muscles, tendons and bone, thereby involving all layers of the integument. Thus plastic surgery remains very broad, often involving combined procedures with other surgical disciplines. The main subcategories within plastic surgery are: treatment of congenital malformations (cleft lip and palate, craniofacial, hand, hypospadias), reconstruction following tumour ablation (breast, head and neck), hand surgery, burn injuries, care of soft tissue trauma and cosmetic surgery. This chapter will attempt to convey some of the main principles and offer a flavour of the speciality.

METHODS OF WOUND CLOSURE

Basic principles

The surgeon has a choice of methods of wound cover but a successful outcome in terms of subsequent scarring and cosmetic result is dependent on adherence to basic plastic surgical principles. These involve correct planning, accurate approximation of skin edges, measures to minimise wound haematoma, minimal handling of the skin edges, avoidance of excess tension on the skin edge and prevention of unnecessary wound contamination. Factors beyond the surgeon's control that may cause a poor scar are the age of the patient, the site and also direction of the wound. In general, apart from scars in infants (1–3 months), which often heal as fine lines, children's scars remain erythematous and harder for a longer duration than in adults and in addition, children are more prone to developing hypertrophic and even keloid scars (see below).

The physical properties of skin depend mainly on the patterns of the fibrous weave of the dermis. These properties can be divided into four groups:

1. skin tension, which if excessive in sutured wounds leads to hypertrophic or stretched scars

2. skin extensibility, that allows for movement across joints and closure of simple skin defects and is maximal in infancy but with age gives way to skin laxity

3. directional variations, that give rise to Langer's lines

4. viscoelastic properties which are creep and stress relaxation.

Creep occurs in the first few minutes when a constant force is applied to skin, causing it to stretch. It is clinically important in that it is utilised to close defects that appear initially just too large for primary closure. Skin can be load cycled; that is, repeated attempts at stretching will increase the stretch. The phenomenon is thought to be due to the realignment of dermal fibres and displacement of tissue fluid and ground substance from the dermis. Stress relaxation is the corollary of creep and is the measured force when skin is stretched a constant distance. Within a few minutes, the measured stress declines as the skin stretches.

Stress relaxation explains why a flap that appears too tight immediately after the operation may look satisfactory later on.

The size of the anticipated skin defect influences the surgeon's choice of wound cover. Obviously, small wounds are closed directly. Larger defects, on the other hand, will require skin flaps and skin grafts. Where it is possible to delay the excision of a lesion, techniques such as serial excision and tissue expansion may be employed.

Direct closure

The vast majority of skin lesions are suitable for excision and direct closure. In general, lesions are excised as an ellipse. When planning elliptical incisions, one is generally taught that the length of the ellipse will be equal to three times the diameter of the lesion and this is a useful guide when explaining to patients (Figure 12.1). However, in reality one can make the limbs of the ellipse shorter, thus decreasing the length of the final scar. The longitudinal axis of the ellipse should be designed to lie along or parallel to a line of skin tension to make it less conspicuous and this becomes particularly noticeable on the face.

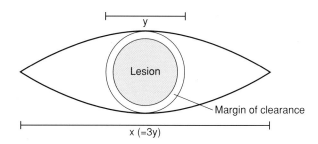

Figure 12.1 If a lesion with an appropriate margin is excised as an ellipse, the length of the final scar is about three times the size of the defect. One tries to shorten the scar by shortening the ellipse, but there may be more bunching ('dog ears') to the skin.

The existence of lines of tension in the skin was first noted by Dupuytren in 1832 and subsequently investigated by Karl Langer, Professor of Anatomy at Joseph's Academy in Vienna. Although some of Langer's lines run across natural creases, they form the basis of our understanding of lines of skin tension. In the face these lines correspond to wrinkle lines in the elderly where they are also known as lines of facial expression (Figure 12.2). In the neck these lines correspond with the lines of dependency where the effects of gravity produce horizontal creases. Lines of skin tension also lie horizontally in flexion creases and in the limbs where it is difficult to choose the correct line it is preferable to follow the line that falls when the limb is in the relaxed position. In a child's face where skin lines are absent, the excision should be planned so that the scar will eventually lie in a line of facial expression.

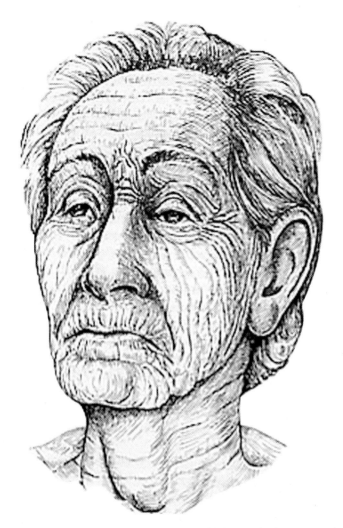

Figure 12.2 The lines of facial expression or wrinkle lines on the face correspond with Langer's lines. Scars are less noticeable if they are along these lines rather than across them.

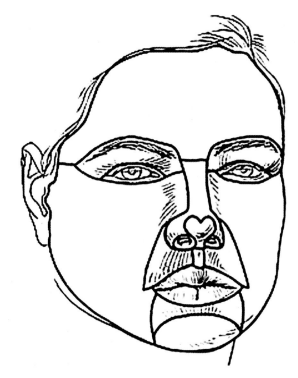

Figure 12.3 The topography of the face can be divided into cosmetic units. Scars are less noticeable if they are at the junction of these units rather than across them.

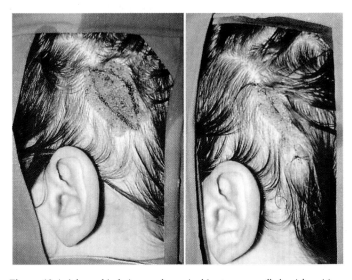

Figure 12.4 A large skin lesion can be excised in stages, so-called serial excision, thereby avoiding grafts or flaps.

When the correct line of excision is in doubt, the lesion itself should be excised and the ellipse planned as the next step depending on how the wound edges lie. Another principle in planning surgical wounds on the face is the appreciation of cosmetic units and the placement of scars at the junction of these units (Figure 12.3). Furthermore, if possible, scars can be hidden in the hair-bearing skin of the scalp or eyebrow. In this instance the skin should not be cut perpendicular to the surface as is the normal teaching, but parallel to the direction of the hair follicles to prevent their disruption and subsequent local balding.

Serial excision

When a large benign lesion has to be removed, it may be possible to excise it in two or more stages (Figure 12.4). This technique utilises the ability of the surrounding skin to 'expand' over time. In each stage of the serial excision the maximum amount of the lesion is excised that will allow the wound to be closed comfort-ably without undue tension. If a wound is closed with excessive tension the scar will stretch, sometimes to a width resembling the size of the original lesion. These staged excisions are planned so that the vertical length of the scar barely exceeds the longest diameter of the lesion. In all but the final stage the excisions are intralesional, as are the suture holes. Although there are variations between patients, often one can plan subsequent stages of excision after a minimum of three months.

Tissue expansion

Skin expansion is seen physiologically in the gravid abdominal skin and has been used for reasons of beauty or tradition by various races, such as the Hottentots who stretch their labia and the women of Chad who stretch their lips.

Tissue expansion as currently practised was first described by Radovan in 1976 and involved the subcutaneous insertion of a silicon bag which was inflated with saline over a period of weeks, thus causing stretching of the overlying skin. The expanded skin can then be used as an advancement or transposition flap to cover any adjacent skin defect.

Experimental data, largely from animal studies, have shown that the thickness of the epidermis remains unchanged by tissue expansion, although there is increased mitotic activity during expansion. Electron micrograph studies have shown that the undulations of the dermal and epidermal junction are unfolded during expansion and there is a reduction in intercellular distance in the epidermis. The skin appendages are compressed during expansion but do not degenerate. There is some evidence of increased melanocytic activity and this has been used to explain the hyperpigmentation of the expanded area that sometimes occurs and which reverses at the end of expansion. The dermis is affected quite significantly and thins during expansion and a fibrous capsule forms around the prosthesis. There is also atrophy of fat. Nerves are largely unaffected and seem to stretch although at certain sites, such as the forehead, distortion can cause considerable pain. Interestingly, there is increased angiogenesis in the expanded skin, much akin to processes occurring in vascular surgical delay, thus allowing long transposition flaps of expanded skin to be designed. When muscle either overlying or beneath the prosthesis is examined, there are features of atrophy but muscle function remains unchanged.

Tissue expansion has been used most successfully in the scalp and for breast reconstruction. Complications are higher when used in limbs but even here, when patient selection is appropriate, the risks are acceptable. Careful planning is required for a successful outcome. As a rule, expanders are placed via radial or V-shaped incisions beneath the galea in the scalp, beneath muscle in breast reconstruction and beneath the skin, but not in a subfascial plane, in the limbs. The selection of implant requires some experience but a useful guide was provided by Joss et al, who explained that the length of the expander should correspond to the length of the defect but the width should be twice the width of the defect (Figure 12.5).

Complications from the use of the expanders include infection, extrusion and failure to cover the required defect which is most often due to poor planning.

Skin grafts

A graft is a piece of tissue that, once transplanted on to a distant site, is dependent on neovascularisation from the host wound bed

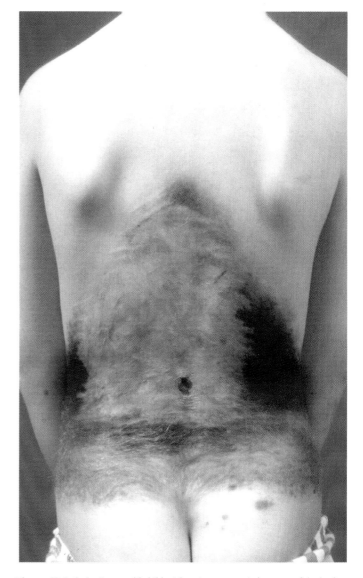

Figure 12.5 A An 8-year-old child with a giant congenital naevus of the back.

for its survival. Skin, bone, muscle and nerve tissue are often transplanted as grafts. Skin grafts offer the simplest method of covering defects that are too large for direct closure.

Skin grafts contain epidermis and variable amounts of dermis. If the entire thickness of dermis is included, they are described as full-thickness grafts, whereas if there is a variable amount of dermis, they are called split-thickness grafts (Figure 12.6). The history of skin grafting dates back to pre-Christian times in India but the skill became lost until rediscovery in the 19th century. In 1804, Baronio of Italy carried out a successful autograft on sheep and in 1817, Sir Astley Cooper in London grafted a full-thickness piece of skin from an amputated thumb onto the stump. In 1822, Bünger first applied a skin graft from the thigh to the nose. Early skin grafts were exceptionally thin and consisted of little more than epidermis alone, but it was the true split-thickness skin graft that allowed larger wounds to be resurfaced. In the 1870s Lawson,

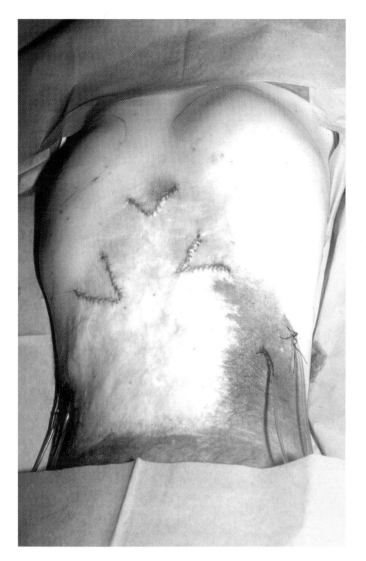

Figure 12.5 B Two crescenteric expanders were placed either side of the midline. The right side became infected and the implant had to be removed. However, the left side was expanded to a volume of 800 ml.

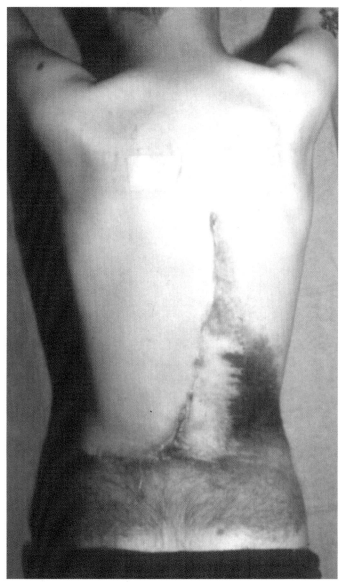

Figure 12.5 C The expanded normal skin was then advanced to the midline. The procedure needs to be repeated on the right side.

Le Fort and Wolfe all used full-thickness skin grafts to treat ectropion, but it is Wolfe, an Austrian ophthalmologist who later settled in Melbourne, Australia, with whom they are most commonly associated.

Differences between split-thickness and full-thickness skin grafts

There are important differences between split-thickness and full-thickness grafts that are relevant when planning surgery. Split-thickness grafts are preferable for covering larger areas. The donor sites heal in 10–14 days by epidermal migration from the wound edge and from foci of epidermal cells in the cut ends of skin appendages. The maximum size of full-thickness grafts is often limited by the ability to obtain primary closure of the donor site.

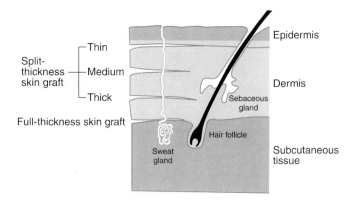

Figure 12.6 Variation in thickness of split-thickness skin grafts and full-thickness grafts.

158

Split-thickness skin grafts are thinner and have lower metabolic requirements than full-thickness grafts and therefore they exhibit better 'take', or survival and are preferable if the wound bed is not well vascularised. Split-thickness grafts contract more than full-thickness skin grafts and in general produce a less favourable cosmetic result because they are less able to correct a greater contour defect, exhibit poorer texture, have unpredictable pigmentation (either hypo- or hyperpigmentation), lower durability and also a more visible donor site. Furthermore, split-thickness grafts in children fail to grow with the child, unlike full-thickness grafts. Hence children with split-skin grafts overlying joints often require scar release as they grow. Finally, the skin adnexae are preserved in full-thickness skin grafts, whereas split-skin grafts are hairless and require long-term use of emollients to prevent drying of their surface.

Split-skin graft storage

Split-skin grafts can be stored wrapped in saline-soaked gauze at 4°C for up to three weeks. Split-thickness skin can also be cryo-preserved for long-term storage in skin banks for later use as a dressing material for patients with massive burns. Non-viable skin that is preserved in glycerol or lyophilised can also be used as a temporary dressing.

Donor sites

Split-thickness skin donor sites usually heal well with minimal scarring but there is always the risk of hypertrophic scarring. The most common donor site for split-thickness skin grafts is the thigh but if only a small graft is required in children, the buttock is a good site as the scar will be hidden. The donor sites for full-thickness skin grafts are more specific. For grafts to the face, the best colour match is obtained from facial skin such as post- or preauricular and the upper eyelids. The supraclavicular fossa is a useful site when large grafts are needed for the face. Large grafts can also be taken from the groin crease.

Biology of skin grafts

When a skin graft is harvested it is very pale and on grafts that are kept exposed, a pink hue is visible after 8–12 hours. At 2–4 days, if grafts are successful, they are bright pink and distended. Some grafts have a bluish tint at this time, probably because the arterial inflow precedes the development of the venous outflow. These observations have attracted much interest but there is still no unifying agreement about the microscopic events.

When a graft is applied to a wound bed, it adheres by a fibrin bond and graft survival is explained by two separate phases. First, there is the phase of serum imbibition during which grafts are nourished by diffusion of metabolites to and from the wound bed across a thin film of serum. During this period grafts gain weight and cell survival is probably dependent on anaerobic pathways.

After day 2, graft survival is maintained by capillary ingrowth from the wound bed, accounting for the bright pink colour of grafts. There is disagreement about whether new blood vessels from the wound bed link directly with the cut vessel on the graft, a process termed capillary inosculation, or more likely, if the capillaries growing from the wound bed forge new pathways into the grafts. Lymphatic growth occurs after seven days.

The delicate bond between graft and wound bed is susceptible to damage from shear forces in the first week and therefore grafts need protection from movement for the first two weeks. Grafts become firmly attached to the wound bed by the ingrowth of connective tissue that forms a scar interface with the grafts and the cellular events resemble those in classic primary healing of opposed skin edges. Graft contracture occurs at this plane and becomes progressive for 3–4 months. Hence when grafts are used to release contractures across flexure creases, the joint should be splinted for that time. It is not known why full-thickness grafts contract less than split-thickness grafts but the ratio of reticular to papillary dermis appears to be important. This is evident from the observation that a split-skin graft will contract more than a full-thickness skin graft even when both are of the same thickness.

Nerves grow into grafts from both the surrounding wound edge and the wound bed. Again, there was debate as to whether nerves follow the neurolemmal sheaths of nerves transferred with the graft or whether they make new pathways. The latter seems more likely led by the release of neurotrophic factors such as nerve growth factor from target cells (hair follicles, sebaceous glands) within a graft. Full-thickness skin grafts acquire a better sensation than split-thickness skin grafts, possibly because of a greater number of target organs. In patients, sensations of pain, light touch and temperature return in that order. However, sensation will never be equal to normal skin as specialised nerve endings such as Merkel cells and Meissner's corpuscles appear to degenerate and so sensation is mediated directly from bare nerve endings.

Surgical technique

With an understanding of the biology of skin graft survival, it is now possible to appreciate four factors essential to achieve satisfactory skin graft take:

1. selection of a vascularised wound bed
2. avoidance of haematoma or seroma
3. perfect graft immobility on the wound bed
4. minimising microbial contamination.

It is essential to apply skin grafts on to a vascularised wound bed. Exposed bone and tendons cannot support overlying grafts but grafts will grow on periosteum and paratenon. By the same token, necrotic debris (slough) must be removed prior to grafting. Haematomas beneath the grafts are the commonest cause of graft failure as they are a barrier to the revascularisation process and it is essential to secure haemostasis on the wound bed before applying the graft. Perforations in the graft may allow small amounts of blood and seroma to drain out. Grafts must be held on the wound bed without any movement for at least seven days to avoid damage to new vessel growth. Tie-over dressings are one way of preventing this movement. Grafts become stable only after 14 days and so if grafts are across joints or directly on muscle, limb splints should be worn for that period. Sometimes dressings can be harmful as they create shear forces between the graft and the wound bed. In such situations, as with grafts on the shoulder or parts of the lower leg, it is often better to expose grafts. Excess pressure (over 30 mmHg) from dressings should be avoided to prevent pressure necrosis of grafts.

Grafts are always contaminated by skin flora and there is a tendency to overstate the importance of infection as a cause of graft failure, as this overlooks other reasons. In practice, only a few bacteria are harmful. *Streptococcus pyogenes* (Lancefield group A) is very harmful to grafts because it produces streptokinase that breaks down the fibrin bond between the graft and the wound bed. *Pseudomonas aeruginosa* is of moderate harm to skin grafts, especially in burn patients where it is a common contaminant. Thus any wound that is more than a few days old should have its bacterial status assessed prior to grafting. The presence of *Streptococcus pyogenes* is a contraindication to grafting and surgery should be postponed until the bacteria is eradicated with systemic antibiotics.

Full-thickness grafts are excised with a scalpel blade. Subcutaneous fat is meticulously removed with scissors to promote maximum contact and minimise the thickness between the skin and wound bed. Split-thickness skin grafts can be taken with a handheld Watson knife (or other modification of the Humby knife) or with a powered dermatome (Figure 12.7). Some experience is required to cut the correct thickness of skin grafts (0.3–0.35 mm). Grafts that are too thin are unstable and significant morbidity is caused from grafts that are too thick because of poor take of the graft and also delayed healing of the donor site, which may lead to hypertrophic scarring. Numerous dressings

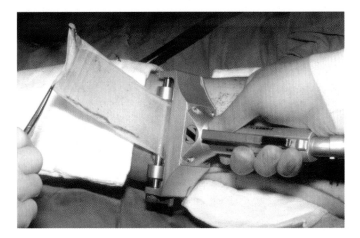

Figure 12.7 A split-thickness skin graft being taken from a patient's thigh using a power dermatome.

have been used for donor sites, but paraffin gauze remains the most common in use. Semiocclusive dressings (Opsite®) have been shown to enhance donor site healing and are good for small wounds. However, the fluid collection beneath the dressing is a potential nidus for infection and regular wound checks with aspiration of the fluid are required. Calcium alginate dressings (Kaltostat®) also promote wound healing and, when impregnated with bupivacaine, provide good postoperative analgesia.[12] Donor site dressings should be left intact until they separate spontaneously once the wound has healed after 10–14 days.

If split-skin graft donor sites are limited, as is often the case in burns, the sheets of split-thickness skin can be meshed so that they can cover a larger area. During healing epidermal cells migrate to fill the interstices of the mesh. However, mesh grafts give a poor cosmetic result as the mesh pattern often persists. Another way of expanding skin is the so-called Chinese method where the split-thickness skin is finely diced and then spread over a large area. Although wound cover is achieved, the new skin is very fragile because of the lack of dermal support, akin to problems with cultured keratinocyte grafts.

Skin flaps

As opposed to skin grafts which are avascular at the time of transplantation, skin flaps are vascularised segments of tissue that are transferred from one site to another. In comparison with skin grafts, local skin flaps provide similar tissue and resurface defects without leaving a contour defect, thus giving a better aesthetic result. In addition, skin flaps can resurface exposed bone or tendons and are also preferable to grafts for cover of vital structures such as major nerves and blood vessels. Furthermore, sensation on skin flaps is better than on skin grafts.

One of the major advances in plastic surgery in the past two decades has been our increased understanding of skin blood supply. Although the subject was studied by Manchot in the 19th century and more recently by Salmon, recent significant contributions have been made by Cormack & Lamberty, and Taylor et al.

The immediate blood supply to the skin is from the subdermal plexus which is fed by one of three systems:

1. perforators from the underlying muscle

2. perforators from the underlying deep fascia

3. a direct cutaneous system.

Skin flaps are described as random or axial pattern dependent on the blood supply. In random pattern flaps the subdermal plexus is fed by perforators from the underlying muscle or fascia. Axial pattern flaps have a direct cutaneous supply that extends to the entire length of the flap.

Skin flaps are also classified by their proximity to the defect. Local flaps arise from the immediate vicinity of the defect, whereas distant flaps arise from an adjacent region of the body. Free flaps are flaps that are transported from one part of the body with their blood supply identified and then reanastomosed using micro-surgical techniques to blood vessels at the recipient site. Skin flaps can also be transferred along with their underlying fascia, muscle or even bone and are described respectively by the terms fascio-cutaneous, musculocutaneous and osseocutaneous flaps.

Local flaps

These skin flaps have a random blood supply and are used for the coverage of small defects. They are used in various parts of the body when direct closure is not possible or when direct closure would cause undue distortion of the local tissue.

Advancement flaps: rectangular and V-Y

In these flaps tissue proximal to the defect is advanced forward. In the rectangular advancement flap, it is often necessary to excise small triangles adjacent to the base of the flap (Burrow's triangle) to facilitate advancement (Figures 12.8, 12.9). The V-Y island flap, so-called because a V-shaped incision is made with final closure in the shape of a Y, is a more straightforward procedure.

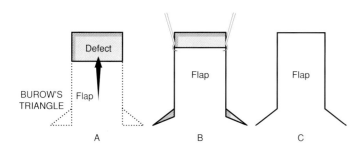

Figure 12.8 A rectangular advancement flap requires the excision of Burrows triangles to facilitate its movement.

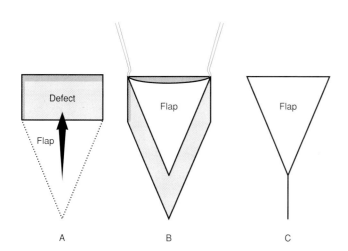

Figure 12.9 A V-Y advancement flap where the flap is designed as a V and, following advancement, the wound is closed in the shape of a Y.

Pivot flaps: transposition and rotation

These flaps have in common a pivot point and an arc through which the flap is rotated. The radius of the arc is the line of greatest tension of the flap and its realisation is important to the planning of these flaps. In transposition flaps (Figure 12.10), a rectangular or square area of skin and subcutaneous tissue adjacent to the defect is moved to cover the defect. In rotation flaps (Figure 12.11), a semicircular area of skin and subcutaneous tissue adjacent to the defect is rotated to fill the defect. In the planning of rotation flaps, the defect first has to be triangulated, and so a small amount of normal skin has to be excised along with the lesion. The triangle will have two equal sides and one shorter side. The tissue movement is based on the arc of a semicircle, the circumference of which may need to be eight times the length of the short side of the triangle. A releasing back cut may be

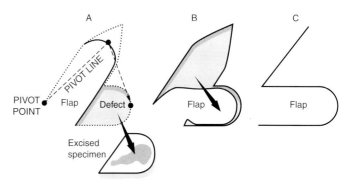

Figure 12.10 A transposition flap, where skin from one site (where there is skin laxity) is transposed on a pivot point to fill an adjacent defect. The defect from where the flap originated is closed directly.

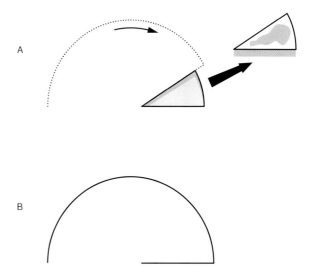

Figure 12.11 A rotation flap can be performed by redistributing skin surrounding a defect in a circular manner.

necessary to facilitate flap movement. The secondary defect may be closed directly or require a split-skin graft.

Rhomboid flap

This is a type of local transposition flap that was originally described in Russian by Limberg. The defect is made into a rhomboid shape and then a transposition flap from any one of the four sides of the rhomboid can be used to fill the defect. The secondary defect from where the flap arose is closed directly, giving this flap the unique property of a moving pivot point (Figure 12.12). There have been some modifications of Limberg's original description, including that suggested by Quaba & Sommerlad[19] which allows for ease of flap design.

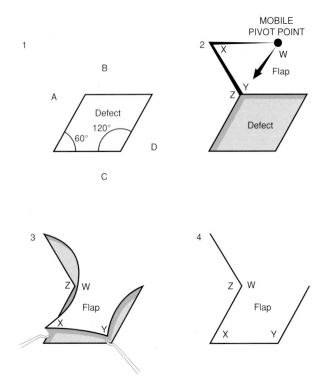

Figure 12.12 A rhomboid or Limberg flap is a type of transposition flap with a unique moving pivot point.

Regional (distant) flaps

These are flaps of skin or other tissue with an axial blood supply that are raised and isolated on their vascular pedicle and transferred to a distant site. The origin of the vascular pedicle is kept intact and serves as the pivot point of rotation of the flap. The defect at the donor site from where the flap originated may be sutured directly or require a skin graft.

Flap design is based on knowledge of the vascular anatomy. The first axial pattern skin flaps were the deltopectoral (Figure 12.13) and groin flaps.[17] Muscle and myocutaneous flaps are also used as

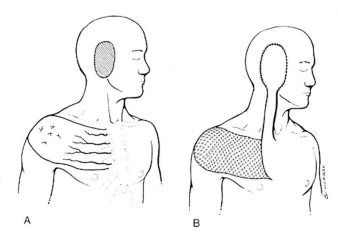

Figure 12.13 The deltopectoral flap was the first axial pattern flap described. It has a blood supply originating from perforators of the internal mammary vessels, particularly from the 2nd, 3rd and 4th intercostal spaces. The flap can be extended on to the deltoid area, but the blood supply is random and unpredictable. The flap is still used in head and neck reconstruction although it has been largely superseded by free flaps.

regional flaps. The latissimus dorsi flap, that was originally described by Tansini in 1895 and rediscovered by Olivari in 1976, is still commonly used in breast and head and neck reconstruction (Figure 12.14). Another early muscle flap was the pectoralis major flap. Ariyan demonstrated its use in head and neck reconstruction and, along with the deltopectoral flap, it remained the major flap in head and neck reconstruction until the advent of free flaps.

With further advances in the anatomy of the skin vasculature, many other regional flaps were discovered. One major advance was the description of fasciocutaneous flaps and more recently flaps based on perforating cutaneous branches of deeper vessels.

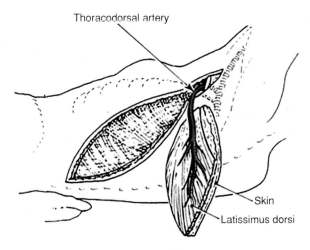

Figure 12.14 Illustration of the left lateral torso showing the latissimus dorsi myocutaneous flap. Its blood supply is from the thoracodorsal vessels which are branches of the axillary vessels.

162

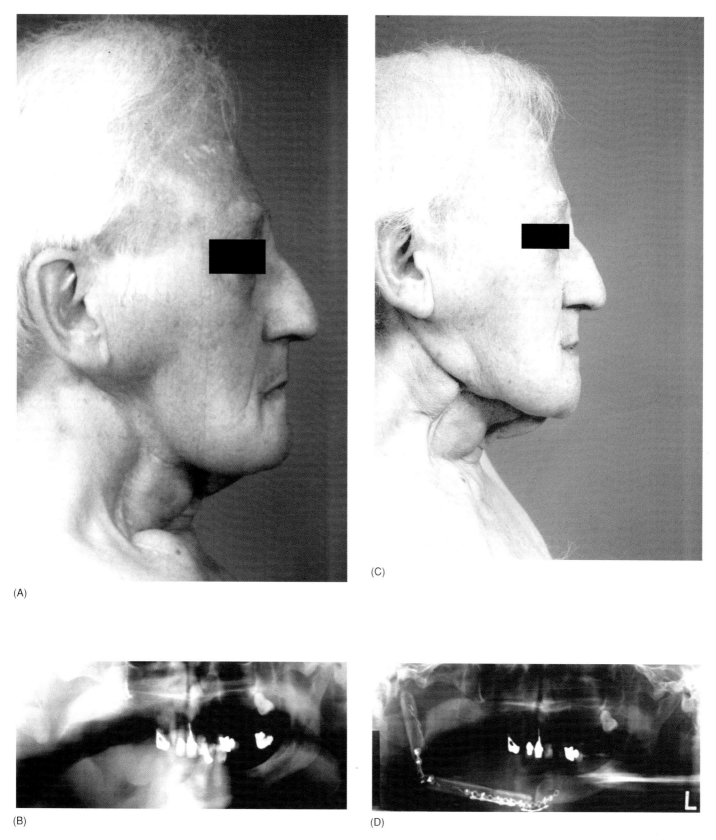

(A)

(B)

(C)

(D)

Figure 12.15 A, B. This 65-year-old man had squamous cell carcinoma involving the right mandible 20 years earlier. The intraoral defect was resurfaced with a fore-head flap, but the mandible was not reconstructed. He presented with increasing difficulty with mastication. **C, D**. After careful preoperative planning the right mandible was reconstructed with a free fibula flap taken from his right leg. His occlusion was improved and he subsequently had osseo-integrated dental implants inserted into the reconstructed mandible.

Free microvascular transfer

These are flaps again with an axial blood supply but, unlike pedicled flaps, the vascular pedicle is divided from its origin and then reanastomosed to an artery and vein at the new recipient site of the flap. Thus free flaps have a much greater versatility of movement than regional flaps and have brought major advances to the surgeon's ability to reconstruct areas of the body following trauma or tumour resection. Since the vessels are only a few millimetres in diameter, microsurgical techniques are used for the anastomosis. Thrombosis at the anastomosis or torsion of the vessels will cause flap failure. A unit with good experience should have a free flap failure rate below 5% and reexploration rate below 15%. Success is based on surgical technique, specific anaesthetic techniques for free flap surgery and postoperative monitoring.

Some examples of free flaps in frequent use are as follows.

Breast reconstruction (see later)

- Transverse rectus abdominis myocutaneous flap or the deep inferior epigastric artery flap.

Soft tissue reconstruction in the head and neck

- Radial forearm flap.
- Latissimus dorsi flap.

Bone reconstruction in the head and neck

- Fibula flap (Figure 12.15).
- Iliac crest based on deep circumflex iliac artery flap.
- Osseocutaneous radial forearm flap.

Pharyngeal reconstruction

- Jejunum.
- Colon.
- Tubed radial forearm flap.

Soft tissue reconstruction in the lower limb

- Latissimus dorsi muscle and myocutaneous flap.
- Radial forearm flap (Figure 12.16).
- Gracilis flap.
- Rectus abdominis flap.

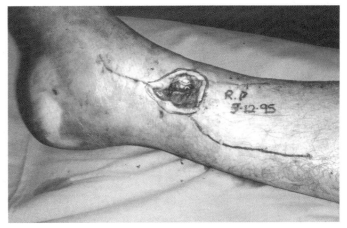

(A)

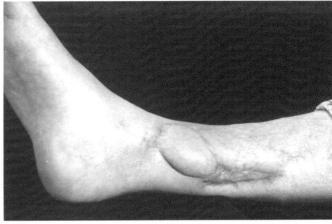

(B)

Figure 12.16 A. This man had a compound fracture of the right tibia and fibula (Gustillo 3B grade). The soft tissue defect exposed the fracture site and the fixation plate and screws. Without cover there would be a risk of osteomyelitis. **B.** The defect was covered with a radial forearm free flap which was anastomosed to the posterior tibial vessels.

Muscle flaps for facial reanimation in facial palsy

- Pectoralis minor flap.
- Gracilis flap.

ABNORMAL SCARS (HYPERTROPHIC AND KELOID)

Clinical features

Although one hopes that all scars will heal perfectly as thin lines, often this is not the case. Abnormal scars may be wide, hypertrophic or keloid. Hypertrophic and keloid scars are both raised, pink in white-skinned individuals and thickened. The distinction between keloid and hypertrophic scars is a clinical one and it is not correct to think of them as the same phenomenon that is quantitatively different.

Hypertrophic scars stay within the boundaries of the original scar and subside over a 2–3-year period. Patients are troubled by the appearance of the scar, intractable itching and contracture. They are less associated with racial origin and have lower familial tendency than keloids. They can occur at any age but are most frequent below the age of 20. Hypertrophic scars develop a few weeks after injury and are prevalent on scars across flexor surfaces and where the wound is under tension (Figure 12.17).

Keloid scars outgrow the boundaries of the original scar, invading surrounding normal tissue. Keloids are most likely in patients of African origin but also in Chinese and Celts. In addition, there may be a familial predilection. They can occur at any age but are most prevalent between 10 and 30 years and are rare in very young children and the elderly. Keloids develop a few months after the wound repair and occur most commonly on the lower face, neck, ear lobes, presternal area and back. They rarely subside and treatment is largely unsuccessful (Figure 12.18).

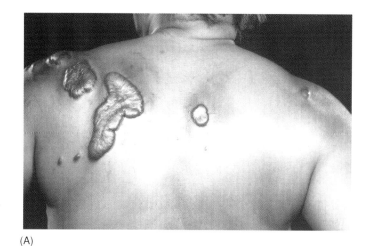

(A)

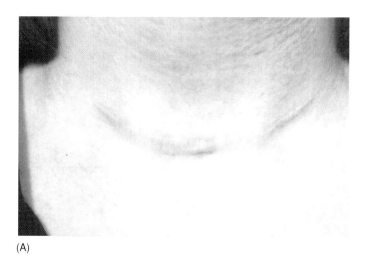

(A)

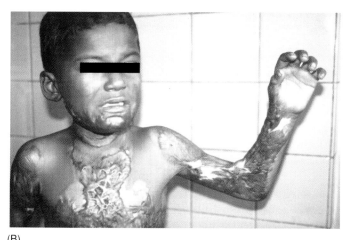

(B)

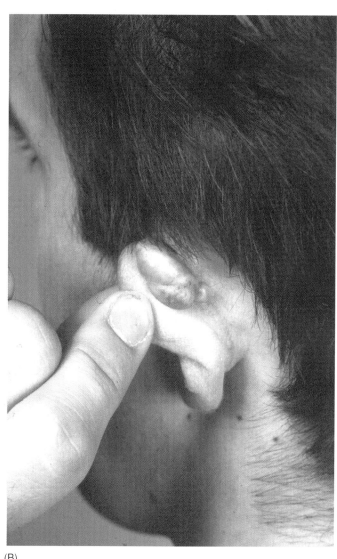

(B)

Figure 12.17 Hypertrophic scars. **A.** In a patient following thyroidectomy. **B.** This child has severe hypertrophic scarring following a burn with associated joint contractures.

Figure 12.18 Keloid scars. Unlike hypertrophic scars, these spread beyond the area of the initial scar. **A.** In a woman following minor skin infections and **B.** in a child following surgery for prominent ear correction.

Hypertrophic and keloid scars are indistinguishable histologically. In both, the pathology is within the dermis where there is dense hyalinised fibrous tissue with excess collagen deposition that is organised as discrete nodules. Frequently the rete pegs in the papillary dermis of the lesions are obliterated. Unlike normal dermis where collagen is arranged in discrete fascicles separated by interstitial space, the collagen nodules in keloids and hypertrophic scars appear avascular and are arranged in a haphazard manner. Keloid nodules are thought to have a glassy appearance compared with hypertrophic scars.

Aetiology

Clues to the aetiology of both hypertrophic and keloid scars lie in some clinical observations. Both types of scars are common in some areas such as the sternum and shoulders. Hypertrophic scars often occur where the axis of the wound crosses natural lines of skin tension rather than parallel to them. This gave rise to the theory that abnormal mechanical stresses are an important trigger of hypertrophic scarring. Hypertrophic scars are very common following a burn injury, particularly in children. Interestingly, they seldom occur in superficial burns that have healed quickly but are likely to form at sites where the burn injury was deeper and the wound slow to heal. Similarly, parts of wounds that dehisced and became infected are also more likely to become hypertrophic than areas of uneventful primary healing.

Other theories for the aetiology of hypertrophic and keloid scars include the suggestion that there were abnormalities of the immune system, but Cohen et al were unable to show any derangement of local or systemic immune factors. Tissue culture and biochemical studies have confirmed the increased production of collagen in keloid scars. Furthermore, fibroblasts that have been isolated from keloid scars continue to overproduce collagen when in culture. Hence it appears that once the fibroblasts have been stimulated to behave abnormally, they continue to do so even when removed from the abnormal environment. Specific collagen studies have shown that the overproduction is mainly of collagen type I and not type III that is seen in wound healing.

One popular concept is that hypoxia may stimulate or be responsible for the propagation of hypertrophic and keloid scars. Kischer et al observed increased occlusion of the microcirculation within lesions due to endothelial cell proliferation. It was hypothesised that perivascular myofibroblast contraction may contribute to microvascular occlusion. The resulting hypoxia could stimulate endothelial hyperplasia, causing further hypoxia which eventually led to excess collagen production.

The symptom of severe itching in hypertrophic scars has attracted some interest and high concentrations of neuropeptides have been shown in hypertrophic scars when compared with normal skin. These nerves may be responsible for the itching but since some neuropeptides are trophic agents, it has been suggested that they may stimulate growth of the abnormal scars.

Treatment

Hypertrophic scars, by their nature, will regress with time. However, at the earliest suggestion that a scar may become hypertrophic, it is advisable to institute preventative measures. The mainstay of management is the use of pressure garments. Quinn introduced the use of silicone gel for hypertrophic and keloid scars. To be effective, silicone gel needs to be applied for at least 12 hours a day. As a practical guide, as soon as a wound is seen to be hypertrophic and in all healed burn wounds, we would advocate use of pressure garments in conjunction with silicone gel which can be worn inside the garment for a minimum period of six months. Children cope very well with this regime, but occasionally some develop an atopic sensitivity to silicone gel.

Intralesional steroid injections can be used for hypertrophic scars and are often very effective. Surgery is not advised in the active phase when scars are red and itchy but thereafter the scar may be excised and the wound resutured although there might be recurrence of the hypertrophic scar. Alternatives are the use of Z-plasty techniques to realign the direction of the scars to lie parallel with the lines of skin tension or to introduce local unaffected flaps to relieve tension and break up the scar.

Treatment of keloid scars is frustrating. Surgical excision alone is unlikely to be successful and the lesions are likely to recur and may be larger than their original size. Intralesional excision is thought to be less harmful as it does not damage normal tissue. Intralesional steroid injections can decrease the size of keloids. It is our practice to use intralesional injections of triamcinolone 10 mg/ml (maximum 1 ml) at six-week intervals. A minimum of three injections is necessary before the benefit of the treatment can be assessed. In young children this may necessitate a general anaesthetic in order to give the injections. If steroid injections are unsuccessful, the next option would be to combine intralesional surgical excision with postoperative steroid injections. Complications of steroid injections such as local fat atrophy and depigmentation are due to extravasation into normal tissue.

Many workers have used radiotherapy following excision of keloids but I do not recommend their use in children due to the risk of future malignancy. However, patients are often willing to take that risk, such is the social stigma of keloids. A summary of various regimes of surgery, radiotherapy and steroids in the treatment of keloids was published by Lawrence. Although quantitative comparison of published data is not possible due to numerous variations in patient cohort and treatment protocols, it nevertheless provides an impression of treatment efficacy. Analysis showed that steroid injections alone had a mean success rate of 66%. Surgery alone had a mean success rate of 28%, that increased to 52% when combined with postoperative steroid injections and 75% with radiotherapy.

BREAST RECONSTRUCTION

Introduction

Breast reconstructive surgery should be within a multidisciplinary breast service. This may comprise surgeons, specialist nurses, radiotherapists/oncologists, radiologists, psychologists and prosthetists (anaplastologists). Both general surgeons and plastic surgeons currently perform breast reconstruction but in the future, a subspeciality of breast surgery encompassing the oncological, reconstructive and aesthetic aspects of the subject may evolve.

Breast reconstruction may be immediate or delayed. Early fears that immediate reconstruction was ill advised on oncological grounds and concerns about masking recurrence have been disproved. Furthermore, there was early evidence that immediate reconstruction improves psychological outcome. Even when the cancer is aggressive reconstruction can be offered in an attempt to optimise remaining quality of life. The percentage of women now choosing immediate breast reconstruction with mastectomy is over 50%.

Appropriate patient and technique selection are the key to success and are based on the following criteria.

● Age, weight, history of smoking and past medical history, including previous surgery, particularly to the abdomen.

● Previous radiotherapy to the chest, which increases the incidence of wound complications with marginal necrosis and low tolerance to tissue expansion.

● Likelihood of requiring postoperative radiotherapy.

● Lifestyle, particularly if they are keen sportswomen.

● Patient preference which is often influenced by the team and family.

● Patient's acceptability for surgery to the opposite breast. This is often necessary either to lift (mastopexy) or augment the opposite breast.

Techniques

The surgeon needs to decide on the amount of skin and breast volume that needs replacing. Extra skin can be either imported from another site (e.g. back or abdomen) or created by expanding the existing skin.

There are three commonly used techniques of breast reconstruction.

Use of implants alone

This is best for delayed reconstruction, where there is good-quality chest skin and when there has been no previous radiotherapy (Figure 12.19). The implant of choice is a tissue expander.

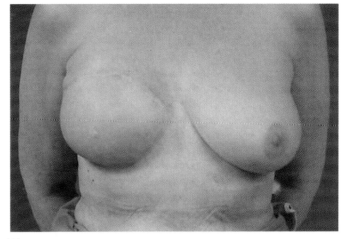

(A)

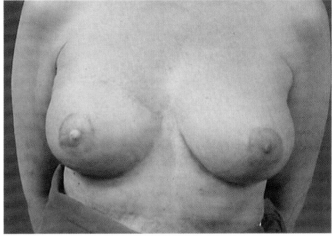

(B)

Figure 12.19 A. This woman had a right mastectomy nine years previously and did not have radiotherapy. She had reconstruction with an expander implant alone. **B**. After 6 months she underwent left breast mastopexy (lift) and right nipple-areolar reconstruction. She went on to have the right areolar area tattooed to achieve a better colour match.

Some expanders are permanent whereas others are removed and replaced with a permanent prosthesis.

Advantages

● A simple procedure that does not compromise other reconstructive options and that satisfies many patients.

● There is no donor site morbidity.

Disadvantages

● Margins of the implant are more discernible than when it is covered with the latissimus dorsi muscle.

● Hard to achieve natural breast ptosis (drooping).

● If the overlying skin necroses or wound margins dehisce, the implant will extrude, become infected and require removal.

The latissimus dorsi muscle or myocutaneous flap

This is used as a muscle-only flap to cover implants during immediate reconstruction and its use decreases the incidence of implant infection and extrusion. It is used as a myocutaneous flap with an ellipse of skin from the back if there is the need for extra skin, especially when there has been previous radiotherapy to the chest (Figure 12.20).

Advantages

● The latissimus dorsi is for most patients an expendable muscle and its loss creates minimum morbidity. Contraindications to

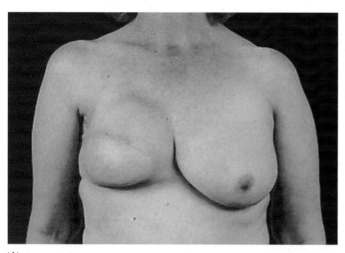

(A)

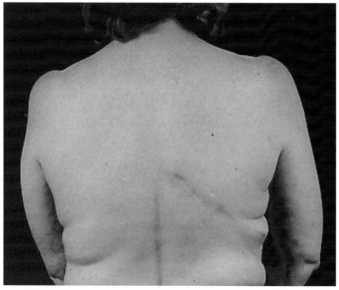

(B)

Figure 12.20 A. This woman had a right mastectomy and immediate reconstruction with a pedicled latissimus dorsi myocutaneous flap and implant. She was readmitted at the time of this photograph for a left breast reduction and right nipple-areolar reconstruction. **B**. Scar on the right side of her back from where the flap was taken.

its use are in keen sportswomen, particularly crosscountry skiers and climbers.

Disadvantages

● There is usually a scar on the back, although in a thin patient where only muscle is needed it is possible to raise the muscle with a short extension to the mastectomy wound. Endoscopic assistance can minimise the need for scars on the back.

● A serous collection often forms at the donor site. Frequent aspiration may be required for several weeks.

● Flap failure can occur if the vascular pedicle of the flap is damaged or anomalous.

● Contraction of the latissimus dorsi muscle on the chest wall can be unsightly and for this reason the thoracodorsal nerve is often purposely divided.

● There is almost always the need for an implant, with its related problems.

The transverse abdominis myocutaneous (TRAM) flap

This flap utilises the lower abdominal skin to replace both skin and volume (Figure 12.21). The rectus abdominis muscle is traditionally included in the flap as a 'carrier' for the vessels that supply the flap. The flap can be transferred to the chest as a pedicled flap based on the vascular supply from the superior epigastric vessels that pass on the deep surface of the rectus abdominis muscle. The alternative is to use it as a free flap where the blood supply is via the inferior epigastric vessels. These vessels are anastomosed to the thoracodorsal or internal mammary vessels using microsurgical techniques. The TRAM flap is a poor choice in patients who are cigarette smokers, overweight or unfit.

A more recent modification is the free deep inferior epigastric perforator (DIEP) flap, where the abdominal skin flap is raised without the underlying rectus abdominis muscle by dissecting the individual perforating vessels as they pass through muscle. This modication minimises abdominal donor site morbidity but is technically more difficult and the incidence of flap failure is initially higher.

Advantages

● Provides autologous reconstruction without the need for implants.

● Breast feels more normal and the aesthetic standard can be high. Natural ptosis often results, reducing the need for a mastopexy (lift) to the opposite breast.

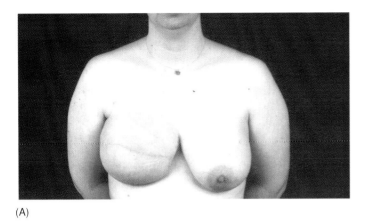

(A)

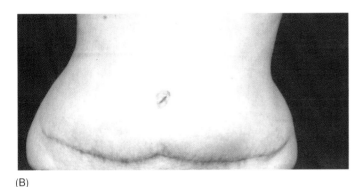

(B)

Figure 12.21 This woman had right mastectomy and immediate reconstruction with a free TRAM flap. The inferior epigastric vessels of the flap were anastomosed to the right internal mammary vessels. A subsequent procedure is planned to reshape the reconstruction, create a nipple–areolar complex and perform a mastopexy on the left breast.

Disadvantages

- In general the complications are higher with pedicled than free flaps.

- There are several complications related to the donor site. There is always a long transverse scar and circular scar around the umbilicus. Abdominal wall weakness has been reported in up to 30% of patients, particularly with pedicled flaps since more muscle is taken. In addition, there can be an incisional hernia and abdominal distension. With pedicled flaps there may be a bulge of rectus muscle beneath the costal margin.

Partial necrosis of the flap can occur and is often due to incorrect patient selection. Skin or fat necrosis has been reported in 30% of patients and is again more common with the pedicled technique.

Less common flaps are the use of the skin and fat over the iliac crest (Ruben's flap) and buttock skin and fat which can be taken with the superior gluteal pedicle or can be perforator based. Both are transferred as free flaps.

Contraindications

There are few absolute contraindications to breast reconstruction. Relative contraindications concern patient fitness for prolonged surgery, conditions that impair wound healing and obesity. Patients with locally aggressive disease and those with breast and chest wall radionecrosis are often in need of chest wall cover, rather than breast mound reconstruction (Figure 12.22).

Subcutaneous mastectomy

A subcutaneous mastectomy is often selected for patients with carcinoma *in situ* and sometimes it is possible to save the nipple. The decision to remove the nipple is based on disease severity and its proximity to the nipple, which takes into consideration the size of the breast. These patients often achieve the best aesthetic results from reconstruction because the breast envelpe is preserved (Figure 12.23).

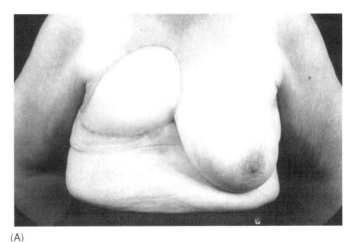

(A)

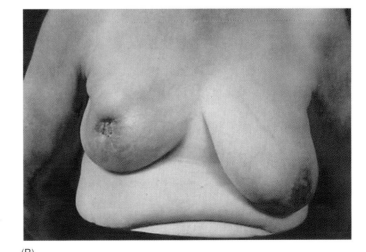

(B)

Figure 12.22 A. This woman had recurrent carcinoma of the right breast following previous lumpectomy and radiotherapy. **B**. A radical resection was done and the chest wall defect was covered with a large latissimus dorsi myocutaneous flap.

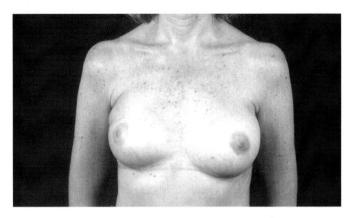

Figure 12.23 This woman had a right breast subcutaneous mastectomy preserving the nipple. An immediate reconstruction was done with a latissimus dorsi muscle flap and expander implant. Subsequently right breast augmentation was done to achieve symmetry.

Nipple-areola reconstruction

The nipple-areola complex can be restored either with a prosthesis or with a local skin flap and skin grafts. Autologous reconstruction usually requires tattooing to achieve the best colour match and even so is not often as good as the prosthesis.

Partial mastectomy defects

The evolution of breast reconstruction has now progressed to the reconstruction defects following local excision. In women with small breasts, extra tissue is needed from local flaps or small latissimus dorsi myocutaneous flaps. In women with large breasts, following tumour excision the remaining breast can be reshaped using techniques used in breast reduction surgery. Simultaneous reduction of the opposite breast may be required to achieve symmetry.

The silicone controversy

Breast implants have a silicone elastomer and a filler material. Silicone gel became a popular filler because it has a consistency similar to body fat and these implants were used for cosmetic breast augmentation and breast reconstruction. Concerns were raised in the early 1990s in North America on the safety of the silicone gel and in the absence of adequate laboratory or clinical data, the US Food and Drug Administration (FDA) banned the use of silicone gel implants for cosmetic augmentation but allowed their use in breast reconstruction. In the UK, the Medical Devices Agency (MDA), which is part of the Department of Health, reviewed the available data and concluded that there was no need to ban these implants. Careful scrutiny of published data shows that there is *no* evidence that silicone gel-filled implants:

- cause an autoimmune-type disease, by silicone acting as a hapten
- cause breast cancer
- delay the detection of breast cancer[54]
- make mammographic detection of tumours more difficult (although patients will need more than the standard views).

In the absence of adequate data confirming their safety, it was recommended that patients having silicone gel implants should with consent be registered in a database, the National Breast Implant Registry. In addition, an Independent Review Group on silicone breast implants was established and its report was presented to the Chief Medical Officer in July 1998. Further literature on the topic should be reviewed by the MDA.

In my practice, patients are given the choice between silicone and saline implants and available data is offered so that they can make an informed choice. Capsule formation is the most common problem with breast implants. The use of textured elastomer as compared with smooth implants has reduced the incidence of severe capsule formation from 30% to 10% at three-year follow-up. Longer follow-up studies are awaited.

All implants can rupture, spilling their contents. Often the spillage is intracapsular but if the silicone becomes extracapsular, silicone granulomas form. These are sometimes painful and are often removed to exclude cancer. The chance of spillage or 'bleed' of the filler through the shell is theoretically less with recent cohesive silicone gels but it is too early to have good follow-up data.

Soya bean oil implants

In the 1990s Trilucent™ breast implants (Lipomatrix Inc./AEI Inc., formerly Collagen Aesthetics International Inc.) were marketed for breast augmentation. These contained soya bean oil which was radiolucent and was therefore thought to be useful for mammography. Also, as a 'natural' product, it was offered as an alternative to silicone.

However, there were adverse reports of breast swelling and discomfort in some women with these implants and in March 1999 the implants were voluntarily withdrawn from sale by the company. Further data to the MDA suggested that the breakdown products of the filler material can include aldehydes. At the reported levels the aldehydes could react with protein and DNA and thus pose a genotoxic hazard. The MDA therefore issued a hazard notice in June 2000 advising women to have the implants removed.

Acknowledgements

My thanks to Mr Neil Rothnie and Mr Mike Salter, consultant surgeons, Southend Hospital, for their help with the section on breast reconstruction and for the use of photographs of patients who have been under our combined care. My thanks also to Mr Peter Weller, consultant maxillofacial surgeon, for the joint care of the patient illustrated in Figure 12.15.

REFERENCES

1 Radovan C. Breast reconstruction after mastectomy using the temporary expander. *Plast Reconstr Surg* 1982; **69**: 195–208

2 Matton GE, Tonnard PL, Monstrey SJ, Van Landuyt SH. A universal incision for tissue expander insertion. *Br J Plast Surg* 1995; **48**: 172–176

3 Joss GS, Zoltie N, Chapman P. Tissue expansion technique and the transposition flap. *Br J Plast Surg* 1990; **43**: 328–333

4 Davis JS. Story of plastic surgery. *Ann Surg* 1941; **113**: 651

5 Hauben DJ, Baruchin A, Mahler A. On the history of the free skin graft. *Ann Plast Surg* 1982; **9**: 242–245

6 Bünger C. Gelungener versuch einer Nasenbildung aus einem völlig getrennten Haustück dem biene. *Jahresbericht Chirurgie Augen-Heilk* 1822; **4**: 569–582

7 Ollier LXEL. Greffes cutanées ou autoplastiques. *Bulletin de l'Académie de Medcine de Paris* 1872; 2 Série, 1: 243–250. In: McDowell F, ed. *Plast Reconstr Surg* 1966; **38**: 98–104

8 Réverdin JL. Greffe épidermique-expérience faite dans le service de M le Docteur Guyon, a l'Hôpital Necker. *Bulletin de la Impéral Société de Chirurgie de Paris* 1869; **10**: 511–515. In: McDowell F, ed. *Silvergirl's Surgery: Plastic Surgery*. Austin, Texas: Silvergirl Inc., pp 3–5

9 Thiersch C. Uber die feineren anatomischen Varänderunger bei Aufheilung von Haut auf Granulationen. *Verhandlungen der Deutschen Gesellschaft fer Chirurgie Berlin* 1874; **3**: 69–75. In: McDowell F, ed. *Silvergirl's Surgery: Plastic Surgery*. Austin, Texas: Silvergirl Inc., pp 12–13

10 Blair VP, Brown J. The use and uses of large split skin grafts of intermediate thickness. *Surg Gynecol Obstet* 1929; **49**: 82–97

11 Kelton PL. Skin grafts. *Select Read Plast Surg* 1992; **7**: 1–25

12 Butler PEM, Eadie PA, Lawlor D, Edwards G, McHugh M. Bupivacaine and Kaltostat reduces post-operative donor site pain. *Br J Plast Surg* 1993; **46**: 523–524

13 Manchot C. *Die Hautarterien des Menschlichen Körpers*. Leipzig, FCW Vogel, 1889. *The Cutaneous Arteries of the Human Body*. Translated by Ristic J, Morain WD. New York: Springer-Verlag, 1983

14 Salmon M. *Les artères de la peau*. Paris: Masson, 1936

15 Cormack GC, Lamberty BGH. *The arterial anatomy of skin flaps*. Edinburgh: Churchill Livingstone, 1987

16 Taylor IG, Palmer JH, McManammy D. The vascular territories of the body (angiosomes) and their clinical applications. In: McCarthy JG ed. *Plastic Surgery*. Philadelphia: WB Saunders, 1990

17 McGregor IA, Morgan G. Axial and random pattern flaps. *Br J Plast Surg* 1973; **26**: 202–213

18 Limberg AA. Design of local flaps. In: Gibson T, ed. *Modern Trends in Plastic Surgery*, 2nd edn. London: Butterworths, 1966

19 Quaba AA, Sommerlad BC. A square peg in a round hole: a modified rhomboid flap and its clinical application. *Br J Plast Surg* 1987; **40**: 163–170

20 Bakamjian VY. A two stage method for pharyngoesophageal reconstruction with a primary pectoral skin flap. *Plast Reconstr Surg* 1965; **36**: 173–184

21 Tansini I. Nuovo processo per l'amputazione della mammella per cancro. *Riforma Medica* 1896; **12**(1): 3–5

22 Hueston JT, McConchie IH. A compound pectoral flap. *Aust NZ J Surg* 1968; **38**: 61–63

23 Ariyan S. The pectoralis major myocutaneous flap. A versatile flap for reconstruction in the head and neck. *Plast Reconstr Surg* 1979; **63**: 73–81

24 Ponten B. The fasciocutaneous flap: its use in soft tissue defects of the lower leg. *Br J Plast Surg* 1981; **34**: 215–220

25 Quaba AA, Davison PM. The distally-based dorsal hand flap. *Br J Plast Surg* 1990; **43**: 28–39

26 Soutar DS, ed. *Microvascular Surgery and Free Tissue Transfer*. London: Edward Arnold, 1993

27 Cohen IK, McCoy BJ, Mohanakumar T, Diegelmann RF. Immunoglobulin, complement, and histocompatibility antigen studies in keloid patients. *Plast Reconstr Surg* 1979; **63**: 689–695

28 Cohen IK, Keiser HR. Collagen synthesis in keloid and hypertrophic scar following intralesional use of triamcinolone. *Surg Forum* 1972; **23**: 509–510

29 Kischer CW, Theis C, Chavapil M. Perivascular myofibroblasts and microvascular occlusion in hypertrophic scars and keloids. *Human Pathol* 1982; **13**: 819–824

30 Crowe R, Parkhouse N, McGrouther DA, Burnstock G. Neuropeptide containing nerves in painful hypertrophic scar tissue. *Br J Dermatol* 1994; **130**: 444–452

31 Larson DL. Contracture and scar formation in the burn patient. *Clin Plast Surg* 1974; **1**: 653–656

32 Quinn KJ. Silicone gel in scar treatment. *Burns* 1987; **13**: S33–40

33 Lawrence WT. In search of the optimal treatment for keloids: report of a series and review of the literature. *Ann Plast Surg* 1991; 27: 164–178

34 Dean C, Chetty U, Forrest AP. Effects of immediate breast reconstruction on psychosocial morbidity after mastectomy. *Lancet* 1983; **1**: 459–462

35 Stevens LA, McGrath MH, Druss RG, Kister SJ, Gump FE, Forde KA. The psychological impact of immediate breast reconstruction for women with early breast cancer. *Plast Reconstr Surg* 1984; **73**: 619–628

36 Bostwick J III, Nahai F, Wallace JG, Vasconez LO. Sixty latissimus dorsi flaps. *Plast Reconstr Surg* 1979; **63**: 31–41

37 Olivari N. The latissimus flap. *Br J Plast Surg* 1976; **29**: 126–128

38 Boyd JB, Taylor GI, Corlett R. The vascular territories of the superior epigastric and deep inferior epigastric systems. *Plast Reconstr Surg* 1984; **73**: 1–16

39 Taylor GI, Corlett RJ, Boyd JB. The versatile deep inferior epigastric (inferior rectus abdominis) flap. *Br J Plast Surg* 1984; **37**: 330–350

40 Hartrampf CR Jr, Bennett GK. Autologous tissue reconstruction in the mastectomy patient. A critical review of 300 patients. *Ann Surg* 1987; **205**: 508–519

41 Holmström H. The free abdominoplasty flap and its use in breast reconstruction. An experimental study and clinical case report. *Scand J Plast Reconstr Surg* 1979; **13**: 423–427

42 Blondeel PN. One hundred free DIEP flap breast reconstructions: a personal experience. *Br J Plast Surg* 1999; **52**: 104–111

43 Koshima I, Soeda S. Inferior epigastric artery skin flaps without rectus abdominis muscle. *Br J Plast Surg* 1989; **42**: 645–648

44 Elliott LF, Hartrampf CR Jr. The Rubens flap. The deep circumflex iliac artery flap. *Clin Plast Surg* 1998; **25**: 283–291

45   Shaw WW. Breast reconstruction by superior gluteal microvascular free flaps without silicone implants. *Plast Reconstr Surg* 1983; **72**: 490–501

46   Blondeel PN. The sensate free superior gluteal artery perforator (S-GAP) flap: a valuable alternative in autologous breast reconstruction. *Br J Plast Surg* 1999; **52**: 185–193

47   Clough KB, Kroll SS, Audretsch W. An approach to the repair of partial mastectomy defects. *Plast Reconstr Surg* 1999; **104**: 409–420

48   Kessler DA. The basis of the FDA's decision on breast implants. *N Engl J Med* 1992; **326**: 1713–1715

49   Medical Devices Agency. *Silicone Gel Breast Implants*. London: Medical Devices Agency, 1998. http://www.medical-devices.gov.uk/silicone.htm

50   Berkel H, Birdsell DC, Jenkins H. Breast augmentation: a risk factor for breast cancer? *N Engl J Med* 1992; **326**: 1649–1653

51   Deapen DM, Pike PHMC, Casagrande JT, Brody GS. The relationship between breast cancer and augmentation mammoplasty. *Plast Reconstr Surg* 1986; **77**: 361–368

52   Deapen DM, Brody GS. Augmentation mammoplasty and breast cancer: a 5 year update of the Los Angeles study. *Plast Reconstr Surg* 1992; **89**: 660–665

53   Deapen DM, Bernstein L, Brody GS. Are breast implants anticarcinogenic? A 14 year follow-up of the Los Angeles study. *Plast Reconstr Surg* 1997; **99**: 1346–1353

54   Carlson GW, Curley SA, Martin JE, Fornage BD, Ames FC. The detection of breast cancer after augmentation mammoplasty. *Plast Reconstr Surg* 1993; **91**: 837–840

55   Independent Review Group. *Silicone Gel Breast Implants: the Report of the Independent Review Group*. London: Medical Devices Agency, 1998. http://www.silicone-review.gov.uk

56   Malata CM, Feldberg L, Coleman DJ, Foo ITH, Sharpe DT. Textured or smooth implants for breast augmentation? Three year follow-up of a prospective randomised controlled trial. *Br J Plast Surg* 1997; **50**: 99–105

57   Medical Devices Agency. *Trilucent™ Breast Implants: Recommendation to Remove*. London: Medical Devices Agency, 2000. http://www.medical-devices.gov.uk/hn2000(05).htm

58   Medical Devices Agency. *Statement on the Safety of Trilucent Breast Implants*. London: Medical Devices Agency, 2000. http://www.medical-devices.gov.uk/tbi-state.htm

Section 2

Critical Care and Applied Physiology

13

Fluid balance

Body water
Functions of the kidney
    Glomerular function
    Tubular function
Diuresis
    Water balance
    Regulation of total body water
Disturbances of total body water content
    Water depletion
    Water intoxication
Electrolyte disorders
    Sodium
    Potassium
Acid–base balance
    Disturbances of acid–base balance
    Interpretation of acid–base changes

Normal fluid and electrolyte requirements
    Fluid balance in the uncomplicated patient
    Changes in fluid and electrolyte requirements
        in response to surgery and trauma
Fluid and electrolyte problems in surgical patients
    Blood and plasma
    Gastrointestinal losses
    Intraperitoneal loss of fluid
    Septicaemia
    Excessive insensible fluid loss
    Renal failure
Oedema and lymphatic function
    Control of flow between plasma and interstitial
        compartments
    Causes of oedema

Andrew T. Raftery

BODY WATER

In healthy adults water constitutes approximately 60% of the body weight. Body water is partitioned into two compartments:

- intracellular
- extracellular.

The latter may be further divided into intravascular and extravascular (interstitial) compartments.

The intracellular compartment is rich in potassium and contains only a small quantity of sodium. Sodium predominates in the extracellular compartment, an active sodium pump mechanism maintaining an ionic gradient by excluding sodium from the cell.

For a 70 kg man there would be approximately 25 l of intracellular water and 19 l of extracellular water. Of the extracellular water, 3 l is in the blood plasma and 15 l in the interstitial fluid with the remaining 1 l being transcellular fluid, e.g. cerebrospinal fluid, peritoneal fluid, intraocular fluid.

Plasma water and interstitial fluid have similar electrolyte compositions but plasma water contains more protein than interstitial fluid. The plasma proteins, chiefly albumin, account for the high colloid osmotic pressure of plasma, which is an important factor in the distribution of fluid between vascular and interstitial compartments as defined by Starling's Law.

Before discussing disturbances of fluid, electrolyte and acid base balance, it will be appropriate to review the functions of the kidney.

FUNCTIONS OF THE KIDNEY

The kidneys have several functions. They contribute to biochemical haemostasis by:

- eliminating waste products.
- regulating fluid and electrolyte balance.
- regulating acid–base balance.

They produce certain humoral agents:

- erythropoietin.
- vitamin D metabolites.
- renin.
- prostaglandins.

The fundamental unit of the kidney is the nephron which is composed of a glomerulus and tubular system. Blood is filtered at the glomerulus, entering Bowman's capsule from whence there is a system of tubules which modifies the filtered plasma. These tubules are the proximal convoluted tubule, the loop of Henle, the distal convoluted tubule and collecting tubules.

Glomerular function

The glomerular filtration rate (GFR) is dependent upon the glomerular capillary arterial pressure (60 mmHg) minus plasma colloid osmotic pressure (30 mmHg) plus the hydrostatic pressure in Bowman's capsule (20 mmHg), i.e. the filtration pressure is 60 − (30 + 20) = 10 mmHg. Arterioles before and after the capillary bed in Bowman's capsule (afferent and efferent arterioles) are capable of adjusting glomerular pressure and hence flow. Constriction of the afferent arteriole decreases capillary pressure and therefore filtration. Constriction of the efferent arterioles increases capillary pressure and increases filtration. GFR may be calculated by measuring the clearance of a substance from the blood into the urine. The substance must have the following properties:

- freely filtered at the glomerulus.
- neither absorbed nor secreted by the tubules.
- does not attach to plasma proteins.
- not metabolised by the kidney.

In clinical practice GFR is measured as creatinine clearance, since creatinine is produced endogenously and does not need to be infused intravenously.

$$GFR = \frac{UV}{P} \ ml/min$$

P = plasma concentration in mg/ml
V = volume of urine in ml/min
U = urine concentration in mg/ml

The normal GFR is approximately 125 ml/min. Approximately 180 l of water is filtered in 24 hours but only about 1.5 l is lost in the urine. Autoregulation of renal blood flow results in a relatively stable glomerular hydrostatic pressure and therefore GFR. However, if arterial blood pressure falls below 60 mmHg, as in shock, glomerular filtration ceases, leading to anuria.

Juxtaglomerular apparatus

The juxtaglomerular apparatus lies adjacent to the vascular pole of the kidney. It secretes renin in response to the following:

- reduced blood volume.
- sympathetic nerve stimulation.
- low sodium concentration in distal tubule.
- circulating catecholamines.
- renal ischaemia.

Renin hydrolyses angiotensinogen to form angiotensin I. Angiotensin I is converted to angiotensin II by converting enzyme, which is found in the kidney and lung. Angiotensin II has the following effects:

- stimulation of Na^+ reabsorption in the proximal convoluted tubule.

- vasoconstriction of efferent arterioles to maintain GFR when blood pressure is low.

- stimulation of aldosterone release from the adrenal cortex.

- stimulation of antidiuretic hormone (ADH) release.

- stimulation of thirst.

Tubular function

The glomerular filtrate, which is isotonic with plasma, has to be modified osmotically so that water and electrolytes are conserved and waste products concentrated for elimination. This occurs in the tubules where 99% of the filtered volume is reabsorbed together with important constituents of the filtrate. The various tubules differ in structure and function.

Proximal convoluted tubule

Approximately 60–80% of the filtered water and sodium is reabsorbed from the proximal tubules per 24 hours. Absorption of potassium, phosphate and glucose also occurs in the proximal convoluted tubule. The tubular cells secrete hydrogen ions and ammonia into the lumen.

Loop of Henle

The loop of Henle is responsible for the development of a high renal medullary osmotic pressure by a countercurrent multiplier system. The active transfer of sodium from the tubular fluid into the interstitium by the cells of the ascending limb creates a hypertonic environment in the interstitium of the medulla. By the time the fluid enters the distal tubule in the cortex it has lost a considerable amount of sodium and has become hypoosmotic to cortical plasma.

Distal convoluted tubule

Sodium chloride is absorbed throughout the length of the distal tubule. The initial part of the distal tubule is impermeable to water but the permeability of its latter part is controlled by ADH, some 10–20 l of water per day being absorbed. Potassium, hydrogen ions and ammonia are secreted into the distal tubule.

Collecting ducts

The collecting ducts run through the hyperosmotic medulla to drain into the renal pelvis. Sodium reabsorption continues in the collecting ducts. ADH exerts its effect primarily on the collecting ducts, the epithelial cells being selectively permeable to water under the effects of ADH. In the absence of ADH, as in diabetes insipidus, the water permeability of the ductal epithelium is very low and little absorption occurs and patients may pass in excess of 20 l of urine a day with an osmolality lower than 50 mosmol/l. With maximal concentrations of ADH, as little as 500 ml of urine is excreted per day with a very high osmolality of 1200 mosmol/l.

DIURESIS

There are two types of diuresis, water and osmotic.

Water diuresis occurs when water is ingested or administered in excess of the body's requirements. ADH secretion is suppressed, the collecting ducts become relatively impermeable to water and the excess water is lost without solute. Thus the kidney can adjust its excretion of water without markedly affecting its handling of solutes.

Osmotic diuresis results when more solute is presented to the tubules than they can reabsorb. Examples of osmotic diuresis include:

- diabetes, where the concentration of glucose in the plasma rises so that the filtered load exceeds the tubular maximum.

- the administration of mannitol which is filtered but is a non-reabsorbable solute.

- inhibition of tubular function, e.g. by drugs which block reabsorption of sodium chloride in one or more parts of the tubule.

Water balance

Normally body water remains constant. Over a 24-hour period, therefore, intake and loss of water must balance exactly.

Intake is composed of drinking fluids, solid food (which may contain as much as 1 l of fluid in 24 hours) and the water of oxidation of metabolites (about 300 ml in 24 hours). Water is lost in the following ways.

• evaporation via the respiratory system	500 ml
• skin (insensible)	400 ml
• faeces	100 ml
• urine (obligatory)	500 ml
Total	1500 ml

Urine water loss is variable. About 600 mosmol of solutes must be excreted each day in the urine. The maximal achievable urinary osmolality is about 1200 mosmol/l and therefore the obligatory volume of urine is about 500 ml per day. In practice, water intake is such that 1.5 l of urine is excreted each day.

Regulation of total body water

Although the movement of certain ions and proteins between the various compartments is restricted, water is freely diffusible.

Consequently the osmolality of all components is identical, being maintained within a narrow range of 285–295 mosmol/L. Control of osmolality occurs by two mechanisms:

- adjustments in secretion of ADH

- thirst-mediated water intake.

If water loss exceeds gain there is a reduction in total body water content and the osmolality of the body fluid increases. This results in two effects:

- thirst, resulting in ingestion of water

- release of ADH so that water is retained by the kidneys.

Conversely excess intake of water dilutes the body fluids, reducing the osmolality. This eliminates thirst and inhibits the release of ADH, thus allowing diuresis and consequent removal of excess water.

In health, both thirst and ADH release are determined by the osmolality of plasma perfusing nuclei in the hypothalamus. The receptors indicating thirst have an osmotic threshold of about 10 mosmol higher than that of the osmoreceptors involved in ADH release. Under normal circumstances, therefore, thirst is not experienced until ADH release has ensured that ingested water will be retained by the kidneys.

Other mechanisms are available for the stimulation of thirst and ADH release. These are important in conditions where circulating blood volume falls. They include:

- reduced arterial blood pressure (signals via carotid and aortic baroceptors)

- reduced central venous pressure (signals via atrial low pressure receptors)

- increased angiotensin II in the brain.

DISTURBANCES OF TOTAL BODY WATER CONTENT

Changes in total body water affect the concentration of solutes in all the body compartments.

Water depletion

Pure water depletion is rare in clinical practice. More usually, it is associated with sodium depletion. Pure water depletion usually results from decreased water intake.

Causes of water depletion include:

- diminished oral intake:
  - exhaustion
  - inability to swallow, e.g. comatose
  - restricted intake after gastrointestinal surgery

- loss of fluid from the lungs
  - hyperventilation with unhumidified air

- diabetes insipidus

- diuretic phase of acute renal failure.

Pure water deficiency is reflected biochemically by hypernatraemia. This is associated with an increase in plasma osmolality, concentrated urine and a low urine sodium concentration despite the hypernatraemia.

Clinical manifestations are usually due to the hypernatraemia which can depress the CNS, leading to lethargy or coma. The plasma sodium is usually in excess of 160 mmol/l. Treatment consists of intravenous administration of water as 5% dextrose in water.

Water intoxication

This is more common in clinical practice. It occurs with the administration of excessively large amounts of water in patients who are unable to excrete it. It is difficult to produce water intoxication in health, the kidneys having a maximal excretory rate of about 750 ml of water per hour.

Causes of water intoxication include:

- impaired renal excretion of water, e.g.:
  - renal failure with excessive intake
  - excessive administration of 5% dextrose in the postoperative period when ADH secretion is high
  - ADH-secreting tumours

- cardiac failure

- liver disease

- hypoalbuminaemia.

The commonest cause of water intoxication in surgical practice is excessive fluid administration in patients with compromised renal function.

Pure water excess is reflected clinically by peripheral oedema, raised JVP and pulmonary oedema.

Treatment depends on the degree of overhydration. If it is associated with gross pulmonary oedema and is life threatening, dialysis or continuous venovenous haemofiltration is indicated. With less severe causes and previous normal renal function, water restriction and the administration of a diuretic will suffice. If cardiac failure is present, digitalization may be indicated. A summary of the disturbances of body water is shown in Table 13.1.

ELECTROLYTE DISORDERS

Sodium

Sodium is the major cation in the extracellular fluid (ECF). In a typical diet 100–300 mmol Na are consumed daily. Almost all of

Table 13.1 Disturbances of body water

	Osmolality of body fluid	Compartment affected	Clinical manifestation
Water excess			
Primary	Reduced	ICF↑ ECF↑	Water intoxication
Secondary to ↑ Na$^+$	Normal	ECF↑	Oedema
Water depletion			
Primary	Increased	ICF↓ ECF↓	Thirst
Secondary to ↓ Na$^+$	Normal	ECF↓	Circulatory collapse

this is absorbed from the gastrointestinal tract, only about 5–10 mmol daily being lost in the faeces. Excretion of sodium is chiefly renal, the only other route in health being from the skin as sweat. The loss of Na$^+$ in sweat is extremely variable. Each litre of sweat contains 30–50 mmol Na so that the loss of a few litres of sweat can cause a significant loss from the ECF.

Regulation of sodium

This occurs by both renal and extrarenal mechanisms.

Renal

Ninety-nine percent of the filtered sodium is reabsorbed, 60% in the proximal tubule, 25% in the loop of Henle and approximately 10% in the distal tubules and collecting ducts. Regulation of sodium balance in the kidney is determined by the GFR, the renin-angiotensin mechanism and several prostaglandins. Angiotensin II has two important intrarenal effects. It stimulates Na reabsorption in most nephron segments and it constricts the glomerular arterioles. These factors favour Na$^+$ retention and restoration of ECF volume.

Extrarenal

These include the renin-angiotensin mechanism via aldosterone and atrial natriuretic peptide (ANP). In addition to its renal function, the renin-angiotensin mechanism has important extrarenal actions. Circulating angiotensin II stimulates release of aldosterone from the zona glomerulosa of the adrenal gland. Aldosterone promotes sodium reabsorption in the distal nephron (distal tubule and collecting ducts) as well as in colonic epithelium and the ducts of salivary and sweat glands.

ANP is released from the cardiac atria in response to stretch. It increases the excretion of Na$^+$ by increasing GFR, inhibiting Na$^+$ reabsorption in the collecting ducts and reducing the secretion of renin and aldosterone.

Sodium excess

Hypernatraemia is usually a sign of water depletion but other causes may be apparent. These are shown in Box 13.1.

Box 13.1 Causes of hypernatraemia

Sodium excess:
Excessive IV sodium therapy, especially postoperatively
Conn's syndrome (primary hyperaldosteronism)
Cushing's syndrome
Steroid therapy
Chronic congestive cardiac failure (CCF)
Cirrhosis of the liver

Water depletion:
Reduced water intake, e.g. coma, confusion
Renal, e.g. osmotic diuresis, diuretic phase of acute renal failure, post-relief of obstructive uropathy, diabetes insipidus
Others, e.g. fever, burns, diarrhoea, fistulae

With sodium retention the osmolality of the ECF increases, resulting in the release of ADH and retention of water in the distal tubules to increase the volume of ECF and restore osmolality to normal.

Clinically, in the presence of sodium excess there is dependent oedema, increase in body weight and eventually pulmonary oedema. Treatment of sodium excess is aimed at reduction of intake together with treatment of the underlying cause, e.g. the use of spironolactone in Conn's syndrome or liver disease and digitalization in congestive cardiac failure. If hypernatraemia is a reflection of water depletion then increase in the water intake by intravenous administration of 5% dextrose will usually suffice.

Sodium depletion

Hyponatraemia may be the result of either water retention or sodium depletion. The causes of sodium deficiency are shown in Box 13.2.

Sodium depletion initially results in a decrease in the osmolality of ECF. So long as osmoregulation continues, loss of Na$^+$ leads to a loss of water at a rate of 1 litre per 150 mmol of Na$^+$. This water loss is shared between the plasma and the extravascular ECF. The consequences are more serious for the circulation than are those of primary water depletion since the ECF and plasma are chiefly affected by the water deficiency. The chief manifestation, there-

Box 13.2 Causes of sodium deficiency

Low intake
    Saline-free intravenous solutions
    Reduced oral intake, e.g. coma, dysphagia

Excessive loss
    Gastrointestinal tract:
        Diarrhoea and vomiting
        Intestinal obstruction
        Fistulas
        Paralytic ileus
Excessive sweating, e.g. fever
Burns
Drainage of ascites
Addison's disease
Diuretics
Inappropriate secretion of ADH:
    Bronchogenic carcinoma
    Head injury

fore, of depletion of body Na^+ is peripheral circulatory failure. Laboratory findings include a raised PCV and eventually urea, creatinine and electrolytes will be disturbed due to a depressed GFR.

Treatment

- Hyponatraemia due to ECF depletion is usually treated with isotonic saline as sodium loss is invariably accompanied by water loss. Infusion of normal saline requires close monitoring with checking of the serum electrolytes and measurement of urinary sodium which increases with adequate sodium repletion.

- Hyponatraemia with an apparently normal or high ECF volume should be treated by water restriction. Avoidance of a diuretic is advisable since this may remove nearly as much sodium as water.

- Severe hyponatraemia (< 119 mEq/l) with clinical symptoms such as fits, confusion or coma should be treated with hypertonic saline.

Potassium

Potassium is the chief intracellular cation, 98% of it being within the cells. The intracellular concentration (150 mmol/l) is not critical but a two- to threefold increase or decrease in the extracellular concentration can paralyse muscle or cause cardiac arrest. Rapid loss of 5% of intracellular K^+ into the ECF would be lethal.

Factors affecting plasma potassium levels include:

- aldosterone, which increases renal excretion by its effects on the distal tubule

- insulin, which promotes entry of K^+ into cells

- acid–base balance, where acidosis results in increased plasma K^+ due to reduced entry into cells and reduced urinary excretion whilst alkalosis causes the opposite effect

- hydration where K^+ is lost from cells in dehydration and returns when the patient is rehydrated

- catabolic states, e.g. trauma, major surgery, severe infection, where K^+ is lost from the cells.

Hyperkalaemia

Hyperkalaemia is a potentially fatal condition of insidious onset. The causes are shown in Box 13.3.

Box 13.3 Causes of hyperkalaemia

Excess administration of potassium, especially rapidly
Renal failure
Haemolysis
Crush injuries
Tissue necrosis, e.g. burns, ischaemia
Metabolic acidosis
Adrenal insufficiency (Addison's disease)

Clinically signs may be difficult to detect and sudden cardiac arrhythmia with cardiac arrest may be the first sign. Laboratory tests will confirm high serum K^+ with acidosis. ECG changes include peaked T-waves, loss of P-waves and widening of the QRS complex. Urgent treatment of hyperkalaemia is required. The following methods are available:

- infusion of calcium gluconate

- infusion of glucose and insulin

- ion exchange resins, e.g. resonium

- haemodialysis

Hypokalaemia

Potassium depletion is usually the result of abnormal losses from the gastrointestinal or renal tract. The causes are shown in Box 13.4.

Clinically fatigue and lethargy are initial symptoms with eventual muscle weakness. Laboratory tests will confirm low serum K^+ together with alkalosis. ECG changes include low broad T-waves and the presence of U-waves. Treatment is by correction of K^+ deficiency with oral supplements or, in severe cases, slow intravenous replacement with careful monitoring.

ACID–BASE BALANCE

During the course of daily metabolism approximately 70 mEq of hydrogen ion is generated into the body fluids. In addition, a large

Box 13.4 Causes of hypokalaemia

Inadequate intake
  Potassium-free IV fluids
  Reduced oral intake:
    Coma
    Dysphagia
Excessive loss
  Renal:
    Diuretics
    Renal tubular disorders
  Gastrointestinal:
    Diarrhoea
    Vomiting
    Fistulas
    Laxatives
    Villous adenoma
  Endocrine:
    Cushing's syndrome
    Steroid therapy
    Hyperaldosteronism (primary and secondary)

amount of carbon dioxide is produced that combines with water to form carbonic acid (H_2CO_3). Efficient methods need to be available to eliminate these acids, otherwise the pH of the body fluids would fall rapidly. Hence buffering systems are required. Buffers are substances which minimise the change of pH for a given addition of acid or alkali. Proteins, haemoglobin, phosphates and bicarbonate are important buffer systems. The bicarbonate system is important in that CO_2 is excreted in the lungs and can be regulated by changes in ventilation. Bicarbonate excretion can also be regulated in the kidney. The lungs are responsible for the excretion of some 15 000 mmol per day of acid while the kidneys excrete only 40–80 mmol per day.

The carbonic acid–bicarbonate system ($H_2O+CO_2 \rightleftharpoons H_2CO_3 \rightleftharpoons H^+ + HCO_3^-$) is catalysed by carbonic anhydrase. The Henderson–Hasselbalch equation is derived from this:

$$pH = pK + \log \frac{[HCO_3^-]}{[H_2CO_3]}$$

The pK for the HCO_3^-/H_2CO_3 system is 6.1. The carbonic acid is more usefully expressed in terms of carbon dioxide and the equation then becomes:

$$pH = 6.1 + \frac{\log[HCO_3^-]}{0.03 \times pCO_2}$$

where 0.03 is the solubility of CO_2 expressed in mmol/l/mmHg and pCO_2 in mmHg.

The equation makes it clear that pH depends on the ratio of $[HCO_3^-]$ to pCO_2, i.e. the buffer pair. HCO_3^- is controlled slowly by the kidneys while CO_2 is controlled rapidly by the lungs. If the CO_2 rises the bicarbonate will also rise to keep the $\frac{HCO_3^-}{pCO_2}$ ratio constant.

Similarly if bicarbonate falls there will be a fall in pCO_2 to prevent a change in pH. If the primary change is an alteration in CO_2 it is called a respiratory acidosis or alkalosis; if it is a primary change in HCO_3^- it is called a metabolic acidosis or alkalosis. A simple way of looking at the Henderson–Hasselbalch equation is:

$$pH = constant + \frac{kidney\ function}{lung\ function}$$

Basically the regulation of pH is achieved through control of:

- excretion of H^+ and reabsorption of HCO_3^- by the kidneys
- excretion of CO_2 by the lungs through regulation of alveolar ventilation
- buffering of H^+ by other buffering systems within the body.

Disturbances of acid–base balance

Major disturbances in acid–base balance are rare in the uncomplicated surgical patient and usually arise in seriously ill patients being managed on high-dependency or intensive care units.

Primary respiratory disturbances cause changes in pCO_2 and produce corresponding effects on the blood hydrogen ion concentration. Primary metabolic disturbances affect the plasma bicarbonate. However, whether the disturbance is primarily respiratory or metabolic, some degree of compensation occurs in either the numerator or denominator of the Henderson–Hasselbalch equation to limit or negate the change in blood pH. Those changes in pCO_2 from respiratory disturbances are compensated for by renal tubular handling of bicarbonate and the metabolic disturbances are compensated for by appropriate respiratory changes.

Box 13.5 Causes of respiratory acidosis (any cause of hypoventilation)

Respiratory depression
  CNS depression:
    Head injury
    Drugs, e.g. opiates, anaesthetics
    Coma
    CVA
    Encephalitis
  Neuromuscular disease:
    Myasthenia gravis
    Guillain–Barré syndrome
  Skeletal disease:
    Kyphoscoliosis
    Ankylosing spondylitis
    Flail chest
Artificial ventilation (uncontrolled and unmonitored)
Impaired gaseous exchange:
  Thoracic injury, e.g. pulmonary contusions
  Obstructive airways disease (acute and chronic)
  Alveolar disease, e.g. pneumonia, ARDS

Respiratory acidosis

Respiratory acidosis is caused by CO_2 retention due to inadequate alveolar ventilation. The causes of respiratory acidosis are shown in Box 13.5. Acute respiratory acidosis occurs when respiration suddenly becomes inadequate. The pCO_2 is elevated but there is little change in plasma bicarbonate concentration (HCO_3^-). Over 80% of carbonic acid resulting from increased pCO_2 is buffered by intracellular mechanisms, e.g. proteins and haemoglobins. Relatively little is buffered by bicarbonate ion and therefore plasma HCO_3 may be normal. Treatment is directed towards the underlying cause and providing assisted ventilation.

Respiratory alkalosis

This occurs when carbon dioxide is lost via excessive pulmonary ventilation. The causes are shown in Box 13.6. The usual cause in surgical practice is prolonged artificial ventilation with inadequate monitoring. Acute hyperventilation lowers the pCO_2 without concomitant changes in plasma HCO_3^-). In the non-ventilated patient, hyperventilation may result from anxiety or fever. Clinical manifestations of respiratory alkalosis include circumoral paraesthesia, paraesthesia in the periphery, carpopedal spasm and a positive Chvostek's sign. These are due to hypocalcaemia which results from a reduced level of ionised calcium in the presence of a raised pH. Treatment is to decrease ventilation, e.g. sedatives in anxiety, rebreathing the same air to decrease CO_2 loss or adjustment in mechanical ventilation.

Box 13.6 Causes of respiratory akalosis (any cause of hyperventilation)

Stimulation of respiratory centre:
    High altitude (hypoxia)
    Pneumonia
    Pulmonary oedema
    Pulmonary embolism
    Fever
    Head injury
    Metabolic acidosis (overcompensation)
Increased alveolar gas exchange:
    Hyperventilation, e.g. hysteria, pain, anxiety
    Artificial ventilation (uncontrolled)

Metabolic acidosis

Metabolic acidosis is caused by increased production of hydrogen ion from metabolic causes or from excessive bicarbonate losses. In either case the plasma HCO_3^- is decreased, producing an increased hydrogen ion concentration. The causes are shown in Box 13.7.

Metabolic acidosis may occur with a normal anion gap or an increased anion gap due to an increased acid pool. For electrochemical neutrality of the ECF, the number of anions must equal

---

Box 13.7 Causes of metabolic acidosis

Excessive production of H^+:
    Diabetic ketoacidosis
    Lactic acidosis secondary to hypoxia
    Septicaemia
    Starvation
Impaired excretion of H^+:
    Acute renal failure
    Chronic renal failure
Excess loss of base:
    Diarrhoea
    Intestinal, biliary and pancreatic fistulas

---

the number of cations. Normally only Na^+, K^+, HCO_3^- and Cl^- are measured in the laboratory. When the normal values of these are added they do not balance, i.e. Na^+ (140) + K^+ (5) = 145; and HCO_3^- (25) + Cl^- (105) = 130. The difference, 15 mEq/l, is known as the anion gap and represents anions that are not usually measured. With excessive bicarbonate loss, e.g. diarrhoea, fistulas, the decrease in plasma HCO_3 is matched by an increase in the serum Cl^- so that the anion gap remains around the normal level. Metabolic acidosis resulting from an increased production of acid is associated with an increased anion gap. Conditions in which this may occur are lactic acidosis secondary to hypoxia, ketoacidosis of diabetes and renal failure. The lungs compensate by hyperventilation which returns the hydrogen ion concentration to normal by lowering pCO_2. Clinically the patient has rapid deep respirations. Arterial blood gas analysis shows the characteristic picture of low pH, low standard bicarbonate and a low arterial pCO_2. Serum K^+ is elevated because of a shift from ICF to ECF.

Treatment is directed at the underlying cause. HCO_3^- loss due to diarrhoea or pancreatic fistulas is treated with appropriate fluid and bicarbonate replacement. Acid retention, i.e. increased anion gap, requires specific therapy for each cause. Diabetic ketoacidosis is treated with insulin and fluid replacement, renal failure with dialysis and lactic acidosis is managed with treatment appropriate to the treatment of shock.

Metabolic alkalosis

Metabolic alkalosis is probably the most common cause of disturbance of acid–base balance in surgical patients. The causes are

---

Box 13.8 Causes of metabolic alkalosis

Excess loss of H^+:
    Vomiting
    Nasogastric aspiration
    Gastric fistula
    Diuretic therapy (thiazide or loop)
    Cushing's syndrome
    Conn's syndrome
Excessive intake of base:
    Antacids, e.g. milk-alkali syndrome

---

shown in Box 13.8. Blood hydrogen ion concentration is decreased as a result of the accumulation of bicarbonate in the plasma. Metabolic alkalosis is usually caused by prolonged vomiting or nasogastric aspiration.

Hydrochloric acid secretion by the gastric mucosa returns bicarbonate to the blood. Gastric acid is subsequently reabsorbed in the small bowel so that there is no net gain or loss of N^+. If H^+ is lost by vomiting there is a net gain of HCO_3^- in the circulation. This is usually excreted by the kidneys but if volume depletion accompanies the loss of H^+, the kidneys preserve fluid by increasing sodium absorption and any anions filtered. Consequently the excess bicarbonate is not excreted and perpetuates the metabolic alkalosis. The kidney attempts to compensate by conserving H^+ at the expense of K^+ lost in the urine. The patient becomes hypokalaemic not only because of excess urinary loss but because K^+ shifts into the cells in response to the alkalosis.

Metabolic alkalosis may also occur due to loss of K^+. Without an adequate K^+ the kidney must exchange H^+ for Na^+, resulting in loss of acid in the urine.

Estimation of electrolytes reveals an elevated HCO_3^- and decreased K^+. Compensation is by hypoventilation to increase pCO_2 and by renal loss of HCO_3^-. Treatment varies with the cause. Loss of acid by vomiting or nasogastric aspiration requires fluid replacement, usually as normal saline. With adequate fluid replacement, the stimulus to tubular sodium reabsorption is diminished and the kidneys can then excrete the excess bicarbonate. Potassium chloride should also be given to correct K^+ deficiency. K^+ loss, usually due to diuretics, requires K^+ replacement.

A summary of disturbances of acid–base balance is shown in Table 13.2.

Mixed acid–base disorders

In many situations mixed disorders of acid–base balance occur. The commonest example in surgical practice is a combination of metabolic acidosis and respiratory alkalosis. This may occur in renal failure, with sepsis and in septic shock. As the two acid–base disorders tend to cancel each other out, the disturbance in H^+ is usually small. Respiratory acidosis and metabolic acidosis may occur together in ARDS, cardiac failure and cardiac respiratory arrest. Respiratory alkalosis and metabolic alkalosis in combination is rare but may occur when overventilating a patient with chronic respiratory acidosis.

Interpretation of acid–base changes

A blood gas analyser usually prints out the variables shown below. The example shows normal values.

Temp	37°
pH	7.35–7.45
pCO_2	4.6–5.8 kPa (35–44 mmHg)
pO_2	10–13 kPa (75–10 mmHg)
HCO_3^- (actual)	22–26 mmol/l
Total CO_2	24–28 mmol/l
Standard bicarbonate	22–26 mmol/l
Base excess	−2 to +2 mmol/l
Standard base excess	−3 to +3 mmol/l
O_2 saturation	>95%
Hb	11.5–15.5 g/dl

As the patient's acid–base status varies, three factors are changing at the same time: pH, pCO_2 and HCO_3^-. These and other variables are measured on a blood gas analyser as indicated above. The actual bicarbonate is calculated from the Henderson–Hasselbalch equation. The standard bicarbonate is a value obtained after correction of the pCO_2 to 40 mmHg (5.3 kPa). This correction is required in order to remove any respiratory component. In other words, it indicates what the bicarbonate would be if there were no respiratory disturbance. The normal standard bicarbonate is 22–26 mmol/l. Values above this range indicate metabolic alkalosis: values below indicate metabolic acidosis.

The base excess (or deficit) is the amount of base or acid required to return the pH to 7.4 at a pCO_2 of 40 mmHg (5.3 kPa) and a temperature of 37°. The base excess indicates the metabolic status of the patient, i.e. a base excess indicates metabolic alkalosis, a base deficit (or negative excess) indicates metabolic acidosis.

The standard base excess takes into account the difference in buffering capacity between the patient's ECF and the patient's blood which was analysed. The interstitial component of the ECF has less protein and haemoglobin and therefore less buffering capacity than blood. Standard base excess is usually greater than the base excess, although in practice, the difference is not important.

Interpretation of blood gas analysis should be performed systematically. First the pH should be noted. This indicates whether the patient is acidotic or alkalotic. Next the pCO_2 is noted. This will indicate the respiratory component, i.e. it will be elevated in a respiratory acidosis and decreased in a respiratory alkalosis. Next, the standard bicarbonate or base excess is noted. Both give the same information,

Table 13.2 Disturbances of acid base balance

Abnormality	Primary disturbance	pH	Base excess	Compensatory mechanism
Metabolic acidosis	HCO_3^- ↓	↓	−ve	↓ pCO_2
Respiratory acidosis	pCO_2 ↑	↓		↑ HCO_3^-
Metabolic alkalosis	HCO_3^- ↑	↑	+ve	↑ pCO_2
Respiratory alkalosis	pCO_2 ↓	↑		↓ HCO_3^-

i.e. the metabolic acid–base status after correcting for the pCO_2. The serum electrolytes should then be checked and the anion gap (see above) calculated. It is normally between 10 and 19 mmol/l and reflects the concentration of those anions present in the serum but not routinely measured, e.g. phosphates, organic acids. The significance of the measurement of the anion gap is that in certain metabolic acidoses, e.g. lactic acidosis and diabetic ketoacidosis, it will be increased by the presence of organic anions while in metabolic acidosis in which chloride replaces bicarbonate, e.g. diarrhoea, fistulas in which bicarbonate is lost, the anion gap will remain normal.

NORMAL FLUID AND ELECTROLYTE REQUIREMENTS

An average adult normally loses between 2.5 and 3 l of fluid in 24 hours, approximately 1 l being lost from the skin and lungs (insensible losses), 100 ml in the faeces and the remainder in the urine. About 100–150 mmol of Na^+ and 50–100 mmol K^+ are lost in the urine each day. This is usually balanced by normal dietary intake.

Fluid balance in the uncomplicated patient

In patients maintained on an intravenous infusion the appropriate amounts of Na^+ and K^+ should be added to the water requirement. In the uncomplicated patient, therefore, 2.5–3 l of intravenous fluid containing 150 mmol of Na^+ and 60 mmol of K^+ should be administered. A suitable fluid regime for 24 hours would therefore be as follows.

500 ml 0.9% sodium chloride + 20 mmol KCL
500 ml 5% dextrose
500 ml 5% dextrose + 20 mmol KCL
500 ml 0.9% sodium chloride
500 ml 5% dextrose + 20 mmol KCL
500 ml 5% dextrose

Each bag of fluid is given over four hours.

Changes in fluid and electrolyte requirements in response to surgery and trauma

Following surgery or trauma certain physiological responses occur in the body. Catecholamines are released and stress stimulates the hypothalamo-pituitary-adrenal axis with an increase in secretion of cortisol and aldosterone. These hormones produce conservation of sodium and water by the kidney, resulting in reduction of urine volume and urine sodium concentration. If renal perfusion falls, e.g. due to haemorrhage or loss of fluid into other spaces, then the renin-angiotensin-aldosterone mechanism is activated. This also promotes reabsorption of sodium and water and more potassium is lost in the urine. ADH secretion from the posterior pituitary gland also leads to water conservation. Despite the loss of potassium in the urine, serum potassium does not usually fall but may even rise, due to release of potassium from tissue damage

caused by trauma or surgery or administration of stored blood containing excessive potassium.

These factors must be taken into account when prescribing intravenous fluids, particularly in the first 24 hours after major surgery. The regime described above for the uncomplicated patient may not be appropriate and an appropriate regime for the first 24 hours postoperatively is indicated below.

500 ml 0.9% sodium chloride
500 ml 5% dextrose
500 ml 5% dextrose
500 ml 5% dextrose

Each bag of fluid is given over six hours.

Fluid and electrolyte balance on subsequent days should be managed according to measured losses and electrolyte estimation. In the elderly and those with cardiac or renal problems, fluid balance is best managed with the aid of CVP monitoring.

In previously fit patients the kidneys are normally able to maintain fluid and electrolyte homeostasis in the face of variations in intravenous administration of fluid and electrolytes. However, the compensatory capacity may be reduced by renal parenchymal disease and chronic renal impairment.

FLUID AND ELECTROLYTE PROBLEMS IN SURGICAL PATIENTS

The common causes of fluid and electrolyte loss in surgical patients are shown in Box 13.9.

Blood and plasma

Blood loss may be rapid, the loss of 1 litre causing hypotension and hypovolaemic shock. Blood loss obviously must be replaced

---

Box 13.9 Causes of fluid loss in surgical patients

Blood
    Trauma
    Surgery
Plasma
    Burns
Gastrointestinal
    Nasogastric aspiration
    Vomiting
    Diarrhoea
    Intraluminal: Intestinal obstruction
                     Paralytic ileus
    Fistulas
    Stomas
Exudate in peritoneal cavity:
    Peritonitis
    Acute pancreatitis (also into the retroperitoneum)
    Septicaemia
Excess insensible loss:
    Fever
    Sweating
    Hyperventilation

Table 13.3 Normal daily gastrointestinal secretion volumes and electrolyte composition

Secretion	Volume (l)	Na$^+$ (mmol/l)	K$^+$ (mmol/l)	Cl$^-$ (mmol/l)	HCO$_3^-$ (mmol/l)
Saliva	1–1.5	20–80	10–20	20–40	20–160
Gastric juice	1–2.5	40–100	5–10	120–140	0
Bile	0.5–1.5	140–200	5–10	40–60	20–60
Pancreatic juice	1–2	130	5–10	10–60	80–120
Succus entericus	2–3	140	5	Variable	Variable

by blood but initially plasma expanders such as gelatin solutions are used until crossmatched blood is available. Less rapid haemorrhage allows time for the loss to be replaced from the extracellular extravascular compartment. Thus greater volumes may be lost slowly before the circulation is compromised. Plasma loss from severe burns is replaced by plasma, the anticipated losses being replaced according to a standard formula.

Gastrointestinal losses

Between 6 and 10 litres of electrolyte-rich fluid are secreted into the upper gastrointestinal tract daily (Table 13.3). Most of this fluid is reabsorbed lower down in the intestine.

Abnormal fluid losses must either be measured or estimated as accurately as possible. With sequestration in the bowel lumen only an estimate can be made but with fistulas the amount can be measured accurately and its electrolyte content assessed.

As a general rule gastrointestinal fluid losses should be replaced with normal saline with the addition of potassium as necessary. Volume replacement is best assessed by measuring the urine output and the CVP. Regular assessment of serum electrolytes will provide information regarding their requirements.

Intraperitoneal loss of fluid

Peritonitis and acute pancreatitis will result in loss of fluid, rich in protein and electrolytes, into the peritoneal cavity and, in the case of acute pancreatitis, the retroperitoneum. These losses should be made good by plasma substitutes and normal saline.

Septicaemia

Septic shock is associated with peripheral vasodilatation causing relative hypovolaemia. There is a large increase in capillary permeability resulting in extensive loss of protein and electrolytes from the circulation into the extracellular space. This loss, combined with peripheral vasodilatation, results in collapse and shock. Fluid replacement is with plasma expanders and normal saline. The exact fluid loss is difficult to estimate but should be monitored by urine output, blood pressure, CVP and often pulmonary wedge pressure monitoring.

Excessive insensible fluid loss

Insensible fluid losses may be greatly increased in the ill patient. Pyrexia increases insensible losses by about 10% for each degree Celsius rise in temperature, the loss being chiefly from the lungs as expired water vapour. Excessive sweating causes loss of sodium-rich fluid, sweat containing about 50 mEq/l Na$^+$. This may easily be overlooked in the pyrexic patient in a hot humid ward in the summer months.

Renal failure

Acute renal failure

Acute renal failure (ARF) is defined as a rapid decline in renal function over hours or days which is of sufficient severity to disturb homeostasis. It may result from impaired renal perfusion (prerenal), intrinsic renal disease (renal) or obstruction to the renal tract (postrenal). A list of causes of renal failure is shown in Box 13.10.

The large majority of ARF cases will fall into the categories of prerenal failure or acute tubular necrosis (ATN). The term prerenal failure is used when renal dysfunction is entirely attributable to hypoperfusion and restoration of renal perfusion leads to resumption of renal function. The term acute tubular necrosis is used to define a sequence of events that comprises:

- circulatory compromise and/or nephrotoxins
- urinary abnormalities suggestive of tubular dysfunction
- recovery of renal function within days or weeks.

Prerenal failure and ATN almost invariably occur in the presence of shock. If the patient has not been in shock then it is unlikely that the cause of their acute renal failure is prerenal failure or ATN due to haemodynamic problems. It is therefore important in this context to look for obstructive (postrenal) or intrinsic renal causes.

Most circumstances predisposing to prerenal failure are invariably associated with secretion of ADH. ADH acts on the collecting ducts to increase tubular reabsorption of water but also of urea. This may explain why the plasma urea increases out of proportion to the creatinine in prerenal failure. The plasma urea may also

Box 13.10 Causes of acute renal failure

Prerenal
    Dehydration
    Haemorrhage
    Burns
    Acute pancreatitis
    Sepsis
    Congestive cardiac failure
Renal
    Renovascular disease:
        Embolus
        Thrombosis
    Parenchymal renal disease:
        Renal ischaemia (acute tubular necrosis)
        Nephrotoxins, e.g. gentamicin, radiographic contrast medium
        Glomerulonephritis
        Interstitial nephritis
        Impaired uric acid metabolism
    Myoglobinuria:
        Crush injury
        Compartment syndrome
    Haemoglobinuria:
        Haemolysis
Postrenal
    Ureteric obstruction, e.g. calculous disease, especially with single kidney
    Prostatic hypertrophy
    Urethral abnormalities
    Pelvic tumours
    Retroperitoneal fibrosis

increase out of proportion to the creatinine with sepsis and in patients on steroids, due to the catabolic effect, and with gastrointestinal haemorrhage due to the absorption of protein, associated with the blood, from the bowel lumen.

The distinction between prerenal failure and ATN due to haemodynamic instability may be difficult. Biochemical analysis of the urine may be helpful. In prerenal failure the urinary electrolytes reflect the response of normal tubules to impaired renal function. There is retention of sodium and water, leading to low urinary sodium with a high urinary urea and creatinine. The urine osmolarity is high. Restoration of renal perfusion leads to a rapid improvement in renal function. With ATN the urinary sodium is elevated and the concentrations of urea and creatinine are low. The urine osmolality is also low. These changes are indicative of tubular dysfunction. Whatever the treatment, renal function rarely improves rapidly. The changes in urinary biochemical indices in prerenal failure and acute tubular necrosis are shown in Table 13.4.

The clinical diagnosis of renal failure is made when plasma urea and creatinine are elevated. Other important biochemical changes include:

- hyperkalaemia
- metabolic acidosis
- hypocalcaemia
- hyperphosphataemia.

Hyperkalaemia is due not only to reduced urinary excretion but also to potassium release from cells, e.g. with extensive tissue damage or increased catabolism as in sepsis, burns or rhabdomyolysis. In ARF the renal buffer systems for excreting acid are impaired and metabolic acidosis occurs, with consequent release of potassium from cells.

In ARF the plasma Na+ is usually normal since deficits of sodium are usually matched by those of water. Hence ECF volume may be reduced but plasma sodium concentration remains the same. However, intake of water may exceed the rate at which it can be excreted and hyponatraemia may result.

Classically three phases of acute renal failure are described:

- oliguric phase
- diuretic phase
- recovery phase.

Oliguric phase

This usually begins within 24 hours of the inciting event. The average duration is 1–2 weeks. If it lasts longer than four weeks,

Table 13.4 Distinction between physiological oliguria and acute tubular necrosis

Urine	Prerenal oliguria	Acute tubular necrosis
Specific gravity	> 1020	< 1010
Osmolality mosmol/kg	> 500	< 350
Sodium mmol/l	< 15	> 40
Urine/serum creatinine	> 40	< 20
Fractional sodium excretion*	< 1	> 2
Renal failure index**	< 1	> 2

*Fractional sodium excretion $= \dfrac{\text{urine sodium} \times \text{plasma creatinine}}{\text{plasma sodium} \times \text{urine creatinine}} \times 100$

**Renal failure index $= \dfrac{\text{urine sodium} \times \text{plasma creatinine}}{\text{urine creatinine}}$

the diagnosis of ATN should be reviewed and consideration given to a diagnosis of acute cortical necrosis, glomerulonephritis or vasculitis. The electrolyte and metabolic consequences of the oliguric phase have been described above.

Diuretic phase

A progressive increase in urine volume is a sign that renal function has started to recover. However, renal function is by no means normal early in the diuretic phase. The persistent reduction in GFR is evident from the failure of plasma urea and creatinine to fall. In patients in hypercatabolic states, plasma urea and creatinine may even continue to rise for several days after the end of the oliguric phase. As GFR increases the levels eventually decline but this may take several weeks.

During the diuretic phase, the kidneys do not have the capacity to modulate sodium excretion in the normal way, such that urinary sodium excretion may be in the range of 50–70 mmol/l. If the urine output is 5 litres a day then around 300 mmol of sodium may be required to prevent negative balance. On occasions the diuretic response may be excessive, i.e. in excess of 5 litres per day. However, such episodes are rare nowadays due to regular dialysis during the oliguric phase preventing overhydration.

Fluid and electrolyte management needs to be as carefully managed during the diuretic phase as during the oliguric phase. The persisting abnormalities of GFR and tubular function may lead to overhydration, underhydration, hypokalaemia or to hyponatraemia or hypernatraemia if oral and intravenous intake are not carefully monitored in the light of urinary losses and estimation of plasma or electrolyte levels.

Recovery phase

Renal function continues to improve from three to 12 months after an episode of ATN. Only in a minority of patients does the GFR return to normal. In addition to persistent minor reductions in GFR, there is evidence that tubular dysfunction may persist with maximum concentrating capacity being permanently impaired in many patients.

Chronic renal failure

In chronic renal failure (CRF) there is a progressive loss of nephrons causing permanently impaired renal function. The first sign of CRF is diminished renal reserve which is detected as a decrease in GFR. When GFR has reached 5 ml/min end-stage renal failure is present and there is a need for dialysis. In CRF compensatory mechanisms maintain acceptable health until the GFR is about 10–15 ml/min. Life-sustaining excretory and homeostatic mechanisms continue until the GFR is less than 5 ml/min.

Water

Inability to concentrate urine in the presence of dehydration is often the first symptom of CRF. This results in the symptoms of polyuria, nocturia and thirst occurring when the GFR is about 30 ml/min. Defective urine concentration is due to increased solute load in surviving nephrons. Thirst accompanies polyuria and water balance is maintained provided that there is access to fluid intake. Careful attention to fluid balance is required in the presence of surgery, fever and other sources of extrarenal loss of water if dehydration, hypotension and consequent further impairment of renal function are to be avoided. Urine dilution is maintained until late in CRF but large water loads are excreted more slowly than in healthy subjects and excess fluid intake results in hyponatraemia with cerebral oedema, the latter causing confusion and convulsions.

Sodium

As renal function decreases, normal mechanisms increase the fraction of filtered sodium excreted so that sodium balance and ECF volume are maintained until the GFR is less than 10 ml/min. As renal failure progresses these adaptive mechanisms are lost and total body sodium increases and, with water to maintain osmotic equilibrium, results in fluid overload, hypertension and oedema.

Potassium

Most patients maintain a normal K^+ until the GFR is less than 5 ml/min but the capacity to excrete potassium is limited. Hyperkalaemia may therefore result from a sudden reduction in GFR, an increase in dietary potassium, the administration of potassium-sparing diuretics, e.g. spironolactone, administration of potassium-containing intravenous fluids, surgery, trauma and hypercatabolic states. Acidosis raises serum potassium by transferring it out of the cells and by interfering with renal excretion.

Acid–base balance

The kidney is the principal organ maintaining acid–base balance by reabsorption of bicarbonate, acidification of urinary buffers and excretion of ammonia. As CRF progresses, intact nephrons increase absorption of bicarbonate and excretion of H^+. Together with intracellular buffers and respiratory compensation, these prevent acidosis until the GFR is less than 20 ml/min. As the GFR falls below 10 ml/min, net acid production exceeds the excretory capacity of the remaining nephrons, diminished tubular function impairs bicarbonate regeneration and ammonia synthesis and acidosis progresses.

As a result of these changes in fluid and electrolyte homeostasis, the following clinical features occur:

- hypertension

- peripheral oedema

- hyponatraemia due to fluid retention

- salt retention

- metabolic acidosis

- hyperkalaemia.

OEDEMA AND LYMPHATIC FUNCTION

Oedema is an increase in the volume of interstitial fluid above normal levels.

Control of flow between plasma and interstitial compartments

A hydrostatic pressure difference across the capillary endothelium results in flow from vessel to tissue space. The retention of plasma proteins within the vasculature is an opposing force, i.e. the plasma oncotic pressure. The Starling equilibrium describes the relationship between hydrostatic pressure, oncotic pressure (colloid osmotic pressure) and fluid flow across the capillary membrane. The blood pressure (hydrostatic pressure) at the arteriolar end of a capillary is about 32 mmHg and at the venular end about 12 mmHg. The hydrostatic pressure in the interstitial fluid is approximately 0 mmHg. The interstitial colloid osmotic pressure (tissue oncotic pressure) varies but averages around 5 mmHg.

According to the Starling equilibrium:

> Capillary hydrostatic pressure plus tissue oncotic pressure (pressure tending to drive fluid out of the capillary) = interstitial fluid pressure plus plasma oncotic pressure (pressure tending to hold fluid into the capillary).

At the arterial end, the net intracapillary hydrostatic pressure, i.e. 32 mmHg, exceeds the net oncotic pressure (i.e. plasma oncotic pressure (25 mmHg) − tissue oncotic pressure (5 mmHg) = 20 mmHg) by 12 mmHg, driving fluid out of the capillaries. The intracapillary hydrostatic pressure at the venous end falls to 12 mmHg and is exceeded by the net oncotic pressure (plasma oncotic pressure − tissue oncotic pressure, i.e. 20 mmHg − 12 mmHg = 8 mmHg inward pressure) and reabsorption begins. Thus filtration is favoured at the arterial end of the capillary while absorption is favoured at the venous end (Fig 13.1). Any fluid not reabsorbed from the interstitium by the capillaries is returned to the circulation by the lymphatic system.

Causes of oedema

The causes of oedema are:

- increased capillary hydrostatic pressure, e.g. chronic right heart failure, venous obstruction, increased fluid volume (overtransfusion)

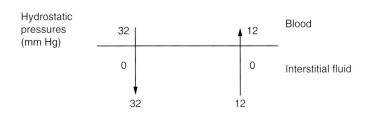
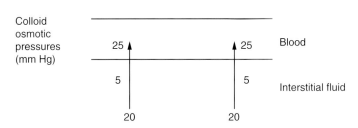
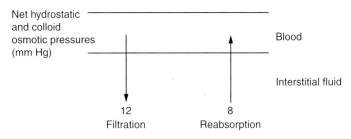

Figure 13.1 The Starling equilibrium across the capillary.

- decreased plasma oncotic pressure due to hypoproteinaemia (e.g. starvation, cirrhosis, nephrotic syndrome)

- increased capillary permeability, e.g. inflammatory or allergic reactions

- increased tissue oncotic pressure, e.g. lymphatic blockage, protein accumulation in burns.

Obstruction to lymphatics (lymphoedema)

The lymphatics remove protein and excess fluid which has been filtered at the arterial end of the capillary and has not been reabsorbed at the venous end. If lymphatic obstruction occurs this fluid cannot return to the vascular system and accumulates behind the obstruction, causing oedema.

Lymphatic obstruction may occur due to lymph node pathology as a result of the following:

- metastatic tumours

- surgical removal, e.g. with mastectomy or block dissection

- irradiation

- filariasis.

14

Blood and reticuloendothelial system

Blood components
Anaemia
  Deficiency of haematinics
  Haemolytic anaemias
  Defective red cell production
  What is a safe haemoglobin level in patients
    undergoing surgery?
Coagulation and bleeding disorders
  Congenital bleeding disorders
  Acquired coagulation disorders
  Thrombocytopenia
  Vascular abnormalities causing bleeding
  Assessment of a patient with bleeding
Thrombotic disorders
  Arterial thrombosis
  Venous thrombosis
  Thrombophilia
  Referral for specialist tests
  Treatment of thrombosis
  Prevention of venous thromboembolism

Blood transfusion
  Blood donation
  Crossmatching blood
  Maximum blood-ordering schedules (MBOS)
  Blood and blood products
  Complications of transfusion
  Hospital transfusion committee
  The Serious Hazards of Transfusion (SHOT)
    scheme
  Autologous transfusion
  Blood substitutes
  Surgery in Jehovah's Witness patients
Immunology
  Immune response to infection
  Allergies
  Transplantation
  Malignant lymphomas
  Biopsy of lymph nodes

J. A. Copplestone, A. L. G. Peel

The anatomy and physiology of blood have been extensively reviewed in the chapter 'Haemopoietic and lymphoreticular systems' in *Fundamentals of Surgical Practice*. This chapter will concentrate on the surgical principles relating to the abnormalities of the blood and the therapeutic use of blood, its components and blood substitutes. It concludes with a section on the surgical aspects of immunology and malignant lymphomas.

BLOOD COMPONENTS

Peripheral blood is composed of fluid and cellular components. The fluid component is important functionally to the surgeon in terms of the intravascular volume, fluid interchanges between the intravascular, interstitial and intracellular spaces, the stable biochemical components with anion and cation ratios, acid–base balance, trace elements and the complex protein fractions. The latter are important in maintaining osmotic pressure, nutritional, haemostatic and immune (antibody) functions.

The cellular components include:

- erythrocytes, responsible for oxygen carriage and delivery to the tissues
- platelets, important in primary haemostasis by plugging endothelial defects and initiating and localising the coagulation cascade to the site of injury
- leucocytes, including both granulocytes and mononuclear cells responsible for host defence.

ANAEMIA

Deficiency of haematinics

Iron

In men and postmenopausal women the most common cause of iron deficiency anaemia is chronic blood loss. In premenopausal women, heavy prolonged menstruation is a frequent cause. Dietary deficiency is rare but iron absorption, never an efficient process, may be further compromised by gastroduodenal disease or surgery. A combination of iron deficiency anaemia and positive faecal occult blood indicates that the site of blood loss is the gastrointestinal tract.

- A full history and clinical examination should be performed, including a rectal examination.
- Before giving oral iron, a full blood count (FBC) should be performed. The peripheral blood film shows microcytic hypochromic red cells. Measurement of the serum iron (low) and total iron-binding capacity (high) or ferritin level (low) gives additional information and helps exclude anaemia of chronic disorder. Rarely, when the state of iron stores remains uncertain, a marrow aspirate can be helpful.

The common causes of iron deficiency associated with gastrointestinal disease are:

- gastric or duodenal ulcer
- gastric carcinoma
- colonic (especially caecal) carcinoma
- inflammatory bowel disease
- coeliac disease.

Other important causes of iron deficiency include:

- reflux oesophagitis
- haemorrhoids
- aspirin or non-steroidal antiinflammatory drugs.

However, the more serious conditions listed above should be excluded before attributing an iron deficient anaemia to such conditions.

Treatment of iron deficiency

- Treat the underlying cause.
- Treat the deficiency with oral iron (ferrous sulphate 200 mg bd in adults), monitoring the reticulocyte response and the haemoglobin level which should rise by 1 g/dl/week. Total dose intravenous infusion may be used when oral iron is not tolerated or ineffective, but may cause anaphylactic reactions. Intramuscular iron is less often used (painful, leaves skin staining). An intravenous formulation of ferric sucrose complex is available for patients not able to take oral preparations.
- Iron treatment should be continued for three months after the haemoglobin has returned to normal and longer if blood loss is continuing.

Folate

Folate deficiency causes a macrocytic anaemia with a low red cell folate level and a megaloblastic marrow indicating a maturation defect in the production of the erythrocyte. The causes of folate deficiency are shown in Box 14.1.

Treatment

Dietary deficiency may be made good by the addition of vegetables or with folic acid tablets. Routine folic acid supplement in the diet eliminates the deficiency in pregnancy which is important in the prevention of fetal abnormalities, especially neural tube defects. Bacterial overgrowth requires broad-spectrum antibiotics and mucosal abnormalities have specific remedies. Folic acid alone should not be given unless the vitamin B_{12} level is known to be normal.

Box 14.1 Causes of folate deficiency

- Increased physiological demands: pregnancy, lactation, prematurity
- Dietary deficiency, especially elderly and alcoholics
- Malabsorption: mucosal abnormality – coeliac disease, gluten enteropathy, tropical sprue
- Drug induced: chemotherapeutic agents (antimetabolites), anticonvulsants
- Increased cell turnover: haemolytic anaemias, myelofibrosis, carcinoma, lymphoma, myeloma
- Other: inflammatory bowel disease, psoriasis, rheumatoid arthritis, tuberculosis

Vitamin B$_{12}$ (cobalamin)

In addition to a macrocytic anaemia, usually thrombocytopenia and neutropenia are present. In pernicious anaemia, neurological disorders, peripheral neuritis and subacute combined degeneration of the spinal cord may occur.

Treatment

Hydroxycobalamin 1 mg by intramuscular injection should commence as soon as blood levels have been taken. Patients usually have a dramatic symptomatic response within 24 hours and there should be a significant reticulocytosis after seven days. On occasions hypokalaemia can occur after treatment. Blood transfusion should be avoided as it may precipitate cardiac failure. A faltering response may be due to concomitant iron deficiency. Schilling's test for vitamin B$_{12}$ absorption should be delayed until the megaloblastosis has resolved. In patients receiving three-monthly maintenance treatment, blood levels of vitamin B$_{12}$ are always high and no further tests are indicated.

Box 14.2 Causes of vitamin B$_{12}$ deficiency

- Pernicious anaemia – an autoimmune condition with atrophic gastritis and deficiency of or blocking antibodies to intrinsic factor
- Total or partial gastrectomy
- Disease (Crohn's disease) or resection or the distal ileum (60 cm)
- Small bowel bacterial overgrowth and utilisation, e.g. diverticulum, blind loop syndrome, strictures, e.g. Crohn's disease
- Nutritional, e.g. vegans.

Other causes of macrocytic red cells include:

- alcohol
- liver disease
- hypothyroidism
- reticulocytosis

- cytotoxic drugs
- aplastic anaemia
- pregnancy
- myelodysplastic syndromes
- myeloma
- neonatal red cells.

Haemolytic anaemias

Haemolytic anaemias are due to an increased premature destruction of red blood cells. Compensatory reticulocytosis occurs if there is an adequate supply of haematinics. The increased Hb breakdown causes jaundice and reduced serum haptoglobins. The causes of haemolytic anaemia are classified as:

- hereditary disorders: Rbc membrane, enzymes, haemoglobin
- acquired disorders: immune autoimmune, alloimmune, drug related, Rbc fragmentation syndromes, infections, chemicals.

Red cell membrane disorders

Hereditary spherocytosis is the most common inherited membrane disorder and is usually due to spectrin abnormality causing increased red cell fragility. Anaemia and jaundice can occur at any age and if severe, can be ameliorated by splenectomy. Ideally this is delayed in childhood because of the risk of overwhelming postsplenectomy infection. Patients often have pigment gallstones and require cholecystectomy.

Other forms of membrane abnormality include hereditary elliptocytosis which has a similar clinical picture to hereditary spherocytosis.

G6PD deficiency

Glucose-6-phosphate dehydrogenase is an important enzyme as it is the only source of NADPH within the red cell. The gene is located on the X chromosome and a wide variety of abnormalities have been reported, mainly affecting males from West Africa, the Mediterranean, the Middle East and South-East Asia. Heterozygote females have a resistance to falciparum malaria.

Infections, acute illnesses, drugs or fava (broad) beans can cause rapid intravascular haemolysis with haemoglobinuria. This can be self-limiting but some cases need blood transfusion.

Haemoglobinopathies

These common inherited diseases are broadly divided into structural abnormalities of haemoglobin, e.g. sickle cell anaemia, and imbalance of globin chain synthesis, the thalassaemias.

Sickle cell anaemia

This disease is caused by a single nucleotide base change in the DNA leading to substitution of valine for glutamine at position 6 of the beta chain of haemoglobin (HbA → HbS). When exposed to low oxygen tension, HbS forms insoluble crystals which polymerise into long fibres and cause the characteristic sickle red cells. These block the microcirculation, causing infarcts, leading to painful crises. Homozygote patients (HbSS) have 90–100% HbS in their red cells but the clinical expression of the disease is very variable. Crises can be painful, visceral, aplastic or haemolytic. Other features include splenomegaly and leg ulceration.

Painful vascular-occlusive crises may be precipitated by:

- dehydration
- hypoxia (anaesthesia)
- vascular stasis.

The pain is severe and often requires opiate analgesia and therefore the possibility of surgical pathology can be difficult to assess. Treatment involves rehydration and adequate analgesia and some patients require red cell exchange transfusion.

Sickle cell trait is due to heterozygote HbAS, where the red cells contain 24–40% HbS. It is a benign condition but crises can still occur in severe stress such as anoxia (anaesthetics) or severe infection.

Sickle Hb can occur in combination with other Hb abnormalities (HbC, HbD, HbE) or with thalassaemias. These tend to affect the red cell sickling disease in different ways, e.g. HbSC patients have an increased risk of venous thromboembolism.

Thalassaemias

In affected individuals, the production of alpha or beta chains of the haemoglobin molecule is imbalanced, giving rise to a microcytic, hypochromic anaemia.

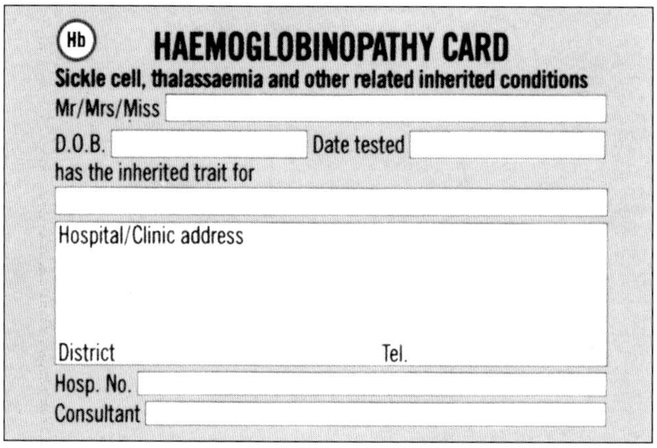
(Hb) HAEMOGLOBINOPATHY CARD
Sickle cell, thalassaemia and other related inherited conditions
Mr/Mrs/Miss
D.O.B. Date tested
has the inherited trait for
Hospital/Clinic address
District Tel.
Hosp. No.
Consultant

Figure 14.1 Haemoglobinopathy card (Crown copyright material is reproduced with the permission of the Controller of Her Majesty's Stationery Office).

Patients with thalassaemia major require red cell transfusion from childhood to prevent skeletal and growth abnormalities. They also need iron chelation.

Patients with thalassaemia trait (thalassaemia minor), however, are usually symptomless. The condition can be suspected from the FBC which shows a low mean cell volume and high red cell count. Confirmation is by Hb electrophoresis, globin chain synthesis or Hb DNA testing. Accurate diagnosis is important for antenatal testing and genetic counselling. Thalassaemia trait patients should not be given iron therapy unless they are shown to have low iron stores.

Immune haemolytic anaemias

These haemolytic anaemias are due to the presence of antibodies directed against red cells. This is detected in the direct antiglobulin (or Coombs) test. They are divided into warm or cold types according to whether the antibody reacts better at 37°C or 4°C. Autoimmune antibodies react against the patient's own red cells and can cause a problem in trying to identify crossmatched blood. Alloimmune antibodies react against foreign red cells, which is most likely to occur following red cell transfusion, but haemolytic disease of the newborn due to Rhesus antibodies is another example. Some drugs such as methyldopa or (large doses of) penicillin can cause immune-mediated haemolysis in the presence of the drug.

Other causes of haemolysis

Red cell fragmentation syndromes occur following physical damage to red cells on artificial heart valves or arterial grafts. In disseminated intravascular coagulation (DIC) cells are damaged by strands of fibrin. The peripheral blood film will show schistocytes and red cell fragments.

Severe burns can damage red cells. Some drugs cause an oxidative haemolysis with Heinz body formation (e.g. dapsone, salazopyrine). Chemical poisoning can cause severe haemolysis with copper (Wilson's disease), lead, chlorate or arsenic. In *Clostridium perfringens* infection and malaria, intravascular haemolysis may occur (blackwater fever).

Defective red cell production

Anaemia arising from marrow failure is not uncommon and may be caused by:

- marrow replacement by metastatic carcinoma, from primary breast, prostate, kidney, bronchus and thyroid carcinomas which typically spread to the marrow bones. This often produces a leucoerythroblastic anaemia, i.e. nucleated red cells and myelocytes are seen in the peripheral blood film
- haematological conditions such as leukaemias, lymphomas, myeloma, myelodysplastic syndromes, aplastic anaemia

- chronic diseases with anaemia of chronic disorder: rheumatoid arthritis, connective tissue disorders (SLE), renal failure (impaired erythropoietin response).

What is a safe haemoglobin level in patients undergoing surgery?

The critical function of haemoglobin is to carry oxygen via the circulation to the tissues where oxygen is consumed. Traditionally, a level of 10 g/dl triggered the need for transfusion. Recently, with the increasing knowledge of the hazards of homologous blood transfusion, particularly transmissible agents, this figure has been lowered to between 7 and 8 g/dl. Other variables are important in the consideration of organ and tissue oxygen consumption, especially the oxygen tension at the venous end of the capillary, reduced blood viscosity, and peripheral vasodilatation. In chronic anaemia, better oxygen delivery is associated with an increase in 2,3-diphosphoglycerate and a shift in the oxygen dissociation curve. How well patients can tolerate anaemia also depends on their age and the presence of cardiovascular and respiratory disease. Some anaemic patients develop episodes of silent myocardial ischaemia detected by continuous 'Holter monitoring' ECGs, leading to myocardial hypoperfusion and potentially lethal adverse cardiac events.

Whilst clinical studies have shown that elevation of the haemoglobin to around 11 g/dl in the critically ill surgical patient allows increased oxygen delivery, experience with Jehovah's Witnesses and renal transplant patients shows that lower levels of Hb are tolerated. A recent randomised trial in critically ill patients showed that a restrictive transfusion policy (maintaining Hb 7–9 g/dl) resulted in lower in-hospital mortality than a more liberal policy (Hb 10–12 g/dl).

Although there is no statistically derived haemoglobin level to trigger transfusion, consider:

- lost circulating volume
- red cell transfusion is not indicated if actual or anticipated Hb >10 g/dl.
- red cell transfusion is always indicated if Hb <7 g/dl. Transfuse according to red cell loss.
- patients with Hb 7–10 g/dl are in a grey area
- in patients who will tolerate anaemia poorly, e.g. age over 65 years, the presence of cardiovascular or respiratory disease, consider raising the level at which transfusions are indicated to 8 g/dl
- risk of further bleeding from disordered haemostasis.

COAGULATION AND BLEEDING DISORDERS

Injury to the vascular endothelium breaches its integrity, permitting extravasation of blood into the extravascular space. This is limited by local vasoconstriction. Platelet adhesion to the damaged endothelium in the presence of von Willebrand factor, with release of the contents of the platelet granules, causes the formation of a platelet plug. The activation of coagulation factors on receptors on the platelet membrane initiates the coagulation cascade at the point of endothelial damage (Figure 14.2). Finally, after a series of enzymatic reactions, the unstable platelet plug becomes a stable fibrin clot.

At the same time as the coagulation system is activated, plasminogen is converted to plasmin by tissue plasminogen activator and to some extent by factors XIIa and kallikrein. Thrombin also binds to thrombomodulin on the endothelial cell surface and activates protein C which, with protein S, destroys activated factors VIIIa and Va, thus preventing further thrombin generation.

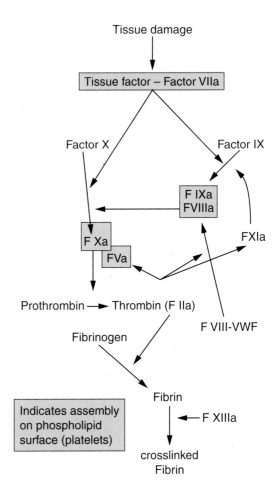

a = activated factor

Figure 14.2 The coagulation cascade.

Congenital bleeding disorders

Haemophilia A and B are caused by deficiencies of factors VIII (FVIII) and IX respectively. The prevalence of haemophilia A is 1 in 10 000 of the population and the prevalence of haemophilia B (Christmas disease) is 1 in 50 000.

Clinical presentations of haemophilia include painful haemarthrosis (resulting in progressive arthropathy), muscle haematomas and prolonged bleeding after trauma or surgery. The severity of bleeding depends on the level of factor: <1 iu/dl severe, 1–5 iu/dl moderate, >5 iu/dl mild. Both forms are X-linked recessive disorders which affect males carrying the mutant allele on a single X chromosome. The daughter of a haemophiliac will be an obligate carrier and the son of a haemophiliac will be normal. For a female carrier there is a 50% chance of a son being a haemophiliac and a 50% chance of a daughter being a carrier. Not all patients have a family history as new mutations occur.

Treatment is by factor concentrate – recombinant DNA manufactured protein for children and derived from plasma for adults. Some patients can develop inhibitors (antibodies) which make treatment difficult and expensive. In all cases of surgery involving a haemophiliac patient, close cooperation with a haematologist is essential to ensure adequate supplies of factor concentrate and appropriate monitoring of the factor level. All patients likely to need blood products should receive immunisation with hepatitis A and B virus vaccines.

Von Willebrand's disease

This is a heterogeneous condition arising from qualitative or quantitative disorders of the von Willebrand factor (VWF) gene, which has been mapped to chromosome 12. It is approximately five times more common than haemophilia. Bleeding is usually mild to moderate and is commonly mucosal or associated with excessive bruising, but haemarthrosis and postsurgical bleeding can occur. The diagnosis can be difficult if FVIII and VWF levels are within the normal range. Patients can often be managed with DDAVP (a vasopressin analogue) and tranexamic acid, but tachyphylaxis occurs. For severe cases or major surgery, VWF concentrate may be required. In one variety (type IIb) which also has thrombocytopenia, DDAVP is not used.

Acquired coagulation disorders

These are caused by:

- clotting factor deficiencies
- peripheral consumption of clotting factors
- platelet abnormalities
- vascular abnormalities.

In many clinical situations, several abnormalities are present at the same time.

Vitamin K deficiency

Vitamin K is required to complete the manufacture of factors II (prothrombin), VII, IX and X, protein C and protein S in the liver. The precursor forms of the proteins are converted to biologically active forms by gamma-carboxylation of glutamic acid which can bind calcium ions when complexed with phospholipid. Warfarin inhibits the recycling of vitamin K in this reaction. Vitamin K is a fat-soluble vitamin obtained from green vegetables and bacterial synthesis in the gastrointestinal tract. The causes of deficiency are:

- poor dietary intake
- malabsorption syndromes
- obstructive jaundice
- drugs – warfarin, phenindione, nicoumalone.

The prothrombin time or INR (international normalised ratio, a ratio of the patient's prothrombin time to that of a normal individual) and the APTT (activated partial thromboplastin time) are prolonged. Treatment depends on the cause and whether oral vitamin K will be absorbed. Correction of the INR occurs after six hours but may take up to two days because of the varying rates of production of the clotting factors affected.

Oral anticoagulants and surgery

Warfarin is increasingly being used in the treatment and prevention of thromboembolic disease and in patients with atrial fibrillation. This means that it is not uncommon for patients requiring surgery to be taking anticoagulants or to present with symptoms which could arise from haemorrhage.

- Management of the patient depends on the indication for the anticoagulation. In some situations, e.g. metal prosthetic heart valves, some form of anticoagulation is required and the patient will need to be changed to heparin.

- Elective surgery – warfarin may need to be stopped three days prior to admission and the INR should be below 2.5 It can be recommenced at the usual daily dose postoperatively as soon as the patient has an oral intake, provided there is no excessive bleeding.

- Warfarin can be reversed using vitamin K, fresh frozen plasma, prothrombin complex depending on the urgency of surgery and the risk of bleeding (Box 14.3).

- Many drugs can alter the effect of warfarin, especially antibiotics, and the INR should be carefully monitored and warfarin dose adjusted appropriately. Drug interactions are listed in books such as the British National Formulary.

Liver disease

In acute and chronic liver disease, the bleeding disorder is multifactorial.

Box 14.3 Recommendations for management of bleeding and excessive anticoagulation in patients on warfarin

INR 3.0–6.0 (target 2.5) INR 4.0–6.0 (target 3.5)	Reduce warfarin dose or stop. restart warfarin when INR < 5.0
INR 6.0–8.0 no or minor bleeding	Stop warfarin restart when INR < 5.0
INR > 8.0 no or minor bleeding	Stop warfarin restart warfarin when INR < 5.0 if other risk factors for bleeding give 0.5–2.0 mg vitamin K po
Major bleeding	Stop warfarin give FFP 15 ml/kg or prothrombin complex 50 u/kg give 5.0 mg vitamin K iv/po

- Impaired vitamin K absorption leading to the synthesis of functionally inactive vitamin K-dependent clotting factors.

- Hypersplenism.

- Defective platelet function.

- Functional abnormalities of fibrinogen.

- Disseminated intravascular coagulation – often low-grade and chronic due to failure to clear activated clotting factors from the blood.

- Oesophageal varices.

Massive blood transfusion

This is usually defined as transfusion of over 10 units of blood within 24 hours. It is often associated with abnormalities of other systems (e.g. hepatorenal failure). Coagulation factors and platelets are consumed at the site of bleeding and replacement of stored blood has a further dilutional effect. In some situations, DIC may also be present.

Renal failure

In the presence of uraemia, platelets have abnormal function. Patients with nephrotic syndrome excrete coagulation factors, antithrombin and plasminogen into the urine and not uncommonly develop a thrombotic tendency.

Disseminated intravascular coagulopathy (DIC)

In this clinical syndrome there is unregulated thrombus generation at the site of endothelial injury resulting in the release of thrombin into the circulation. Widespread thrombosis in the microvascular circulation leads to tissue ischaemia and damage.

Consumption of coagulation factors and activation of fibrinolysis occur in the systemic circulation, leading to the clinical manifestation of thrombosis and bleeding.

The clinical presentation varies according to the aetiology but in acute DIC there is usually hypotensive shock, bleeding from wounds, venepuncture and line sites, bleeding from respiratory and gastrointestinal tracts and spontaneous bruising and petechiae. In addition, there may be evidence of thrombosis with venous thromboembolism, digital ischaemia, skin necrosis and gangrene and multiorgan failure (renal, liver, cerebral, respiratory and cardiovascular systems).

Box 14.4 Causes of DIC

Acute disseminated intravascular coagulopathy
- Infections (greater than 50% of cases) especially Gram-negative organisms (endotoxin) and meningococcal septicaemia (increased risk in patient without a functional spleen)
- Trauma
- Liver disease (acute hepatic necrosis)
- Transfusion with ABO incompatible blood
- Obstetric complications including placental separation and amniotic fluid embolus
- Anaphylaxis

Chronic disseminated intravascular coagulopathy
- Carcinomatosis, especially mucin-secreting adenocarcinoma
- Liver disease
- Retained dead fetus
- Aneurysm or vascular malformation

Treatment of DIC

- Treat the underlying cause (if possible).

- Maintain the blood pressure with adequate quantities of crystalloid and red cells.

- Monitor the FBC, platelet count, INR, APPT and fibrinogen level. The presence of FDPs (fibrin degradation products) and fragmented red cells on the film helps to make a diagnosis of DIC but is not useful in monitoring treatment.

- Replace the deficiency of platelets and coagulation factors with platelet concentrates and fresh frozen plasma according to the abnormalities of laboratory tests. If the fibrinogen level is very low, replacement with cryoprecipitate may be necessary.

- In severe DIC, replacement with antithrombin or protein C concentrate has helped patients with marked thrombotic problems. Heparin is occasionally used but can exacerbate bleeding.

- Fibrinolytic inhibitors should not be used as they can worsen thrombotic end-organ failure.

Coagulation inhibitors

Some patients can develop antibodies against coagulation factors, so-called 'inhibitors'. Their presence is suspected when a long INR or APTT is not corrected with normal plasma (which will replace missing factors). Specific assays will confirm the presence of an inhibitor and its titre. This can occur in patients receiving factor concentrates but acquired factor VIII inhibitors also occur in other patients. Surgery should not be attempted in these patients unless absolutely necessary because bleeding can be difficult to control and very expensive to treat.

Thrombocytopenia

Bleeding due to abnormal platelet number or function is characterised by skin purpura (often appearing first on the ankle and shin) or prolonged bleeding after trauma. Provided platelet function remains normal, levels have to fall significantly (below $20 \times 10^9/l$) before spontaneous bleeding occurs. Many drugs, especially aspirin and non-steroidal antiinflammatory drugs, will inhibit platelet function and lead to bruising at higher platelet counts.

Pseudothrombocytopenia

When thrombocytopenia is unexpected, artefactual thrombocytopenia should be considered. It arises from poor venesection technique, with clotting occurring within the specimen bottle, and some patients develop platelet clumping in the presence of EDTA. The platelet count can be checked using citrate as an anticoagulant or a fresh blood film can be examined.

Box 14.5 Causes of thrombocytopenia

Failure of platelet production
- Megakaryocyte depression – drugs, chemicals, viral infection
- Marrow failure – cytotoxic drugs, radiotherapy, leukaemias, marrow infiltration, myeloma, myelodysplastic syndromes, megaloblastic anaemia, HIV infection

Increased consumption of platelets
- Immune – autoimmune thrombocytopenic purpura (AITP)
- Immune thrombocytopenia may also occur secondary to drugs – gold, penicillins, diuretics
  Systemic lupus erythematosus
  Chronic lymphocytic leukaemia
  Infections – HIV
  Heparin
  Post-transfusion purpura
  Neonatal (isoimmune) purpura
- Disseminated intravascular coagulopathy
- Thrombotic thrombocytopenic purpura

Abnormal distribution of platelets
- Splenomegaly

Dilutional loss
- Massive transfusion

Treatment

In the treatment of thrombocytopenia, platelet transfusions are usually effective but in some conditions, platelets are ineffective or contraindicated. Four such conditions are listed below.

Autoimmune thrombocytopenia (AITP)

AITP is acute and self-limiting in childhood. Patients with acute AITP often have a previous viral infection. Adults are more likely to have a chronic form of AITP and this disease often affects women in the 20–50 age group. Treatment is aimed at controlling bleeding symptoms rather than normalising the platelet count. Some patients with mild thrombocytopenia may simply be observed. Others require treatment with steroids, splenectomy, high-dose intravenous immunoglobulins (IVIgG) or immunosuppressive drugs.

Heparin-associated thrombocytopenia (HAT)

HAT occurs 5–10 days after starting heparin and is associated with a fall in platelet count. A few patients develop severe arterial and venous thrombi. Diagnosis is difficult because rapid, specific tests are not generally available. Heparin of all forms should be stopped immediately and in the presence of thrombosis, treatment with danaparoid or a thrombin inhibitor (hirudin or lepirudin) should be considered.

Thrombotic thrombocytopenic purpura (TTP)

TTP (Moschcowitz syndrome) is characterised by fever, microangiopathic haemolytic anaemia, thrombocytopenia, renal failure and neurological dysfunction. Although rare, it is increasingly being seen after bone marrow transplantation and in HIV infection. Patients require fresh frozen plasma often combined with plasmapheresis.

Post-transfusion purpura

This is a rare but potentially lethal condition where severe thrombocytopenia develops 5–12 days after a blood transfusion. It is due to a platelet alloantibody. The recipient is usually homozygous for human platelet antigen HPA1b and makes anti-HPA1a which reacts initially with transfused platelets and later with the patient's own platelets. Affected patients also have tissue type HLA DR 52a.

Platelet transfusion should not be used and the treatment is high-dose IVIgG and steroids.

Vascular abnormalities causing bleeding

These disorders usually cause bruising and bleeding from small vessels. Standard clotting tests are often normal.

- Hereditary haemorrhagic telangiectasia (Osler–Weber–Rendu syndrome) is an autosomal dominant condition where telangiectasia develops in the skin, mucous membranes and internal organs. Chronic iron deficiency can result from recurrent gastrointestinal bleeding.

- Simple bruising.

- Senile purpura.

- Steroid medication.

- Infections: dengue, viral or associated with DIC.

- Henoch–Schonlein purpura in children.

- Scurvy.

- Connective tissue disorders: Ehlers–Danlos syndrome (a hereditary collagen disorder).

Assessment of a patient with bleeding

When reviewing a patient with bleeding, consider the following.

History

- Recent bleeding problems.

- Type of surgery and anaesthetics.

- Past experience with any surgery.

- Drug therapy including self-medication with aspirin and NSAIDs.

- Family history of bleeding.

- Other medical conditions.

Examination

- Sites of bleeding: wounds, drains, mucosal surfaces, joints, muscle, intracavity, etc.

- Degree and type of bleeding: arterial, venous, generalised ooze.

- Bleeding from multiple sites, e.g. line access.

- Presence of purpura or skin infarcts.

Investigations

- FBC: Hb, platelets, film.

- Prothrombin time (INR).

- Activated partial thromboplastin time (APTT).

- Thrombin time.

- Fibrinogen level.

- Fibrin degradation products (FDPs).

In difficult cases of perioperative bleeding or in the preoperative assessment period, consult with your haematologist, who can arrange further assays if necessary. The delivery of appropriate blood product replacement can also be expedited.

As well as considering the possibility of a blood dyscrasia, the surgeon must remember that the most common cause of postoperative bleeding is bleeding vessels arising from failure of haemostasis at the time of surgery. Further operation may be necessary to control the bleeding.

THROMBOTIC DISORDERS

Surgery predisposes patients to thrombosis and underlying diseases may increase this risk. It is therefore not surprising that thrombotic disorders represent a significant proportion of the problems encountered in surgical patients.

Arterial thrombosis

This is often associated with platelet thrombi and atherosclerosis. The risk factors are:

- positive family history

- male sex

- hyperlipidaemia

- diabetes mellitus

- gout

- polycythaemia

- cigarette smoking

- ECG abnormalities

- elevated factor VII levels

- elevated fibrinogen levels.

Venous thrombosis

The major factors predisposing to thrombosis are reduced venous flow and increased coagulability of the blood. The risk factors are listed in Box 14.6.

Thrombophilia

This generic term is used to describe conditions in which there is an increased tendency to thrombosis, usually due to inherited abnormalities in coagulation inhibitors. Currently an abnormality can be identified in approximately 50% of patients with recurrent

Around 4% of young patients with thromboembolism have protein C deficiency.

Some patients with protein C deficiency can develop widespread haemorrhagic skin infarction (warfarin-induced skin necrosis) shortly after starting warfarin. This is thought to be due to differing half-lives of the vitamin K-dependent factors. Protein C falls rapidly, leaving a prothrombotic state. These patients should not receive loading doses of warfarin and heparin can be given until a stable state has been achieved.

Protein S deficiency

Like protein C (see above), this is also a vitamin K-dependent protein and is a co-factor for APC on phospholipid surfaces. The clinical features are similar to protein C deficiency. Protein S deficiency represents approximately 8% of cases with venous thrombosis before the age of 45 years.

Factor V Leiden

This abnormality was discovered by the finding that some patients with recurrent thrombosis did not have a longer APTT when activated protein C was added. This activated protein C resistance (APCR) has now been discovered to be an arginine-to-glycine mutation (R506Q) in factor V, which slows the inactivation of factor V. Specific DNA tests are available. This abnormality occurs in approximately 7% of the Caucasian population and 25% of young patients with thrombosis, especially after oral contraception and pregnancy.

Prothrombin abnormality

Recently a G-to-A mutation at position 20210 in the promoter region of the prothrombin gene has been described. This leads to increased levels of prothrombin being expressed. This abnormality is present in 3% of the general population.

Homocystinuria and hyperhomocysteinaemia

Homocystinuria is a rare condition caused by an inborn error of metabolism, cystathione synthetase deficiency, and is associated with marked venous and arterial thrombosis even in childhood. Population studies have shown that increased homocysteinaemia levels are associated with both venous and arterial thrombosis. This may be due to combination of inherited factors and vitamin B6, cobalamin and folate deficiency.

Other abnormalities

Other factors have been described and include:

Box 14.6 Risk factors of venous thrombosis

- Age
- Obesity
- Sepsis
- Malignancy
- Major trauma
- Immobility
- Dehydration
- Oestrogren therapy, pregnancy
- Nephrotic syndrome
- Pelvic mass or obstruction
- Varicose veins
- Polycythaemia, hyperviscosity
- Thrombocytosis
- Lupus anticoagulant, anticardiolipin antibodies
- Antithrombin deficiency
- Protein C deficiency
- Factor V Leiden abnormality
- Protein S deficiency
- Prothrombin abnormality
- Abnormal fibrinogen
- Abnormal plasminogen
- Raised factor VIII levels
- Raised fibrinogen levels
- Paroxysmal nocturnal haemoglobinuria

thrombosis and it is important to remember that normal 'thrombophilia screen' tests do not exclude a prothrombotic state; the clinical and family history must be taken into account. As more abnormalities have been described, it has been realised that the presence of multiple defects gives a much higher risk of thrombosis.

Antithrombin deficiency

Antithrombin (formerly called antithrombin III) is a protein which binds and inactivates thrombin and anti-Xa. Its activity is increased 1000-fold by heparin and patients who have antithrombin deficiency can be heparin resistant. Heterozygote deficiency causes venous thromboembolism, especially after surgery, immobilisation or pregnancy. It occurs in 0.02% of the general population but in 2–5% of young patients with thrombosis.

Protein C deficiency

Protein C is a vitamin K-dependent protein that is activated by thrombin and complexed with thrombomodulin which is a vascular endothelial cell surface receptor. Activated protein C (APC) then, along with a co-factor protein S, inhibits activated factors V and VIII. Thrombosis occurs in the deep limb veins and also in the cerebral and splanchnic circulations.

- elevated factor VIII levels

- plasminogen deficiency

- factor XII deficiency

- fibrinolytic defects.

The association of these abnormalities with familial thrombosis has not always been fully established. It is likely that new genetic abnormalities will be described, as many cases with a clear family history have normal results on the currently available thrombophilia tests.

Lupus anticoagulant and antiphospholipid syndrome

The lupus anticoagulant (LA) is a misnomer as it is due to the presence of an antibody which prolongs the APTT but which is associated with thrombosis rather than bleeding, as its name suggests. LA and closely related anticardiolipin antibodies are antiphospholipid autoantibodies which give rise to the antiphospholipid syndrome (APS). Patients with these antibodies develop arterial and venous thrombosis, recurrent fetal loss and immune thrombocytopenia. About 10% of patients with systemic lupus erythematosus can develop a lupus anticoagulant, but it can occur in association with other autoimmune diseases, after viral infection or after drug exposure (hydralazine, chlorpromazine).

Referral for specialist tests

As thrombosis occurs with increasing frequency with advancing age, it is often difficult to decide which patients should be investigated for an underlying thrombophilia. These are expensive tests and, if possible, testing should be avoided in the acute postthrombotic stage. Heparin can reduce the antithrombin level and proteins C and S are reduced in patients receiving anticoagulants. Where patients have been shown to have a thrombophilic defect, family studies may need to be performed but tests should only be carried out when the individual has considered all the implications of testing.

Thrombophilia investigations should be considered in patients who have:

- experienced venous thromboembolism before the age of 45 years

- recurrent venous thrombosis or thrombophlebitis

- thrombosis in an unusual site (e.g. mesenteric vein, cerebral vein, etc.)

- unexplained neonatal thrombosis

- skin necrosis, especially on warfarin

- experienced arterial thrombosis before the age of 30 years

- relatives with thrombophilic abnormality

- a clear family history of venous thrombosis

- unexplained prolonged APTT

- recurrent fetal loss, ITP or SLE.

Treatment of thrombosis

In all but especially vascular, cancer and orthopaedic surgery, thrombotic conditions represent a large proportion of the problems encountered. Suspected thrombotic postoperative complications should be confirmed by radiological investigation, as clinical diagnosis is inaccurate and the presence of thrombosis affects the subsequent management of the patient. Where thrombosis is shown to be present, a number of treatments are available.

Physical removal of thrombus

This can be performed when the thrombus involves a large vessel and is often the result of embolism of the clot. It must be combined with measures to prevent further thrombosis.

Bypass of thrombotic block

This is the principle of much of coronary and vascular surgery. The success of surgery depends largely on the patency of the vascular bed, and reversal of the thrombotic process. Increasingly, angioplasty techniques are being developed, often with introduction of stents to maintain vessel patency.

Thrombolysis

In recent arterial thrombosis and where large fresh venous thrombi are present, fibrinolytic activators such as streptokinase, tissue plasminogen activator (TPA) and urokinase can be used. Recent surgery is, however, a contraindication (Box 14.7).

In large venous thrombi affecting the legs or central veins, extended periods of infusion may be necessary. The fibrinogen level should be monitored. At the end of the infusion, patients must be switched immediately to heparin to prevent rebound thrombosis.

Heparin

Conventional unfractionated heparin is a mixture of acidic mucopolysaccharides and acts by potentiating antithrombin which inactivates thrombin (IIa) and factors IXa, Xa and XIa. Heparin also inhibits platelet function. It has to be given by intravenous infusion and has a half-life of around one hour. Its effect is

Box 14.7 Contraindications to fibrinolytic drugs

Absolute contraindications
- Active gastrointestinal bleeding
- Aortic dissection
- Head injury or CVE in past 2 months
- Neurosurgery in past 2 months
- Intracranial aneurysm or neoplasm
- Proliferative diabetic retinopathy

Relative contraindications
- Traumatic cardiopulmonary resuscitation
- Major surgery in the past 10 days
- Past history of gastrointestinal bleeding
- Recent obstetric delivery
- Prior arterial puncture
- Prior organ biopsy
- Serious trauma
- Severe arterial hypertension (>200/110)
- Bleeding diathesis

monitored using the APTT (therapeutic range 1.5–2.5 times normal) and the thrombin time. If bleeding occurs, the infusion should be stopped. Rarely heparin needs to be neutralised by protamine but excessive quantities of protamine can also act as an anticoagulant. Prolonged courses of heparin increase the risk of heparin-associated thrombocytopenia (see above). Longer courses also cause osteoporosis, especially in pregnancy.

Low molecular weight heparins (LMWH)

These forms of heparin have a lower molecular weight and greater activity against factor Xa than thrombin and platelets. They can be administered by subcutaneous injection, have a longer half-life (eight hours) and monitoring, if required, is by an anti-Xa assay. The dose varies with the preparation and is based on the patient's weight. Doses differ dependent on whether the LMWH is being given for treatment of established thrombosis or prophylaxis. They are more expensive than unfractionated heparin but the ease of administration is leading to increased use, especially in the treatment of venous thromboembolic disease and acute coronary syndromes.

Hirudins and other thrombin inhibitors are now available but are not yet in current clinical use.

Oral anticoagulants

Warfarin, phenindione and nicoumalone are all vitamin K antagonists and therefore affect the biological activity of vitamin K-dependent factors II, VII, IX and X and proteins C and S. The factors all have differing half-lives, varying from eight to 72 hours, leading to the prolonged action of warfarin. The dose is controlled by monitoring the prothrombin time, in the INR, with different target values dependent on the risk of thrombosis. Warfarin crosses the placenta and is teratogenic, so should not be used in the first trimester of pregnancy. Many drugs interact with oral anticoagulants; when drugs are started or stopped, the INR should be monitored. A full list is available in the British National Formulary. Bleeding can occur in these patients and reversal of oral anticoagulants is discussed above (see Box 14.3). Where haemorrhage occurs in patients whose INR result is in the therapeutic range, a local cause of bleeding should be considered; it is not uncommon for an early carcinoma affecting the urinary or gastrointestinal tracts to present in this way.

Aspirin

Aspirin irreversibly inhibits platelet cyclooxygenase, reducing the production of platelet thromboxane A2. In doses of 75–300 mg per day, it is used in the secondary prevention of thrombotic cerebrovascular events and other arterial cardiovascular disease. Other antiplatelet agents include clopidrogel, dipyridamole, abciximab (a monoclonal antibody used in coronary angioplasty) and epoprostenol (used in renal dialysis).

Prevention of venous thromboembolism

Postoperative thromboembolism is a major cause of morbidity and mortality. The Thromboembolic Risk Factor (THRiFT) Consensus Group has made recommendations regarding the prophylaxis of thromboembolism in hospital patients.

All medical and surgical patients should be assessed for their risk of DVT with respect to their medical history, existing conditions and investigations (see Box 14.6). The risks can be categorised as follows.

Risk rate of	DVT	Proximal DVT	Fatal PE
Low risk	<10%	<1%	0.01%
Moderate risk	10–40%	1–10%	0.1–1%
High risk	40–80%	10–30%	1–10%

Patient groups falling into these categories will be as follows.

Low risk

- Minor surgery <30 minutes.
- Major surgery <30 minutes; age <40 years and no other risk factors.
- Minor trauma or medical illness.

Moderate risk

- Major general, urological, gynaecological, cardiothoracic, vascular or neurological surgery; age >40 years or other risk factor.

- Emergency caesarean section in labour.

- Major medical illness: heart or lung disease, cancer, inflammatory bowel disease.

- Major burns or trauma.

- Minor surgery, trauma or illness in patients with previous DVT, PE or thrombophilia.

- Hip and knee replacement.

- Lower limb paralysis.

High risk

- Major pelvic or abdominal surgery for cancer.

- Major surgery, trauma or illness in patients with previous DVT, PE or thrombophilia.

- Full limb paralysis.

- Major limb amputation.

- Hip and knee replacement.

For patients with a low risk of thromboembolism, early mobilisation and graduated compression stockings are sufficient. For moderate and high-risk patients, measures include early mobilisation, graduated compression stockings, heparin, foot impulse technology or intermittent pneumatic compression. Specific local protocols should be in place. For some patients at highest risk, prophylaxis may need to be continued after discharge from hospital.

In orthopaedic surgery, LMWH is better than unfractionated heparin but attention must be given to the timing of the injection to prevent perioperative bleeding. The use of mechanical methods needs to be compared with LMWH in larger numbers of patients. Other factors, such as the early postoperative mobilization of patients, are also important.

BLOOD TRANSFUSION

Blood donation

A blood donor can donate 450 ml of whole blood, up to three times a year. Every donor is interviewed to exclude anyone whose blood might harm a recipient, for example by transmitting infection. In the UK, every donation is tested to determine the ABO and Rh D group, antibodies to hepatitis B virus, hepatitis C virus, HIV-1, HIV-2 and syphilis, and polymerase chain reaction (PCR) tested for HCV RNA. From November 1999, all units have been leucodepleted to reduce the theoretic risk of transmission of variant Creutzfeldt–Jakob disease (vCJD). From mid-1998, plasma for fractionation (factor concentrates, albumin, immunoglobulin) has been prepared using non-UK plasma, mainly from the

USA. This measure was also taken by the government to reduce the risk of transmission of vCJD by transfusion. Platelets are prepared from four donor pools of platelet-rich plasma or from donors who undergo regular plateletpheresis. Some blood products undergo further testing: for CMV antibodies, detailed red cell phenotypes (e.g. CcEe rhesus, Kell, Duffy, Kidd, Lewis blood group systems), HLA and HPA type for platelet donors and anti-A, anti-B titre in group O donors.

Crossmatching blood

The purpose of crossmatching blood is to prevent haemolytic reactions which usually involve the donor red cells and antibodies in the recipient. Immediate reactions cause intravascular haemolysis, shock, renal failure and involve mainly, but not exclusively, the ABO blood system. Delayed reactions causing premature destruction of transfused red cells and boosting of the antibody levels also occur.

The provision of blood varies depending on the urgency of the clinical situation.

Group O Rh D negative emergency blood

This is stored in high-risk areas, e.g. labour wards or operating theatres. Blood can be used in life-threatening bleeding without crossmatching.

Group-specific blood

Blood of the same or compatible ABO group as the patient is dispatched and crossmatched whilst the bags are in transit.

Crossmatched blood

Donor red cells and patient's serum are incubated and then tested for the presence of antibodies on the surface of the red cells (indirect antiglobulin or Coombs test). Blood is issued if the test is negative.

Group and antibody screen

The patient's blood is ABO and Rh D grouped (usually by automated techniques) and the serum or plasma is screened for antibodies using three different red cell pools containing the majority of different red cell antigens. When reactions occur, larger panels of typed red cells are used to identify the specificity of the antibody. If the screen is negative, there are unlikely to be problems with subsequent crossmatching and blood can be issued relatively quickly.

Box 14.8 An example of a maximum blood-ordering schedule

General surgery		Radical pelvic surgery	2 units
Amputation	Group and save	Repairs	Group and save
Anal fissure	No provision necessary	Termination	Group and save
Appendix	No provision necessary	Hysterectomy	Group and save
Breast lump	No provision necessary		
Cholecystectomy	Group and save	**Orthopaedics**	
Colonic resection	Group and save	Fractured femoral neck	2 units
Colostomy	No provision necessary	Laminectomy	Group and save
Endoscopy	No provision necessary	Nailing/plating (open	
Exploration CBD	2 units	without tourniquet)	2 units
Haemorrhoids	Group and save	Open reduction	Group and save
Hiatus hernia	Group and save	Spinal fusion	2 units
Laparotomy	Group and save	Surgery to elbow/shoulder	No provision necessary
Liver biopsy	Group and save	Total hip replacement	3 units
Lymph node biopsy	No provision necessary	Total knee replacement	2 units
Mastectomy	Group and save		
Mediastinoscopy	2 units	**Neurosurgery**	
Pilonidal sinus	No provision necessary	Cerebral aneurysm	3 units
Portocaval shunt	2 units	Arteriovenous malformation	Group and save
Pyloroplasty	Group and save	Craniotomy for meningioma/	
Rectal resection	2 units	possible meningioma	2 units
Small bowel – resection	Group and save	Posterior fossa craniotomy	Group and save
Splenectomy	Group and save	Other craniotomy	Group and save
Sympathectomy	Group and save	Extradural haematoma	2 units
Thyroidectomy	Group and save	Laminectomy (except	
Total gastrectomy	2 units	for tumour)	Group and save
Vagotomy	Group and save	Shunts	Group and save
Varicose veins	No provision necessary	Spinal tumour	2 units
Whipple's operation	4 units	Subdural haematoma	No provision necessary
Vascular surgery		**Thoracic surgery**	
Aortic surgery (elective)	2 units	Mediastinoscopy/	
Carotid endarterectomy	Group and save	thoracoscopy	2 units
Non-aortic surgery	2 units	Pleurectomy	2 units
		Thoracotomy	2 units
ENT/oral surgery		Oesophagectomy	4 units
Bi-maxillary osteotomy	Group and save	Video-assisted thoracoscopy	2 units
Block dissection	2 units		
Commando	2 units	**Urology**	
Laryngectomy	2 units	Cystectomy	2 units
		Cystoscopy	No provision necessary
Plastic surgery		Hydrocoele	No provision necessary
Block dissection	2 units	Nephrectomy	2 units
Cleft palate	1 unit	Orchidopexy	No provision necessary
Commando	2 units	Transplant	2 units
Mammoplasty – reduction	2 units	TURP	Group and save
MAX/FAX surgery	2 units		
Micro case surgery	6 units	**Cardiac surgery**	
		Routine CABG/valve replacement	2 units
Obstetrics/gynaecology		Emergency CABG/valve surgery	4 units
Caesarean section	Group and save	Re-do surgery	4 units
Colposuspension	Group and save	Thoracic aortic aneurysm	4 units
Cone biopsy	No provision necessary	Pericardectomy	4 units
Ectopic pregnancy	2 units	Acute aortic dissections	6 units
Large tumours	2 units		
Caesarean section of			
placenta praevia	2 units		

Electronic crossmatching

This is a step further where the blood groups are confirmed as compatible by computer providing the patient has been ABO grouped on more than one occasion and no antibodies have been found when the serum has been screened.

Maximum blood-ordering schedules (MBOS)

Crossmatching and blood grouping techniques have evolved which keep up with the demands on blood banks. By examining the ratio of blood crossmatched to blood used, it is possible to predict blood usage for most operations. MBOS are developed by seeking agreement between anaesthetists, surgeons and blood banks to reduce the amount of blood unnecessarily crossmatched and tied up awaiting transfusion. A typical MBOS is shown in Box 14.8

In many laboratories, group and screening are automated but this can often mean that samples are processed in batches in the normal working day. Crossmatching is often performed by using gel or glass bead columns. The speed with which blood can be provided should not lead to complacency; in complicated cases with autoimmunity or the presence of antibodies, further investigation and the provision of suitable blood can take a considerable time – such patients need blood standing by for elective surgery. In an emergency situation, the risk of red cell haemolysis will have to be balanced against the risk of delaying surgery.

Following the development of a red cell antibody, levels eventually fall and become undetectable. If the patient is transfused, the level is boosted and in the presence of the red cell antigen, haemolysis occurs. It is for this reason that blood banks will require a fresh sample if the patient has been transfused within the previous week.

After transfusion of large amounts of blood, further blood is issued without formal crossmatching (group specific).

Blood and blood products

Red cells

Red cells are suspended in citrate, phosphate, dextrose and adenine (CPDA) or sodium, adenine, glucose and mannitol (SAGM) to maintain their condition for the 35-day shelf life. They contain fewer than 5×10^6 leucocytes. Whole blood is rarely used, as the coagulation factors V and VIII and platelets within it are labile.

Composition of red cell packs

	CPDA	SAGM	Whole blood
Volume	280 ml	350 ml	450 ml
Haematocrit	0.55–0.75	0.50–0.70	0.35–0.45

Platelets

Platelets are prepared from single plateletpheresis donors or from four donor pools. One adult therapeutic dose (ATD) contains 2.4×10^{11} platelets and $<0.5 \times 10^6$ leucocytes. 0.25 ATD packs are available for children. Platelets are stored at 22°C and expire after five days.

The indications for platelet transfusion include:

- thrombocytopenic bleeding due to bone marrow failure associated with disease, cytotoxic therapy and irradiation

- prophylaxis in thrombocytopenia due to marrow failure ($<10 \times 10^9/l$)

- platelet function disorders prior to surgery (after correction of antiplatelet drugs, consideration of DDAVP and correction of the haematocrit)

- after massive transfusion, cardiac bypass and acute DIC.

Platelet transfusions should not be used in thrombotic thrombocytopenic purpura (TTP) and are only used for major haemorrhage in immune thrombocytopenias and are often ineffective.

Although bone marrow aspiration and biopsy can be performed, even in patients with severe thrombocytopenia, the count should be raised to $50 \times 10^9/l$ for lumbar puncture, epidural anaesthesia, insertion of arterial and venous lines, liver biopsy and laparotomy. For operations in critical sites, such as the brain or eyes, the platelet count should be raised to $100 \times 10^9/l$.

Fresh Frozen Plasma (FFP)

Plasma is frozen at −30°C within six hours of blood collection and can be stored for 12 months. When thawed, it contains high levels of all the coagulation factors and should be used within four hours. The dose varies but 12–15 ml/kg is a generally accepted starting dose. The response should be measured using the prothrombin time (INR), APTT or specific assays to guide use.

The definite indications for its use are:

- specific factor deficiencies where factor concentrate is not available

- immediate reversal of warfarin effect (see Box 14.3)

- vitamin K deficiency

- acute DIC

- TTP often in conjunction with plasma exchange

- inherited deficiencies of inhibitors of coagulation in the absence of specific concentrates

In the presence of bleeding and with appropriate coagulation monitoring, FFP is indicated in:

- massive transfusion

- liver disease – there is no agreement of a safe level of INR; 1.6–1.8 is probably realistic prior to surgery

- post cardiopulmonary bypass surgery.

Recently, solvent detergent treated pooled FFP has become available. It has the advantage of having increased protection against viral contamination but the disadvantage of being a pooled product (more donor exposure) and is roughly twice the cost of FFP.

Another product, single donor methylene blue treated FFP, may be available soon.

Cryoprecipitate

Cryoprecipitate is made from thawed FFP and is rich in fibrinogen, factor VIII, von Willebrand factor, FXIII and fibronectin. It is useful in bleeding disorders associated with low fibrinogen.

Albumin

Human albumin solution comes in two strengths. 4.5% human albumin solution (HAS) is used for volume replacement. Increasingly crystalloid, gelatin and starch solutions are being used instead of albumin solutions. 20% HAS is hyperoncotic and will draw fluid into and expand the plasma volume. It is important to monitor circulatory status during the infusion.

Immunoglobulins

Immunoglobulin preparations are made by cold ethanol fractionation of pools of human plasma. Preparations which have high-titre IgG-specific antibodies to Rhesus D antigen, tetanus, measles, hepatitis B, varicella zoster, human rabies, cytomegalovirus and rubella viruses. They must be given intramuscularly. Intravenous IgG (IVIgG) is also available and is used as immunoglobulin replacement or as an immunomodulatory agent.

Factor concentrates

An increasing number of factor concentrates are now available and include FVIII, FIX, FVa, VWF, antithrombin, protein C and C1 esterase inhibitor. Most are expensive and should be used in close cooperation with a haematologist.

Price of blood

The collection, processing and testing of blood and its products are expensive and the resources devoted to transfusion in a hospital are considerable. The approximate costs of these products, excluding crossmatching, are as follows.

- Red cells – £85 per unit
- Platelets – £150 per ATD
- FFP – £20 per unit
- HAS 4.5% – £40 for 500 ml
- HAS 20% – £35 for 100 ml
- IVIg – £80 for 5 g

Complications of transfusion

Acute haemolytic or bacterial reactions

Serious but rare, these are due to red cell incompatibility or bacterial contamination. The most common cause of red cell incompatibility is poor sample or patient identification.

Late haemolytic reactions

These are due to red cell antibodies and can vary in severity but patients often develop anaemia and jaundice.

Non-haemolytic febrile transfusion reactions (NHFTR)

NHFTR due to cytokines in the transfused blood which have been released from white blood cells. Their incidence should fall with the introduction of leucodepleted blood.

Allergic reactions

Urticaria and itching may occur shortly after the transfusion starts and can be treated with antihistamines. Anaphylaxis can occur rarely due to the presence of antibodies in patients with IgA deficiency.

Fluid overload

This can occur after the infusion of large volumes, causing pulmonary oedema.

Infections

Although donors are screened to reduce the risk of infections transmitted by transfusion, some still occur. In the UK, the risk of infection is approximately:

- bacterial infection – 1 in a million
- HIV – 1 in a million
- HBV – 1 in 100 000
- HCV – 2 in a million
- HTLV1 – 1 in a million.

CMV infection is not uncommon but is usually asymptomatic or causes a glandular fever-like illness 3–4 weeks after transfusion. However, some immunocompromised patients are particularly at risk of CMV infection. Leucodepletion will reduce the risk of CMV infection but CMV seronegative blood products are recommended for:

- CMV seronegative bone marrow and stem cell patients
- HIV patients who are CMV seronegative.

PRINCIPLES OF SURGICAL PRACTICE

Iron overload

Red cell transfusion-dependent patients develop haemosiderosis over a period of years. In younger patients, chelation therapy with desferrioxamine is required.

Transfusion-associated graft versus host disease (TA GVHD)

This is rare and is caused by donor T lymphocytes. The following groups of patients should receive irradiated blood products to prevent TA GVHD.

● Intrauterine transfusion and subsequent exchange transfusion.

● Congenital immunodeficiency states.

● Bone marrow and stem cell transplantation.

● Hodgkin's disease.

● Recent purine analogues (used for lymphoma treatment).

● HLA matched platelets.

● Donations from first- or second-degree relatives.

Immunosuppression

Immunosuppression was recognised first in renal transplant patients and is thought to account for a higher tumour recurrence rate in cancer patients who are also transfused and for a higher postoperative infection rate in patients who have been transfused. The incidence of these effects should fall with the introduction of leucodepletion.

Transfusion-related acute lung injury (TRALI)

This causes acute respiratory distress and is due to donor plasma containing antibody to the patient's leucocytes.

Hospital transfusion committee

This is a multidisciplinary committee which helps to ensure safe transfusion practice within a hospital. Its functions include:

● maintaining an up-to-date transfusion policy within the hospital

● auditing transfusion practice and providing clinicians with feedback on their own performance (e.g. the rate of blood used to blood crossmatched)

● ensuring all staff dealing with transfusion samples are adequately trained

● investigating critical or near miss incidents and adjusting the transfusion policy if necessary

● providing assurance reports to the hospital clinical governance board.

The Serious Hazards of Transfusion (SHOT) scheme

The SHOT scheme was set up in 1996 to collect data on the serious sequelae of transfusion. Over half the cases reported until 1998 related to the wrong blood component being transfused. In many cases the crossmatch samples were taken from the wrong patient and the report recommended that prelabelled sampling tubes should not be used. Other episodes involved lack of a formal identity check at the bedside.

Autologous transfusion

The use of a patient's own blood rather than homologous transfusion is becoming more popular but still remains a small percentage of blood transfused.

Predeposited blood can be taken up to four weeks prior to elective surgery. The patient must be fit enough to donate blood (one unit per week) and current guidelines state that the blood must be tested in the same way as donor blood. Anaemia is prevented by treatment with iron and erythropoietin. Surgery must take place as planned as the blood will expire. Predeposited blood is suitable for operations that are likely to use 2–4 units of blood. Any unused blood cannot be used for other patients.

Haemodilution, where a unit of blood is taken in the anaesthetic room prior to surgery and returned to the patient at the end of the operation, is popular because of its simplicity. It is important to adhere to strict labelling and patient identification criteria, especially if the procedure is taking place in adjacent theatres.

Cell salvage is often used in vascular and cardiac surgery. Red cells are collected by suction, washed and returned to the patient. It is important to monitor platelet and clotting tests as these factors are gradually depleted. In orthopaedic surgery, devices are available to reuse blood collected from wound drains.

Blood substitutes

Two types of blood substitutes are currently being used in early clinical trials. Haemoglobin-based oxygen carriers are macromolecules formed by stabilisation of the Hb tetramer. They last several hours but some cause a rise in arterial and pulmonary pressures. Perfluorocarbons (PFC) are synthetic hydrocarbons which increase the amount of oxygen dissolved in plasma. PFCs are insoluble in water and are emulsified with surfactant. Particles are removed by the reticuloendothelial system after several hours. These blood substitutes are likely to find a place in resuscitation and perioperative haemodilution. Coagulation factors are not replaced. Artificial platelet substitutes are also undergoing clinical evaluation.

Surgery in Jehovah's Witness patients

Jehovah's Witness patients do not accept blood transfusions and believe that all hope of eternal life will be forfeited if transfusion is accepted. The courts have consistently upheld adults' decisions to refuse transfusion but in the case of children, legal recourse is available and can transfer responsibility for medical decisions from the parents to the courts. Strategies to cope with surgery in Jehovah's Witness patients include good surgical haemostasis, replacement of iron, recombinant erythropoietin treatment, intra-operative blood salvage and haemodilution with reinfusion as long as the blood remains in continuous contact with the circulation.

IMMUNOLOGY

Fundamentals of Surgical Practice contains information on the cells of the immune system and details of the immune response, including antibody structure and function.

Immune response to infection

A number of immunological responses are needed to combat infections.

- T lymphocytes – protect by killing infected cells
- Antibodies – protect by killing, opsonising or neutralising bacteria or neutralising toxins
- Neutrophils – protect by phagocytosing and killing bacteria
- Complement – protect by opsonisation, inflammation and cell lysis

Immunocompromised patients

Where patients lack or have an abnormal immune response, different clinical problems occur.

- T cell defects (e.g. primary immune deficiency or secondary to immunosuppressive drugs): risk of viral, fungal and opportunistic infections.
- Antibody defects (e.g. common variable immunodeficiency): risk of bacterial infections.
- Neutrophil defects (e.g. neutropenia or chronic granulomatous disease): risk of staphylococcal skin infections or fungal infections.
- Complement defects (deficiency in terminal C5–C9 components): risk of neisserial infections; gonorrhoea, meningitis.

Splenectomy

Since the spleen is the major source of antibody production against encapsulated organisms, splenectomy is associated with a risk of overwhelming postsplenectomy infection (OPSI) by pneumococci, *Haemophilus influenzae*, etc. The risk is thought to be reduced by:

- vaccinating with Pneumovax, Hib and meningococcal vaccine (ideally prior to splenectomy but better late than never)
- prophylactic antibiotics (low-dose amoxycillin).

There are no national guidelines as to when revaccination should be carried out but tests for antibody levels are available. In splenectomy for trauma, some residual spleen is often left and can be functionally very effective. However, splenunculi can cause relapse of the disease when splenectomy is performed for autoimmune or phagocytic diseases.

After splenectomy, patients should be issued with a splenectomy card (Figure 14.3).

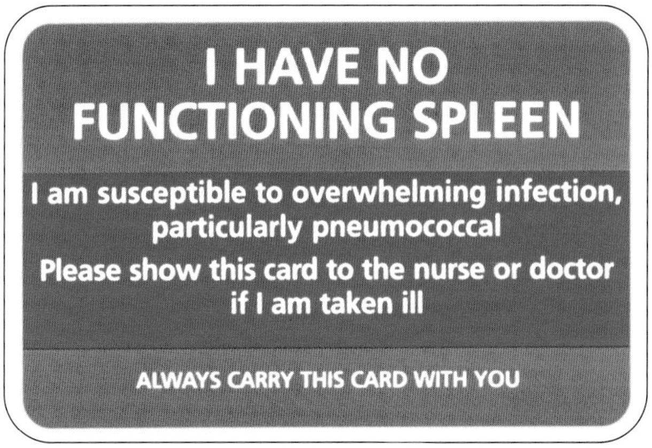

I HAVE NO FUNCTIONING SPLEEN

I am susceptible to overwhelming infection, particularly pneumococcal

Please show this card to the nurse or doctor if I am taken ill

ALWAYS CARRY THIS CARD WITH YOU

Figure 14.3 Splenectomy card (Crown copyright material is reproduced with the permission of the Controller of Her Majesty's Stationery Office).

Allergies

Latex allergy

Two types of latex allergy occur. Type I hypersensitivity is mediated by IgE antibodies and is the type which can be associated with anaphylaxis. Type I latex allergy can be confirmed by RAST or skin prick testing.

Type IV hypersensitivity is mediated by T cells and is associated with contact dermatitis which is unpleasant but not life-threatening. Type IV latex allergy can be confirmed by patch testing (usually performed by dermatologists).

Hereditary angioedema

This is a very rare condition, which is usually familial. Patients lack C1 esterase inhibitor which controls excess complement activation. Such patients are particularly at risk of acute angioedema causing respiratory obstruction following intubation during surgery, obstetric manipulations (e.g. forceps) and dental extraction. Prior to such procedures patients should receive IV prophylactic C1 esterase inhibitor concentrate. Acute attacks in children are rare but can manifest only as abdominal pain (mesenteric angioedema) which can be misdiagnosed as acute appendicitis. Treatment of acute attacks should be with C1 esterase inhibitor concentrate and not with adrenalin, antihistamines or hydrocortisone.

Transplantation

Genetic organisation of HLA system

The major histocompatibility complex (MHC) or human leucocyte antigen (HLA) region in man is located on chromosome 6 and consists of three regions: class I, class II and class III.

- Class I codes for HLA A, B and C genes.

- Class II for HLA DR, DQ and DP genes.

- Class III for TNF (tumour necrosis factor) and complement genes.

The class I and class II genes code for the HLA A, B and C and HLA D molecules which are crucial in transplantation.

A high degree of genetic polymorphism is present and therefore a large number of potential HLA antigens exist within a species. Thus there is considerable difficulty in matching donors and patients.

Structure and function of HLA molecules

HLA class I molecules, A, B and C, consist of a single chain coded for by the MHC, linked to beta-2 microgobulin. They are present on the surface of every nucleated cell in the body and their role is to present peptides derived from viruses or other intracellular organisms to helper T cells which in turn stimulate cytotoxic T cells to kill the infected cells.

HLA class II molecules, DR, DQ and DP, consist of two chains coded for by the MHC. They are only present on a specialised population of cells termed antigen-presenting cells, i.e. macrophages, dendritic cells. Antigen-presenting cells are actively phagocytic and continually 'probe the extracellular environment'. Their role is to present peptides derived from bacteria or other extracellular organisms to helper T cells which in turn stimulate B cells to make antibody against the offending organisms.

Mechanisms of alloreactivity

HLA-mismatched grafts are rejected and HLA-mismatched bone marrow can cause fatal GVHD. These are examples of alloreactivity (reactivity to foreign antigens). The alloreactive response is extremely vigorous and is due to the very large number of T lymphocytes which can recognise foreign HLA molecules (alloreactive T cells). The reason for the existence of such a large number of alloreactive T cells is not to frustrate transplant surgeons but is simply due to viral or bacterial-reactive T cells which are also recognising the foreign HLA molecules, i.e. crossreactivity.

Mechanisms of rejection

There are three types of rejection following organ transplantation. Hyperacute rejection is due to preformed antibodies against HLA antigens on the graft (e.g. from blood transfusion, pregnancy or a previous transplant). Acute rejection is T cell mediated; both helper and cytotoxic T cells play a role but other cells are involved, such as macrophages. Chronic rejection is less clear but is probably also T cell mediated, possibly by a delayed-type, hypersensitivity-type process.

HLA matching

Both serological and DNA methods are currently used for HLA typing. Gradually the serological typing is being superseded by DNA typing which is more sensitive and able to detect differences not recognised by serology.

There is now clinical and laboratory evidence that HLA B and DR matching is more important than HLA A, C, DQ and DP matching. Good HLA matching is crucial for bone marrow transplantation and important, but less crucial, for organ transplantation because of new immunosuppressive drugs.

MALIGNANT LYMPHOMAS

Malignant lymphomas (ML) are broadly divided into two categories: Hodgkin's disease (HD) and all the others under the term non-Hodgkin's lymphoma (NHL). This latter group represents many different diseases. There have been many attempts to classify ML using histopathological criteria, modified by increasing knowledge of lymphoid differentiation and molecular causes of lymphoma. This has led to a bewildering number of terms. The most recent, the WHO Classification, is shown in Box 14.10.

Hodgkin's disease

In 1832, Thomas Hodgkin of Guy's Hospital described seven patients and in 1856 Sir Samuel Wilks added more cases and established the entity Hodgkin's disease. The characteristic Reed–Sternberg cells (Figure 14.4) were described in 1898. It has only recently been accepted that these are B lymphocytes.

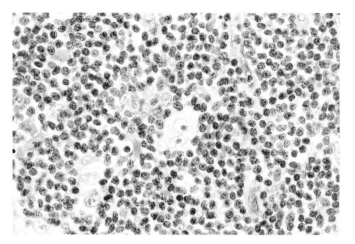

Figure 14.4 Reed–Sternberg cells in Hodgkin's Lymphoma.

The disease affects young adults but older patients can also develop HD. It causes lymphadenopathy and spreads to adjacent nodes and the spleen. In the later stages, other organs such as bone marrow and liver are affected. There is spread through soft tissue in plaques along the body cavities. Patients often have fever, weight loss, night sweats and occasionally have generalised pruritus. Signs of superior vena caval obstruction from a mediastinal mass are not uncommon at presentation.

The diagnosis requires biopsy of affected nodes. Following this, staging investigations give a picture of the extent of disease (Box 14.9). Lymphangiograms and staging laparotomy with splenectomy were an important advance in treatment in the 1970s, but with modern CT, MRI, gallium and PET scanning, neither is needed these days. Staging is used to identify patients with truly localised disease that will benefit from radiotherapy.

Treatment involves radiotherapy for localised disease. HD was one of the first cancers to be shown to be curable by combination chemotherapy. The first regimen was MOPP (mustine, vincristine, procarbazine and prednisolone). Currently derivatives of MOPP such as ChlVPP (chlorambucil, vinblastine, procarbazine and prednisolone) are used along with other drugs. An alternative regimen is ABVD (adriamycin, bleomycin, vinblastine, DTIC). With these chemotherapy regimens approximately 80% of patients achieve a complete remission and half to two-thirds of these have remained without relapse. Residual lymphoid masses at the end of chemotherapy receive radiotherapy. In patients who relapse or progress, treatment with BEAM (BCNU, etoposide, cytarabine and high-dose melphelan) with peripheral blood or bone marrow stem cell support will be considered. This procedure is also termed an autologous stem cell transplant. In patients with progressive disease it may be possible to extend survival for several years using palliative single-agent chemotherapy or small doses of radiotherapy.

Long-term complications of treatment include infertility and second malignancy, including secondary leukaemia. Sperm storage should be considered before treatment if appropriate. It has recently been recognised that young women who received mantle radiotherapy have a high risk of breast cancer and annual mammograms after 10 years have been recommended. Hypothyroidism can develop in patients who received mantle radiotherapy.

Non-Hodgkin's lymphoma

NHL represents many different diseases and they can be broadly divided based on their clinical behaviour into high-grade (aggressive) or low-grade (indolent) types. Paradoxically, high-grade NHL is potentially curable with treatment, whereas low-grade disease tends to relapse and gradually progress as the disease becomes resistant to chemotherapy.

In NHL there is painless generalised lymphadenopathy and involvement of extranodal sites is more frequent than in HD. Patients tend to be older, although NHL occurs at any age. The incidence is increasing and is currently 10.9/100 000 per annum.

A number of cytogenetic abnormalities have been identified in NHL. They often involve bringing oncogenes in close proximity to the immunoglobulin gene. As well as providing an insight into the pathogenesis of lymphoma, these translocations can be used diagnostically, prognostically and to monitor progress in eradicating minimal residual disease.

The treatment of NHL is similar to HD and depends on staging and histology (see Figures 14.5 and 14.6). Localised indolent lymphoma is potentially curable by involved field radiotherapy. For patients with advanced low-grade disease, cure is more remote and median survival is around seven years with around 30% surviving 10 years.

Treatment may be delayed until symptoms occur and is commonly with a chlorambucil-based regimen. Recently purine analogues such as fludarabine and cladrabine have been used. High-dose regimen with stem cell support have been disappointing and have not prevented relapse. Approximately one quarter to

---

Box 14.9	Ann Arbor staging system (Cotswold classification)
• Stage I	Disease in one lymph node area only
• Stage II	Disease in two or more lymph node areas on the same side of the diaphragm
• Stage III	Disease in lymph node areas on both sides of the diaphragm (the spleen is considered to be nodal)
Stage III$_1$	Involvement of splenic, coeliac or portal nodes
Stage III$_2$	Involvement of paraaortic, iliac or mesenteric nodes
• Stage IV	Extensive disease in liver, bone marrow or other extranodal sites
• Substage E	Localised extranodal disease
• A symptoms	Absence of fevers, sweats or weight loss
• B symptoms	Unexplained fever > 38°C, drenching night sweats, weight loss of >10% in the last 6 months
• Definition of bulky disease	Mediastinal mass >one-third of the maximum diameter of the chest, nodal mass >10 cm

one half of patients will in time transform to a high-grade histology and rebiopsy is advisable at the time of relapse or associated with an unusual clinical picture.

For aggressive lymphoma, 90% patients with stage I can be cured with radiotherapy. Relapsing patients can be treated with chemotherapy. For stages II–IV, combination chemotherapy is used. Using CHOP (cyclophosphamide, adriamycin, vincristine and prednisolone) around 55–60% of patients will achieve a complete remission and 60% of these will remain disease free. Relapse is likely to occur within the first two years after treatment. In younger patients with relapse or progressive disease, salvage regimen, including BEAM autologous stem cell transplant, would be considered.

Diffuse large B cell NHL (Figure 14.6) represents the most common form of lymphoma. Some have developed from follicular lymphoma. In this disease there is often a chromosomal translocation t(14;18)(q32;q21) between the heavy chain locus and the BCL2 gene. BCL2 protein is increased and protects the

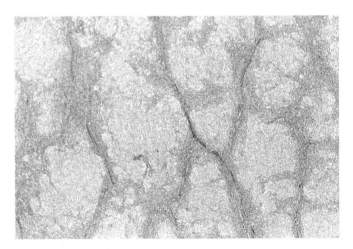

Figure 14.5 Low power view showing follicular pattern in low-grade NHL.

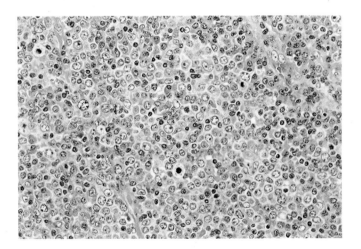

Figure 14.6 High power view of high-grade NHL showing diffuse pattern and numerous blast cells.

Box 14.10	WHO classification of lymphomas

Hodgkin's lymphoma
Nodular sclerosis
Mixed cellularity
Lymphocyte depletion
Lymphocyte-rich (classical)
Nodular lymphocyte predominance

Non-Hodgkin's lymphoma
B cell
Precursor B lymphoblastic leukaemia/lymphoma
B cell chronic lymphocytic leukaemia/small cell lymphocytic lymphoma
B cell prolymphocytic leukaemia
Lymphoplasmacytic lymphoma
Mantle cell lymphoma
Follicular lymphoma
Marginal zone B cell lymphoma of MALT
Nodal marginal zone B cell lymphoma
Splenic marginal zone B cell lymphoma
Hairy cell leukaemia
Plasma cell myeloma/plasmacytoma
Diffuse large B cell lymphoma
Burkitt lymphoma

T cell and NK cell neoplasms
T lymphoblastic leukaemia/lymphoma
Precursor T cell prolymphocytic leukaemia
T cell granular lymphocytic leukaemia
Indolent NK cell large granular lymphoproliferative disorder
Sezary syndrome
Mycosis fungoides
Peripheral T cell lymphomas
Subcutaneous panniculitis like and T cell lymphoma
Hepatosplenic gamma/delta T cell lymphoma
Angioimmunoblastic T cell lymphoma
Aggressive NK cell lymphoma
Nasal and other extranodal NK/T cell lymphoma
Enteropathy type T cell lymphoma
Adult T cell lymphoma/leukaemia (HTLV1 positive)
Anaplastic large cell lymphoma (ALCL)
Primary cutaneous CD30 positive T cell lymphoproliferative disorders

---

lymphocyte from apoptotic cell death, prolonging survival. Another lymphoma, mantle cell lymphoma, has recently been recognised as a distinct entity with a poor prognosis. It has a translocation between the heavy chain locus and BCL1 gene t(11;14)(q13;q32) and causes overexpression of cyclin D1, a key controller of the cell cycle. In Burkitt's lymphoma, the oncogene c-MYC at chromosome 8q24 is translocated to the genes of heavy 14q32 or light chain (2p12, 22q11) rearrangement sites, resulting in uncontrolled expansion of the B cell clone. In Africa, Burkitt's lymphoma occurs in association with Epstein–Barr virus and is seen in areas of endemic malaria.

Gastrointestinal lymphomas are not common (4–9% of NHL) but will present to surgeons. Many are thought to arise from mucosa-associated lymphoid tissue (MALT). In the stomach these tumours are associated with the presence of *Helicobacter pylori*. If only low-grade dysplasia is present, they can respond to

Helicobacter eradication therapy, although a response may take several months to occur. Some gut lymphomas are T cell and occur in patients with previous coeliac disease.

Biopsy of lymph nodes

Whereas fine needle aspirate (FNA) is increasingly being used for the identification of metastatic carcinoma, lymph node biopsy is required for the diagnosis of lymphoma. A negative FNA does not exclude the possibility of lymphoma.

When nodes are excised they can be sent fresh to the histopathology department immediately or outside normal working hours should be incised with a new scalpel blade and placed in a large quantity of formalin for fixation and subsequent microscopic examination. Full clinical details are needed. There should be a local protocol available as these are important specimens and accurate diagnosis is necessary to guide treatment. Often the histology report will take longer as special stains will need to be performed (Box 14.11). Clonality for B cells is demonstrated by showing restriction of light chains and can be confirmed using polymerase chain reaction (PCR) techniques to show that all the cells have the same immunogobulin heavy chain gene rearrangement. For T cells, clonality is harder to prove but similar tests can be performed using T cell receptor gene rearrangement.

Box 14.11 Monoclonal antibodies used in the diagnosis of lymphomas

(CD = cluster of differentiation, a defined antigen to which different monoclonal antibodies react)

CD3	T cell specific
CD4	T helper cells
CD5	T cell marker but also found on B cell CLL and mantle cell lymphoma
CD8	T cytotoxic/suppressor cells
CD10	B lymphoblastic leukaemia and follicular lymphoma
CD20	B cell specific
CD21	Follicular dendritic cell marker
CD30	Marker of Reed–Sternberg cells and anaplastic large cell lymphoma
CD31	Megakaryocyte, platelet and endothelial marker
CD45	Leucocyte common antigen
CD79a	B cell specific
Cyclin D1	Marker of mantle cell lymphoma

Acknowledgement

We are grateful to Dr E.R. Kaminsky for helpful advice on the immunology section and Dr. M Smith for providing figures 14.5–7.

FURTHER READING

1   Aljafri AM, Kingsnorth AN (eds). *Fundamentals of Surgical Practice*. London: Greenwich Medical Media, 1998

2   Baglin TP, Rose PE for the Haemostasis and Thrombosis Task Force for the British Committee for Standards in Haematology. Guidelines on oral anticoagulation. *Br J Haematol* 1998; **101**: 374–387

3   Contreras M (ed). *ABC of Transfusion*, 3rd edn. London: BMJ Books, 1998

4   Cotton DWK. *Synopsis of General Pathology for Surgeons*. Oxford: Butterworth-Heinemann, 1997

5   Hoffbrand AV, Pettit JE *Essential Haematology*, 3rd edn. Oxford: Blackwell Science, 1993

6   Hoffbrand AV, Lewis SM, Tuddenham EGD. *Postgraduate Haematology*, 4th edn. Oxford: Butterworth Heinemann, 1999

7   McClelland B. *Handbook of Transfusion Medicine*, 2nd edn. London: HMSO, 1996

8   Second Thromboembolic Risk Factors (THRiFT II) Consensus Group. Risk of and prophylaxis for venous thromboembolism in hospital patients. *Phlebology* 1998; **13**: 87–97

9   Harris NL et al. WHO Classification of Neoplastic Diseases of the Haemopoietic and Lymphoid Tissues. *J. Clin Oncol* 1999; **17**: 3835–3849

15

Gastrointestinal system

Introduction
  The third compartment
  Fluid balance
Gastrointestinal fluid and electrolyte loss
  Gastric outlet obstruction
  Intestinal obstruction
  Diarrhoea and ileostomy loss
  Small bowel fistulas
  Biliary fistulas
  Acute pancreatitis

Nutritional failure and nutritional support
  Nutritional failure
  Nutritional support
Jaundice and hepatic failure
  Jaundice
  Hepatic failure
Further reading

Craig W. Vickery, Derek Alderson

INTRODUCTION

The principles of fluid balance and nutritional support have already been discussed in Chapter 13 of this book and Chapter 4 of *Fundamentals of Surgical Practice*. This chapter focuses on the specific gastrointestinal causes of abnormal fluid and electrolyte loss, nutritional failure and hepatic disease and the management of gastrointestinal complications in the critically ill patient.

The third compartment

The concept of the third compartment or transcellular fluid arose following the observation that patients with inflammatory disease or after surgical trauma exhibited significant weight gain when fluid overloaded, without developing frank oedema. This fluid was sequestered in the third compartment.

The volume of the third space is normally small, approximately 1 l, and is found in the cerebrospinal fluid, gastrointestinal tract, biliary tree, secretory gland ducts and pleural and peritoneal cavities. In severely ill patients, this volume may rapidly expand as the third space absorbs up to 2–3 l from the ECF in less than 12 hours. This most commonly occurs in ileus fluid, pleural effusions and ascites.

Fluid balance

Maintaining water and electrolyte balance relies on careful assessment of patients' fluid requirements before and during treatment. Requirements for water and electrolytes may be considered in terms of maintenance and replacement (for more detail refer to Chapter 13).

Maintenance

Water and electrolytes are required daily to maintain internal homeostasis in all human beings. Fluid is required to replace insensible losses in expired air, faeces and sweat (approximately 500 ml) and to produce an adequate diuresis to excrete the daily solute load (1.5–2 l). Normal daily electrolyte requirements are shown in Box 15.1.

Box 15.1	Normal daily electrolyte requirements (mmol/kg)		
Sodium	1	Phosphate	0.2
Potassium	1	Calcium	0.1
Chloride	1	Magnesium	0.1

Replacement

It is necessary to consider losses occurring at three possible stages.

1. Patients may exhibit significant *deficits* at the time of presentation, which may be estimated by the duration and severity of fluid loss, initial examination and blood tests. Except in extreme emergencies, resuscitation should be completed in the preoperative phase.
2. *Intraoperative* losses of ECF and evaporation of water from exposed bowel should be estimated, aided by a review of the anaesthetic chart, to ensure they are replaced.
3. An estimate of *continuing* losses may be made by clinical assessment, accurate fluid balance charts and regular serum electrolyte measurements. Significant volumes of fluid sequestered as a result of ileus, diarrhoea or vomitus should be taken into account, as well as nasogastric aspirates and losses via drains and fistulas. Table 15.1 shows the average daily volume and composition of gastrointestinal secretions.

GASTROINTESTINAL FLUID AND ELECTROLYTE LOSS

Box 15.2 shows the causes of abnormal fluid losses from the gastrointestinal tract. It is important to remember that many are associated with nutritional problems, which must also be taken into account when planning treatment.

Gastric outlet obstruction

Infantile hypertrophic pyloric stenosis

Harald Hirschsprung described the clinical and pathological features of infantile hypertrophic pyloric stenosis (IHPS) in 1888. Boys are affected four times more commonly than girls with an incidence among Caucasians of 2–3 per 1000 live births. The pylorus is increased in both length and diameter due to hypertrophy and hyperplasia of the circular muscle layer.

IHPS is classically associated with non-bilious projectile vomiting beginning at 3–6 weeks of age and is uncommon beyond three months. Typically the baby feeds hungrily and vomits towards the end of a feed. In a minority of cases severe dehydration is present on admission with signs of a depressed fontanelle, sunken eyes and dry skin or mucous membranes.

Clinical diagnosis is based on carefully conducted test feeds, observing visible gastric peristalsis and a smooth but firm palpable 'tumour' around the left lateral margin of the rectus abdominis muscle. In the absence of such a tumour an ultrasound scan, measuring the length or diameter of the enlarged pylorus, will establish the diagnosis.

Table 15.1 Mean volume and composition of gastrointestinal secretions compared to normal ranges for plasma and urine

	Volume (ml/24hr)	Sodium (mmol/l)	Potassium (mmol/l)	Chloride (mmol/l)	Bicarbonate (mmol/l)
Plasma		135–145	3.5–5.5	95–105	24–32
Urine		70–160	40–120		
Salivary	1500	10	25	10	30
Stomach	1500	50	15	110	–
Duodenum	500–2000	140	5	80	–
Pancreas	500	140	5	75	115
Bile	800	140	5	100	35
Ileum	3000	140	5	100	30
Colon	Minimal	60	30	40	–

Box 15.2 Causes of gastrointestinal fluid loss

Gastric outlet obstruction
- Infantile hypertrophic pyloric stenosis
- Acquired

Intestinal obstruction
- Neonatal
- Acquired
- Paralytic obstruction

Diarrhoea and ileostomy loss

Small bowel fistulas

Biliary fistulas

Acute pancreatitis

Box 15.3 Causes of acquired gastric outlet obstruction

Benign
- Benign chronic peptic ulceration
- Gastrointestinal stromal tumours (GIST)
- Mucosal diaphragm
- Heterotopic or annular pancreas

Malignant
- Adenocarcinoma of the gastric antrum
- Gastric lymphoma
- Adenocarcinoma of the duodenum
- Pancreatic carcinoma

Others
- Infections – tuberculosis, trypanosomiasis (Chagas disease)
- Crohn's disease, Behçet's disease

Acquired gastric outlet obstruction

Gastric outlet obstruction may occur in the distal antrum, pyloric sphincter or proximal duodenum and therefore this term should replace the more commonly used pyloric stenosis (Box 15.3). Clinically the diagnosis is based on non-bilious vomiting that is typically projectile and may contain recognizable food from the last meal. Although the patient may experience a dull epigastric pain, the colicky pain of small bowel obstruction is absent. On examination, the distended stomach may be palpable, gastric peristalsis visible or a succussion splash audible.

Metabolic disturbance

The severity of the metabolic disturbance depends on the degree of obstruction and its duration but is generally characterised by a hypochloraemic metabolic alkalosis, hypokalaemia and dehydration. Vomiting of gastric secretions causes large losses of HCl and to a lesser extent losses of sodium and potassium. Depletion of ECF and sodium results in reabsorption of sodium by the kidneys, balanced by excretion of H^+ and potassium. Due to depletion of Cl^- electroneutrality is maintained by renal reabsorption of HCO_3^- which augments the metabolic alkalosis.

Management

After establishing the diagnosis, the patient must be resuscitated prior to surgery, which can be delayed until this is complete. A nasogastric tube is inserted for gastric decompression and estimation of the gastric losses. Plasma urea, electrolyte and bicarbonate levels should be measured and restored to normal. Traditionally a combination of 0.45% saline and dextrose containing 10 mmol of potassium chloride per 500 ml was recommended in infants, as they are more prone to hypoglycaemia. Normal saline with potassium supplementation is usually sufficient in adults. The most important aspect of management is close monitoring of the response to fluid resuscitation.

Continuing nasogastric losses should be replaced with normal saline, which enables the kidneys to excrete bicarbonate and correct the alkalaemia. Definitive treatment should be tailored to the individual patient according to aetiology.

Intestinal obstruction

The aetiology of intestinal obstruction may be divided into those that occur in paediatric and adult populations.

Neonatal intestinal obstruction

The causes of neonatal intestinal obstruction have been discussed in detail in Chapter 21 of *Fundamentals of Surgical Practice*. They can be classified as intrinsic, extrinsic or functional. The intrinsic causes may be subdivided into intraluminal, such as meconium ileus, or intramural, such as duodenal, jejunal or ileal atresia. Extrinsic causes include annular pancreas, malrotation or hernias. Functional causes include necrotising enterocolitis.

The clinical picture depends on the level of the obstruction. High obstructions present either *in utero* with polyhydramnios or within a few hours of birth with bilious vomiting. As the level of obstruction moves distally in the small bowel, there is increasing abdominal distension and occasionally jaundice. Colonic conditions such as meconium ileus present after 1–2 days with increasing distension, vomiting and failure to pass meconium.

The management involves a careful assessment of fluid and electrolyte balance. A nasogastric tube should be inserted and resuscitation commenced to replace deficits and correct imbalances. The infant should then be transferred to a specialist unit for definitive treatment of the underlying condition.

Intestinal obstruction in adults

In adults, more than 80% of intestinal obstruction occurs in the small bowel. Obstructions of the small bowel are classified either as mechanical or paralytic.

Mechanical obstruction

- *Luminal* – foreign bodies, faecoliths, bezoars, gallstones, parasites

- *Intramural* – atresia, inflammatory strictures, tumours

- *Extraluminal* – adhesions, hernias, volvulus, intussusception, bands, inflammatory or neoplastic masses

The commonest causes of obstruction in the West are adhesions and hernias, which account for over 80% of cases.

Paralytic obstruction

Paralytic obstruction is due to a failure of the intestinal contents to pass along the lumen of the bowel secondary to peristaltic failure. It may occur in the postoperative phase or secondary to peritonitis, pancreatitis or metabolic disturbances, i.e. hypokalaemia or uraemia.

Metabolic disturbance

The proximal small bowel has a largely secretory role, whereas the distal small bowel is mainly for absorption. Approximately 7 litres of fluid is secreted and reabsorbed through the intestine each day. Any interference with this results in fluid sequestration in the bowel lumen and fluid and electrolyte imbalance. As the bowel becomes distended with gas and large quantities of isotonic fluid, the magnitude of this imbalance will increase. A further proportion of fluid will be lost as vomitus. The overall effect is a loss of neutral, isotonic fluid from both the intravascular and extravascular fluid compartments. In response to the loss of salt, potassium and water, the kidneys conserve salt and water, resulting in oliguria. Blood pressure is maintained in the early stages by fluid shift from the interstitial space but eventually hypovolaemia occurs, which may be profound enough in untreated small bowel obstruction to cause death.

A secondary event is the proliferation of anaerobic bacteria in the accumulated stagnant fluid producing the characteristic smell of faeculent vomitus. As the bowel becomes progressively more distended, the rise in intraluminal pressure impairs venous drainage from the bowel wall. Mucosal oedema increases intraluminal fluid loss and intraperitoneal inflammatory exudate forms. Bacterial translocation across the mucosa may contribute to the infective complications associated with intestinal obstruction.

Critical impairment of the arterial supply or venous drainage of the bowel wall occurs when there is strangulation, for example in a hernial sac or in a closed loop obstruction. Infarction of the bowel wall causes bleeding into the lumen, translocation of bacteria across the bowel wall and ultimately perforation.

Clinical presentation

The clinical picture depends on the level and duration of obstruction. The usual presentation is a combination of abdominal pain, vomiting and abdominal distension. A prolonged history of vomiting and abdominal distension will result in higher accumulated water and electrolyte deficits. High jejunal obstruction is characterised by early, profuse bilious vomiting with minimal distension and fewer distended bowel loops on radiographs. Low ileal obstruction is characterised by colicky abdominal pain, followed later by bilious and faeculent vomiting. Large bowel obstruction leads to distension and constipation before progressing to pain and vomiting several days later. Closed loop obstruction of the large bowel can occur when the ileocaecal valve remains closed or when there is a colonic volvulus.

Management

The treatment of intestinal obstruction should be considered in two parts: resuscitation of the patient and treatment of the underlying cause.

The state of hydration may be estimated from the length of the history, physical signs and blood tests (haematocrit, urea and electrolyte concentrations). Resuscitation should commence with intravenous normal saline and supplemented with potassium if indicated on the basis of electrolyte results. A nasogastric tube will alleviate nausea and vomiting and decompress the bowel. Fluid lost from the aspirate should be replaced with normal saline. The response to resuscitation should be monitored by observation of pulse, BP and urine output through the insertion of a urinary catheter. In patients with associated cardiac co-morbidity, central venous pressure measurement will facilitate adequate rehydration without precipitating heart failure. Analgesics may be required and if there are clinical features of sepsis, antibiotics should be started. Signs of strangulation (persistent pain due to ischaemia) and its consequences (peritonitis) imply a greater degree of urgency regarding both resuscitation and definitive treatment.

Surgery is indicated in those where the cause of obstruction is clear and will not resolve spontaneously, e.g. hernias, intussusception and primary malignant obstruction. Conservative therapy may be indicated in early postoperative obstruction, adhesions or intraperitoneal metastases. Resuscitation should be combined with regular clinical review to identify signs of deterioration or impending strangulation. The period over which conservative therapy can be continued is not defined. The old saying 'The sun should never set on obstructed bowel' may no longer hold true with increasing numbers of patients presenting with adhesions. Around 50% of such cases will resolve over a period of several days without surgical intervention. In this situation regular review of the patient is essential and any suspicion of bowel ischaemia should be acted upon by immediate operation.

Paralytic ileus

Peristalsis relies on coordinated contraction of the gastrointestinal smooth muscle. After an abdominal operation, the whole of the gastrointestinal tract has altered motility but for periods that vary with the anatomy of the intestine. The shortest is in the small bowel, lasting only a few hours; in the colon it is 1–2 days and the longest is in the stomach, lasting up to 3–4 days. The metabolic disturbance is identical to other causes of obstruction, with severe fluid and electrolyte depletion due to loss of secretions into the bowel lumen and nasogastric aspiration. It is treated by supportive measures but if prolonged, may require parenteral nutrition.

It is important to distinguish paralytic ileus from postoperative mechanical obstruction. If high nasogastric volumes persist for more than four days in association with colicky pain, the latter should be considered.

Diarrhoea and ileostomy loss

The mucosa of the gastrointestinal tract is unique since it can both absorb and secrete water and electrolytes. When the absorptive capacity of the colon is exceeded, an excessive amount of fluid will be excreted, resulting in diarrhoea. Therefore, diarrhoea may result from excess secretion, impaired absorption or both.

Water and electrolyte transport across the mucosa is influenced by endogenous factors (cortisol, VIP, gastrin, acetylcholine) and exogenous factors (enterotoxins, bile acids, carbohydrates). Water moves across the mucosa down an osmotic gradient secondary to the transport of solutes. In the gallbladder, ileum and colon this movement is largely the active transport of sodium and chloride

and in the jejunum, the passive absorption of carbohydrates and amino acids. The volume of water transported is proportional to the magnitude of the osmotic gradient and the conductance of the mucosal barrier to water.

The causes of diarrhoea, which act by interfering with this physiological mechanism, are discussed below.

Infectious diarrhoea

Infectious organisms may cause diarrhoea by producing enterotoxins or by direct mucosal damage. The resulting dehydration may be exaggerated by vomiting or paralytic ileus. The common infectious agents that cause diarrhoea are shown in Box 15.4.

> **Box 15.4** Causes of infectious diarrhoea
>
> *Vibrio cholerae*
> *Escherichia coli*
> Rotaviruses
> Campylobacter
> Shigella
> Salmonella
> *Giardia lamblia*
> *Clostridium difficile*
> Schistosomiasis
> *Entamoeba histolytica*

The different strains of *Escherichia coli* are the most common cause of acute travellers' diarrhoea. Enterotoxigenic *E. coli* produce toxins which provoke intestinal secretion without tissue damage whereas enteroinvasive *E. coli* invade the epithelial cells and cause histological damage. The mechanism of cholera toxin is well known. After colonisation and adhesion of the vibrios to the mucosal surface, the enterotoxin, also known as 'choleragen', is delivered to the epithelial cells. This stimulates secretion of water and electrolytes from the intestinal crypts through an increase in intracellular levels of cAMP. The net effect is a massive outpouring of isotonic fluid, classic secretory diarrhoea.

Most cases of infectious diarrhoea are self-limiting and antibiotics are only required in resistant cases.

Inflammatory bowel disease

Ulcerative colitis most commonly occurs between the ages of 15 and 40 years with a prevalence of 40 per 100 000. It is a relapsing and remitting mucosal disease, which almost invariably involves the rectum and then spreads proximally. Inflammation is confined to the mucosa except in severe exacerbations, which distinguishes it from Crohn's disease, which tends to be transmural. The most common presenting symptom is bloody diarrhoea in an otherwise healthy individual. In severe cases there may be constant diarrhoea, resulting in anaemia, water and electrolyte depletion and malnutrition.

Treatment involves resuscitation by fluid replacement in conjunction with steroids to induce remission. In acutely ill patients nutritional support may be required. Indications for surgery include perforation, severe haemorrhage, toxic dilatation or failure of conservative therapy.

Bile acid-induced diarrhoea

Interruption of the normal enterohepatic circulation of bile acids results in bile acid malabsorption. The presence of bile acids in the colon induces watery, secretory diarrhoea. As the majority of bile acids are absorbed in the terminal ileum the commonest causes are Crohn's disease of the terminal ileum, resection or bypass of the ileum. It may also occur in patients who have undergone cholecystectomy or vagotomy. The postcholecystectomy mechanism is thought to be an excess of bile acids escaping ileal reabsorption. Vagotomy is thought to increase the bile acid load in the colon by accelerating intestinal transit.

Bile salt diarrhoea can be treated effectively by cholestyramine, which binds to the bile acids in the gut lumen, abolishing their action as secretagogues of salt and water.

Hormonally induced diarrhoea

Abnormal levels of circulating hormones that affect gastrointestinal function may be associated with paraneoplastic syndromes. In Zollinger–Ellison syndrome, diarrhoea is the second most common clinical feature after peptic ulceration. Gastrinoma increases acid secretion and induces diarrhoea mainly by inactivation of small bowel enzymes; it disappears with antisecretory drugs.

Carcinoid syndrome and medullary thyroid carcinoma produce a number of humoral messengers, including serotonin, prostaglandin E and somatostatin, that cause flushing and diarrhoea. The mechanism is thought to involve secretory diarrhoea and increased intestinal transit. The mainstay of treatment is long-acting somatostatin analogues; occasional patients may benefit from surgery.

Iatrogenic diarrhoea

Laxatives such as sodium picosulphate are routinely used to prepare the bowel prior to investigation or surgery. In the elderly or infirm, fluid supplementation with intravenous saline should be considered.

Treatment of diarrhoea

The treatment of patients with diarrhoea aims to correct dehydration and replace continuing losses while the underlying cause is either treated directly or spontaneous resolution occurs. Fluid and electrolyte replacement are required to prevent the complications of hypovolaemia secondary to isotonic fluid loss, to correct the metabolic acidosis due to loss of bicarbonate and to minimise the risk of dysrhythmias due to

potassium loss. If the overall deficit is severe, resuscitation should be commenced with intravenous fluids. Oral rehydration may be appropriate in less severe cases or where intravenous fluids are less readily available.

As previously mentioned, water is absorbed by facilitated diffusion in the gastrointestinal tract, the major solutes being sugars and amino acids in the jejunum and chloride in the gallbladder, ileum and colon. Based on the average electrolyte composition of diarrhoeal stool, an oral rehydration solution (ORS) requires sugar and salt. The World Health Organisation recommends a solution consisting of the following solutes:

Sodium	90 mmol/l
Potassium	20 mmol/l
Chloride	80 mmol/l
Bicarbonate	30 mmol/l
Glucose	111 mmol/l

Improved sanitation and vaccination, however, have achieved the greatest impact on infectious types of diarrhoea in the last century.

Ileostomy loss

After ileostomy formation, the loss of colonic absorptive functions renders the patient susceptible to salt and water loss. The normal colon absorbs approximately 1 l of water and 100 mmol of sodium chloride daily, with a maximum capacity of 5 l per day. Therefore, even a healthy ileostomy has higher obligatory losses of fluid and electrolytes. Table 15.2 shows the average daily faecal losses of a healthy conventional ileostomy.

These losses are higher in the early postoperative phase. With time, the volume reduces to approximately 200–650 ml, which is considerably less than the normal daily ileocaecal flow of 1–2 litres. This represents adaptation by the small bowel, a function that is lost if more than 10 cm of the distal ileum is resected.

A patient with an ileostomy is at greater risk of diarrhoea which in acute, severe episodes may be life threatening. Diarrhoea in a patient with a conventional or continent ileostomy can be best defined as a faecal output of more than 1 litre per day. Ileal resection and terminal ileal disease can also lead to salt and water depletion and vitamin B12 deficiency. Pouchitis is a phenomenon that occurs in the ileal reservoir of patients who have undergone restorative proctocolectomy. It usually develops in the first year after surgery with malaise, high-output watery or bloody diarrhoea and discomfort. Bacterial overgrowth in the proximal bowel has been implicated in its aetiology.

The treatment of ileostomy diarrhoea relies on the same principles of rehydration and treatment of the underlying cause. Codeine phosphate or loperamide provides symptomatic relief. Metronidazole may be of benefit in diarrhoea associated with bacterial overgrowth.

Table 15.2 Daily faecal losses with an intact bowel and postileostomy

	Water (ml)	Sodium (mmol)	Potassium (mmol)	Chloride (mmol)
Intact bowel	100–150	1–5	5–15	1–2
Post ileostomy★	200–650	81	6	34

★ Kelly DG, Branon ME, Phillips SF, Kelly KA. Diarrhea after continent ileostomy. *Gut* 1980; **21**: 711–716

Small bowel fistulas

A gastrointestinal fistula is an abnormal communication between one hollow organ and another or between a hollow organ and the skin that permits the passage of fluids or secretions. Fistulas may occur anywhere in the small bowel, may drain internally or externally and may be of high (>1 l/day) or low output. Low output or distal fistulas may have few consequences. High-output duodenal or jejunal fistulas (which may lose up to 6 l daily) or those that bypass long segments of small bowel may have considerable effects upon water and electrolyte balance and nutrition. Replacement should be based on the regular measurement of serum electrolytes aided by assessment of the volume and electrolyte concentration of the secretions.

The modern management of intestinal fistulas is based on the following principles.

- Initial resuscitation to restore circulating volume
- Correction of fluid and electrolyte imbalance
- Control of external fistulas to protect the skin and collect effluent
- Eradication of sepsis by drainage and/or antibiotics
- Nutritional support
- Demonstration of the anatomy of the fistula
- Elimination of any distal obstruction

Biliary fistulas

Biliary fistulas can be spontaneous, traumatic or postoperative and may drain either internally or externally. The most common form of spontaneous biliary fistula is an internal one due to calculus erosion, between either the gallbladder or common bile duct and the duodenum. This can lead to infection, particularly where there is distal obstruction, predisposing to ascending cholangitis. External biliary fistulas are usually iatrogenic. Loss of water and electrolytes, particularly sodium, may present problems when the output is more than 500 ml per day. Long-term fistulas deprive the gastrointestinal tract of bile salts, causing steatorrhoea and loss of fat-soluble vitamins.

Acute pancreatitis

Acute pancreatitis may give rise to local or systemic complications. In the early phase, hypovolaemic shock is the major threat to life. The release of enzymes and the activation of proinflammatory mediators increase capillary permeability, producing peripancreatic oedema and decreases in systemic vascular resistance. Sequestration of up to 6 l of fluid may occur in the first 48 hours, reflected by oliguria. The paralytic ileus that develops may last 2–3 days in mild cases but may be protracted in more severe cases. Intestinal obstruction may be caused by mechanical compression of the duodenum by the inflamed and swollen pancreas or by pseudocyst formation in the later phases of the disease.

Metabolic disturbance

The metabolic disturbances include abnormal glucose tolerance in at least 30% of cases, requiring insulin therapy. Hypocalcaemia is an important complication, reflected by its inclusion in prognostic scoring systems. The fall in ionised calcium levels is largely due to the reduction in serum albumin and bound calcium. Additional calcium is bound to fatty acids in 'calcium soaps' released by the action of pancreatic lipase on body fat. When there is severe hypocalcaemia, serum magnesium should also be measured and corrected.

Treatment

In shocked patients treatment should be commenced with intravenous normal saline or colloids. Treatment of hypocalcaemia is necessary if symptomatic. Urine output and central venous pressure should be monitored and the patient should be transferred to a high-dependency/intensive care unit if multiple organ failure develops. If oral intake has not been established within 3–5 days, nutritional support is indicated. This is discussed in detail in the following section.

NUTRITIONAL FAILURE AND NUTRITIONAL SUPPORT

Nutritional failure

The King's Fund Report, published in 1992, estimated that up to 40% of hospitalised patients are undernourished. It contained guidelines for the routine assessment of all patients on admission to hospital and the provision of nutritional support across all medical disciplines.

Nutritional failure or malnutrition may result from a number of mechanisms, including insufficient intake, altered gastrointestinal motility, inadequate absorption or excessive excretion. It may also occur with an intact gut in cases of severe catabolic stress, where the energy and protein requirements may exceed the maximum possible daily intake. These mechanisms do not occur in isolation and often act in synergy. Patients with hypermetabolic stress due to trauma, burns, infection or extensive operations exhibit an increase in basal metabolic rate, increased use of fatty acids as fuel and an increased production of glucose from proteins. Consequently, they require increased levels of nitrogen and energy. When there is a deficient supply of these substrates or their existing nutritional status is compromised, there is a more rapid depletion of body energy stores and, if untreated, protein depletion weakens the host defence, increasing morbidity and mortality.

The essential components of a healthy dietary intake include not only carbohydrate, protein and fat but also vitamins, minerals and trace elements. Nutritional failure rarely occurs in terms of a single nutrient.

Functional consequences of nutritional failure

Weight loss of more than 15% is associated with a loss of approximately 20% of body protein, resulting in a significant alteration in many physiological processes. This results in a loss of mass of the heart, diaphragm, respiratory muscles, liver, skeletal muscle and haemopoietic organs and reduces the rate of synthesis of many proteins. In surgical patients, this compromises normal gastrointestinal function, the immune response and wound healing.

The effect on the gastrointestinal tract may occur as a result of global malnutrition or through the direct absence of nutrients within the lumen of the bowel. The presence of nutrients within the lumen provides an essential stimulus for mucosal growth and function acting through direct physical contact, the stimulation of trophic GI hormones and enhancement of intestinal blood flow. Standard total parenteral nutrition (TPN) preparations lack gut-essential nutrients such as glutamine, short-chain fatty acids and nucleotides and may exacerbate the consequences on the bowel.

Malnutrition of the gastrointestinal tract is characterised by muscular and mucosal atrophy. Nutrient digestion and absorption is reduced by mucosal oedema, loss of absorptive surface area and reduced brush border enzyme activity. Altered bacterial flora, partly due to decreased gastric acid secretion, metabolises nutrients in addition to blocking their absorption.

The physiological gut barrier function, which normally protects against the translocation of bacteria and their toxins from the bowel lumen into lymphatics and the systemic circulation, is diminished by malnutrition. The components of this barrier are intraluminal (gastric acid, pepsin, bile salts, pancreatic enzymes and IgA), intestinal mucus, intrinsic gut motility, gut-associated lymphoid tissue (GALT) and the normal bacterial flora. Defective wound and anastomotic healing has been linked to reduced serum albumin levels.

Causes of nutritional failure

Nutritional failure may result from a number of conditions (Box 15.5), which have specific mechanisms according to their anatomical sites. These are discussed below.

Box 15.5	Causes of nutritional failure
Defect in	**Examples**
Intake	Dysphagia, starvation, oropharyngeal trauma
Digestion	Pancreatic insufficiency or resection, bile salt depletion
Absorption	Coeliac disease, tropical sprue, intestinal surgery
Transport of nutrients	Alpha-beta-lipoproteinaemia
Storage	Cirrhosis, haemochromatosis, hepatic failure
Metabolism	Phenylketonuria, galactosaemia
Abnormal losses	Fistulas, renal failure, protein-losing enteropathy
Increased requirement	Sepsis, trauma, burns, extensive operations

Oropharynx

Facial trauma or complex oropharyngeal surgery will compromise oral intake and alternative access to the gastrointestinal tract, e.g. gastrostomy, should be considered. The swallow mechanism, which may be initiated either voluntarily or as a reflex action, is dependent on coordinated muscle contraction and relaxation. Oropharyngeal dysphagia results from neuromuscular disorders such as motor neurone disease or multiple sclerosis or after cerebral vascular accidents.

Oesophagus

Oesophageal dysphagia may be caused by benign or malignant conditions. Common benign problems are either inflammatory (e.g. gastrooesophageal reflux disease) or primary motor disorders (e.g. achalasia). Less common causes include autoimmune conditions such as scleroderma, caustic strictures and benign tumours.

Malignant tumours such as squamous cell carcinoma or adenocarcinoma essentially cause mechanical obstruction. As the investigation and treatment process may be prolonged, especially when neoadjuvant regimes are used, it is important to make a careful nutritional assessment of such patients, provide oral liquid supplements and, if severe, take steps to relieve the dysphagia to prevent worsening of the patient's nutritional state.

Stomach

The stomach has a number of functions in addition to the storage of food and the control of its release into the duodenum. Hydrochloric acid kills many ingested bacteria. Intrinsic factor is necessary for the absorption of cyanocobalamin (vitamin B12) from the distal ileum. Gastrectomy, pernicious anaemia or

223

chronic atrophic gastritis can all lead to loss of intrinsic factor. To prevent megaloblastic anaemia, regular three-monthly intramuscular injections of vitamin B12 are required.

Total gastrectomy is associated with other long-term nutritional effects; many patients lose weight because of early satiety, dumping syndrome or reflux symptoms. Diversion leads to altered bacterial flora which metabolise vitamin B12 and bile salts, causing fat malabsorption (steatorrhoea) and depletion of fat-soluble vitamins.

Small intestine

The term intestinal failure is defined as a 'reduction in functioning gut mass below the minimum necessary for the adequate digestion and absorption of nutrients'. The major causes of intestinal failure are shown in Box 15.6.

Box 15.6 Causes of intestinal failure

Coeliac disease
Tropical sprue
Whipple's disease
Intestinal resection
Inflammatory bowel disease
Fistulae
Radiation enteritis
Tumours
Parasitic infections (*Giardia lamblia*)

COELIAC DISEASE

Coeliac disease is a condition that predominantly affects the mucosa of the proximal small bowel, characterized histologically by subtotal villous atrophy and intramucosal inflammatory infiltration. Although the exact mechanism is unknown, an abnormal immune response to alpha-gliadin derived from gluten in the diet is thought to be implicated, which is injurious to the small bowel mucosa.

INTESTINAL RESECTION

Massive intestinal resection (short bowel syndrome) leads to a substantial loss of the mucosal surface area for absorption, resulting in the need for specialised nutritional support. It occurs in infants as a result of trauma or necrotising enterocolitis and in adults secondary to superior mesenteric artery occlusion, inflammatory bowel disease or radiation therapy. There is no exact definition of short bowel syndrome but nutritional problems are likely when more than 75% is lost. An important factor is whether the terminal ileum has been removed.

The physiological consequences include watery diarrhoea, malabsorption of fats and fat-soluble vitamins and depletion of the

enterohepatic pool of bile salts. Despite this, many patients continue to feed orally as a result of intestinal adaptation, in which the surface area for absorption is increased by villous hyperplasia. Adaptation occurs in three phases. Immediately postresection, there is massive diarrhoea and the patient is wholly dependent on TPN. Over the next three months major adaptation allows the gradual introduction of an enteral diet low in fat. Full adaptation occurs only in some patients, when a more normal diet higher in fat may be started. Careful monitoring remains essential to measure levels of fat-soluble vitamins and minerals. Food rich in oxalates should be avoided as they form calcium soaps in the bowel lumen and predispose to oxalate renal stones.

The complications of short bowel syndrome include deficiencies of vitamins A, D, E and K and iron and in addition the complications that arise through the use of TPN. These include cholelithiasis, acalculous cholecystitis and hepatosteatosis (fatty liver). Pharmacological agents such as cholestyramine and loperamide may give symptomatic relief. With recent advances in immunosuppression, small bowel transplantation may be a realistic option for some patients.

INFLAMMATORY BOWEL DISEASE

A significant number of patients with Crohn's disease and ulcerative colitis can become malnourished, especially during acute exacerbations. Crohn's disease may result in nutritional failure by a number of mechanisms. Single, large or multiple resections over time may result in a deficiency of mucosal surface area. Internal (enteroenteric) or external fistulas may result in the bypass of long segments of bowel or extensive losses, which may be exacerbated by a protein-losing enteropathy. Chronic inflammation of the terminal ileum may have a similar effect to resection of the terminal ileum with a loss of active transport of bile salts and vitamin B12.

FISTULAS

Gastrointestinal fistulas allow abnormal diversions of nutrients, digestive juices, water and electrolytes, potentially creating a wide variety of pathophysiological effects. Up to 50% of patients with fistulas are malnourished, the primary causes of death being malnutrition, electrolyte imbalance or sepsis. The role of TPN or enteral supplements in the management of enterocutaneous fistulas is primarily one of supportive care to prevent malnutrition in an already debilitated patient. After initially correcting the blood volume, electrolytes and clotting deficiencies, TPN has been shown to substantially improve the rate of spontaneous fistula closure. Enteral nutrition is preferable in some patients, if substrate delivery can be achieved beyond the fistula.

Pancreas

Severe acute pancreatitis produces major catabolic stress, with rapid loss of muscle proteins. The reluctance to use enteral feeding because it stimulates pancreatic secretory activity has recently been challenged. Enteral nutrition is less expensive than TPN, is less invasive and eliminates a potential source of sepsis. Enteral nutrition prevents villous atrophy and maintains gut barrier function, reducing bacterial translocation, which may be implicated in the development of multiorgan failure. Fewer complications and improvements in disease severity scores occur with the use of enteral feeding.

Patients with chronic pancreatitis or after resection may exhibit endocrine (diabetes mellitus) or exocrine pancreatic insufficiency, requiring insulin therapy or oral pancreatic enzyme supplements.

Nutritional support

There are a number of considerations in the provision of nutritional support. Which patients require it? Do they have a functional gut? What is the appropriate substrate? How can access be obtained and maintained for the delivery of this substrate? It is not within the scope of this chapter to discuss these considerations, as they are outlined in full in Chapter 4 of *Fundamentals in Surgical Practice*. The above information will help the reader to understand the processes involved in the nutritional assessment of patients and in the decision of whether enteral or parenteral feeding is preferable.

A detailed discussion of the role of nutritional support in the perioperative setting is outlined below.

Perioperative nutritional support

The role of nutritional support in patients undergoing major surgery is plagued by a lack of prospective, randomised trials. Although feeding may improve nitrogen balance, many studies have failed to show significant clinical benefit in terms of improved wound healing, reduced infectious complications, enhanced recovery or reduced mortality. As there is a high inci-

dence of malnutrition in patients undergoing gastrointestinal surgery, some studies have examined the role of preoperative nutrition. Early studies that focused on the use of TPN showed that operative morbidity was only reduced when the degree of malnutrition was severe. The benefit in patients with less severe nutritional failure was hidden by a higher rate of infective complications in those receiving TPN.

Unless contraindicated, enteral feeding is preferable, as it is associated with fewer septic complications. The rationale for early postoperative enteral feeding is supported by the observation that ileus recovers quickly in the small bowel, allowing it to absorb nutrients almost immediately after surgery. Early jejunal infusion of nutrients is well tolerated in the majority of patients and has potential benefits in preserving the integrity of the gut mucosa and reducing bacterial translocation, which has been implicated in the development of multiple organ failure. Enteral feeding may also attenuate the acute-phase response to injury.

Perioperative nutritional support may benefit those patients who are severely malnourished prior to surgery, those expected to have a delay in adequate intake for 10–14 days or those who develop complications resulting in delayed intake. Future research into enteral feeds enriched in specific nutrients designed to enhance the metabolic response to trauma or major surgery is ongoing. Those currently being evaluated include arginine, glutamine, omega-3 fatty acids, insulin-like growth factors and growth hormone.

JAUNDICE AND HEPATIC FAILURE

Jaundice

Jaundice becomes clinically detectable when the serum bilirubin level exceeds 30–40 μmol/l. It is classically divided into prehepatic, hepatic and posthepatic types (Box 15.7).

Box 15.7 Causes of jaundice

Prehepatic	Hepatic	Posthepatic
Haemolytic	*Hepatitic*	*Common*
Spherocytosis	Viral hepatitis	Gallstones
Eliptocytosis	Alcohol-induced hepatitis	Carcinoma of the pancreas
Autoimmune haemolytic anaemia	Drug-induced hepatitis	Lymphadenopathy in the porta hepatis
Thalassaemia		
Sickle cell	*Cholestatic disorders*	*Infrequent*
	Primary biliary cirrhosis	Carcinoma of the ampulla
Non-haemolytic	Phenothiazines	Pancreatitis
Gilbert's disease	Pregnancy	Benign strictures
Crigler–Najjar syndrome		Mirizzi's syndrome
		Cholangiocarcinoma
		Biliary atresia
		Choledochal cysts

The diagnosis of the jaundiced patient depends heavily on the history and examination. A family history of jaundice indicates a possible prehepatic aetiology. Chronic alcohol abuse, recent travel or drug addiction may suggest hepatitis. Pruritus, secondary to bile salt deposition in the skin, is a common feature of hepatic or posthepatic cholestasis. Severe, episodic right upper quadrant pain with fever and jaundice suggests biliary sepsis, whereas constant epigastric pain and weight loss are more indicative of pancreatitis or malignant disease. Classically, obstructive jaundice presents with a history of pale stools and dark urine.

On examination, jaundice is most evident within the elastic tissue of the sclerae, face and upper limbs. General examination may reveal the stigmata of chronic liver disease, such as spider naevi, clubbing or gynaecomastia. Splenomegaly and prominent abdominal veins suggest portal hypertension. Tenderness may be elicited in the right upper quadrant or an enlarged liver may be palpable. Size and character of the liver may help, e.g. the irregular liver of malignant disease.

Investigations

Laboratory investigations

Biochemical tests of liver function do not always distinguish between the causes of jaundice. Isolated elevation of unconjugated bilirubin as a result of excessive haemolysis is present with prehepatic jaundice. Hepatic alkaline phosphatase is produced in the epithelium of the biliary tree whereas the cytoplasmic enzymes, aspartate transaminase and alanine transaminase, are released from damaged hepatocytes. While different patterns of liver enzymes may suggest a hepatic or posthepatic cause, there is often a mixed picture. Although the levels of cytoplasmic enzymes are highest in acute liver damage (hepatic jaundice), they may also be elevated in long-standing obstruction and infection. Gamma-glutamyl transpeptidase activity is high in biliary obstruction but is also acutely raised by alcohol intake.

If the history suggests hepatitis or autoimmunity, serological tests should be performed. Synthetic liver function may be estimated from albumin levels but the most sensitive indicator is the prothrombin time, reflecting reduced synthesis of clotting factors. Tumour markers such as CA19-9 may be helpful in distinguishing cholangiocarcinoma from sclerosing cholangitis.

Urine analysis provides additional information. In prehepatic disorders the liver is presented with an excessive load of bilirubin which is unconjugated and, because it is not water soluble, absent from urine. The absence of urinary urobilinogen is indicative that no conjugated bilirubin has reached the gastrointestinal tract. While the history, examination and blood tests provide clues to the cause of jaundice, the precise diagnosis is made by radiological and histological methods.

Transcutaneous ultrasonography

This often forms the first line of investigation, as it is non-invasive. The echogenicity of the liver parenchyma may be altered in cirrhosis or with tumours. Dilated intrahepatic or extrahepatic ducts indicate obstruction and its level. Bile duct stones and pancreatic or porta hepatis masses may be visualised.

Cholangiopancreatography

The biliary tree and pancreatic duct may be visualised by endoscopic retrograde cholangiopancreatography (ERCP) or by magnetic resonance cholangiopancreatography (MRCP). Stones are seen as filling defects within the bile ducts and malignancies as strictures. The advantage of MRCP is that it is non-invasive, avoiding the risks of ERCP (pancreatitis, postsphincterotomy bleeding and perforation). The advantage of ERCP is that it may be therapeutic, stones may be removed by sphincterotomy and/or balloon retrieval or stents inserted across strictures.

Percutaneous transhepatic cholangiography

Percutaneous transhepatic cholangiography (PTC) involves the insertion of a fine needle into a dilated intrahepatic duct under guidance and the antegrade filling of the biliary tree with contrast. It is helpful if ERCP has failed or when MRC is unavailable and provides the opportunity for biopsy or stent insertion. PTC may be used in combination with ERCP to pass a guidewire through a stricture so that a stent may be deployed from within the duodenum.

Spiral computed tomography

Computed tomography (CT) provides highly detailed images of the entire liver, biliary system, pancreas, associated vasculature and surrounding structures. It is essential in planning surgery, particularly when resection and reconstruction are likely. Guided biopsies can be obtained in appropriate clinical circumstances.

Other tests

Endoscopic ultrasound (EUS), laparoscopy with laparoscopic ultrasound and biliary scintigraphy (HIDA) are all required in specific situations. EUS is the most sensitive modality for the detection of small pancreatic neoplasms. Laparoscopy is the only technique that can reliably identify peritoneal metastases and HIDA scanning may be required to demonstrate the functional integrity of liver segments after reconstruction.

Pathophysiological effects of jaundice

The pathophysiological effects of jaundice reflect either parenchymal liver disease or obstruction of the biliary tree. Parenchymal liver disease or hepatic failure results in altered drug and hormone metabolism, defective detoxification processes, reduced glycogen stores and impaired synthesis of proteins such as clotting factors or albumin. The causes of hepatic failure are discussed below.

Obstructive jaundice

In obstructive jaundice there is an absence of bile salts in the gastrointestinal tract, which are essential in the emulsification of fat and its absorption. As a consequence, the stools lack pigment; there may be steatorrhoea and impaired absorption of fat-soluble vitamins. There are also changes in gut flora and a reduction in the binding and clearance of endotoxin by bile salts. Biliary stasis leads to secondary bacterial colonisation, predominantly by coliforms.

Specific complications occur, which are both common and important in surgical patients. These are outlined below.

Infection

The increased incidence of septic complications is due principally to impaired immune function. Acute cholangitis, presenting as a combination of right upper quadrant pain, rigors and fever with jaundice (Charcot's triad), is a serious complication of biliary obstruction in association with ascending infection, nearly always due to bile duct stones. Without prompt decompression of the biliary tree, septicaemia or multiple hepatic abscesses may occur.

Coagulation disturbance

Vitamin K deficiency causes prolongation of the prothrombin time due to impaired synthesis of thrombin which occurs as a result of decreased production of the clotting factors II, VII, IX and X.

Impaired wound healing

Wound healing may be impaired as a direct effect of jaundice but is predominantly associated with the nutritional failure that accompanies it.

Hepatorenal syndrome

Patients with hepatic and obstructive jaundice have a higher incidence of developing renal dysfunction. Various pathophysiological mechanisms have been proposed. It was initially thought to be due to a toxic effect of bile salts or bilirubin on the renal tubules but more recent research has focused on gut-derived endotoxaemia and its effects on systemic and renal haemodynamics.

Several therapeutic strategies have been proposed to reduce the level of endotoxins which occur in the portal circulation as a result of increased bacterial translocation secondary to the absence of intraluminal bile salts. Subsequent spillover into the systemic circulation causes systemic endotoxaemia which results in impairment of the hepatic reticuloendothelial system. The therapeutic strategies have included prophylactic oral replacement of bile salts but prospective trials have failed to demonstrate significant benefit. Preoperative oral lactulose has been shown to reduce endotoxaemia in parenchymal liver disease and obstructive jaundice, protecting against postoperative renal failure. The mechanism is unknown; it may be related to a direct antiendotoxic effect, a reduction in endotoxin availability in the colon because of its laxative effect or alterations in colonic bacterial flora.

Recent research has concentrated on the control of fluid balance. Patients are often fasted for prolonged periods for radiological investigations. This reduced oral fluid intake, together with a reduced ability to concentrate the urine, possibly mediated by atrial naturietic peptide, further depletes the ECF. Cortical blood flow in the kidneys is decreased further by intense intrarenal vasoconstriction. This has led to the concept of adequate volume expansion. Jaundiced patients frequently demonstrate secondary hyperaldosteronism and thus tolerate sodium loads poorly. Intravenous infusion of 5% dextrose with potassium as required has been shown in clinical studies to reduce the incidence of renal dysfunction and renal failure.

When renal failure is established, there is no specific treatment. In severe parenchymal disease, the aim is to support the kidneys while the underlying liver disease resolves or a liver transplant is performed. Haemofiltration or dialysis may help control metabolic changes but the outcome is determined by the degree of liver failure. Preoperative relief of obstruction through stenting or external drainage has not been shown to reduce complications or mortality.

Perioperative management of obstructive jaundice

The incidence of postoperative complications can be reduced by improved perioperative management of patients with obstructive jaundice. The principles of management are summarised in Box 15.8.

Hepatic failure

Hepatic failure commonly occurs either in patients with longstanding hepatic insufficiency who sustain an insult that overwhelms their diminished hepatic reserve, or as a result of acute liver damage. The common causes in surgical patients are discussed below:

Common causes of hepatic dysfunction in surgical patients

Hepatitis

Hepatitis is associated with approximately 70% of all cases of acute hepatic failure. It should be excluded in patients with jaundice

Box 15.8 Perioperative management of patients with obstructive jaundice

- Careful control of fluid and electrolyte balance with hourly monitoring of urine output.
- Preoperative fluid expansion with, e.g., 3 l of crystalloid in 24 hours (including 5% dextrose).
- Antibiotic prophylaxis to patients undergoing percutaneous, endoscopic or surgical procedures (e.g. 750 mg oral ciprofloxacin). Prompt treatment of infection.
- Preoperative assessment of coagulation status and administration of vitamin K or fresh frozen plasma as indicated.
- Avoidance of NSAIDs, ACE inhibitors and tetracyclines; judicious use of diuretics.
- Nutritional assessment supplemented by the insertion of a feeding jejunostomy if a prolonged postoperative recovery is anticipated.

who have a hepatitic enzyme picture, through serological screening. Hepatic failure is most commonly associated with hepatitis B but 30% is related to hepatitis C.

Cirrhosis

There are many causes of cirrhosis but alcoholic, posthepatitic and idiopathic are all common in the West. Clinical manifestations of chronic liver disease and/or portal hypertension vary widely depending on aetiology and the regenerative function in the liver. Cirrhosis does, however, carry significant risks for the surgical patient with an increased incidence of sepsis as well as hepatic decompensation as a result of an impaired response to the trauma of surgery.

Total parenteral nutrition

TPN is often associated with a rise in serum bilirubin, transaminases and alkaline phosphatase, without evidence of extrahepatic obstruction. The cause is still unknown but histological examination often shows fatty infiltration, periportal inflammation and intrahepatic cholestasis. This may lead to secondary bacterial colonisation of the biliary tree. The absence of nutrients within the bowel lumen promotes stasis and reduced gallbladder contraction, predisposing to acalculous cholecystitis.

Hepatic hypoperfusion

Mild to moderate hepatic impairment may result from an ischaemic insult, proportional to the length and severity of the ischaemia time. Common causes include any conditions which lead to the systemic inflammatory response syndrome (SIRS), cardiogenic or haemorrhagic shock, burns and trauma.

Drug induced

Intrahepatic cholestasis, hepatitis or even massive necrosis may result from drug interactions or overdosage. Those commonly

associated are paracetamol or iron sulphate in overdose (10%), NSAIDs, erythromycin, steroids, isoniazid and halothane anaesthesia.

Other rarer causes of hepatic failure include the Budd–Chiari syndrome, fatty liver of pregnancy, haemochromatosis, Wilson's disease and malignant hyperpyrexia.

Clinical picture

Patients with acute hepatic failure exhibit jaundice, hepatic encephalopathy and hepatic fetor but lack signs of chronic liver disease, i.e. spider naevi, palmar erythema, unless the episode represents an acute event in a patient with preexisting liver disease. Ascites and oedema may occur.

Pathophysiology

Histologically, there is massive necrosis of the liver lobules. The liver plays an important role in supplying glucose to the tissues and both the storage and synthesis of glucose may be impaired. There may also be a reduction in the availability of bile salts in the gut lumen. Patients generally metabolise endogenous protein more rapidly, even in the absence of major catabolic stress. This leads to skeletal muscle proteolysis in an attempt to synthesise glucose.

The liver also has a role in the clearance of toxins that accumulate in the body as byproducts of metabolism. A number of toxins normally present in the gastrointestinal tract pass into the portal circulation and are cleared by the hepatic reticuloendothelial system, including endotoxin, bacteria, ammonia, gamma-butyric acid and mercaptans. Hepatic encephalopathy results from the absorption of ammonia and mercaptans from protein metabolism in the bowel that bypasses the normal excretory mechanisms in the liver.

The liver also synthesises a number of 'stress proteins' or acute-phase reactants such as clotting factors, components of the complement cascade and fibronectin, which form an essential part of the host response to critical illness.

Hepatic failure itself may also lead to renal failure (hepatorenal syndrome), increased susceptibility to infection, i.e. spontaneous bacterial peritonitis, and multiorgan failure.

Management

Nutritional support is widely advocated. The goals are similar to those in other critically ill patients. It should provide enough nutrients to prevent the catabolism of body protein, optimise hepatic regeneration and provide adequate amino acids for the synthesis of acute-phase reactants. If oral intake is insufficient, then enteral feeding is preferred because of the risk of sepsis with TPN. Fine-bore feeding tubes should be carefully inserted into the duodenum or jejunum to prevent possible trauma to varices.

The initial diet should restrict protein intake but may be increased if there is no deterioration in mental status. Medium-chain triglycerides have been advocated as a source of energy, because glucose infusions may precipitate fatty change in the liver. Meticulous fluid and electrolyte balance should be observed as patients are intolerant of sodium loads and tolerate hypokalaemia poorly. Clotting abnormalities should be treated with vitamin K or fresh frozen plasma.

Patients who develop encephalopathy may benefit from branched chain amino acid formulas, although the evidence to support this is not strong. Other measures include oral neomycin 0.5–1 g every six hours to reduce ammonia production by colonic bacteria and lactulose 50 ml orally every two hours to act as an osmotic laxative, decreasing bowel transit time and reducing ammonia absorption. Mannitol may be required in cases of cerebral oedema. The use of sedatives should be minimised.

Outcome

The aim of treatment is to support the patient until the liver has regenerated enough to function unaided or until a liver transplant is possible. Bearing in mind the likely aetiologies of liver failure, it is not usually feasible to directly treat the underlying cause. Death is usually due to multisystem organ failure, cerebral oedema, sepsis or haemorrhage.

FURTHER READING

1 Daly JM. The evolution of surgical nutrition: nutrient and anabolic interventions. *Ann Surg* 1999: **229** (1) 19–20

2 Diamond T, Parks RW. Perioperative management of obstructive jaundice. *Br J Surg* 1997: **84**, 147–149

3 Fleming CR, Remington M. Intestinal failure. In: Hill GL, (ed). *Nutrition and the Surgical Patient*. Edinburgh: Churchill Livingstone, 1981: 219–235

4 Lennard-Jones JE. *A Positive Approach to Nutrition as Treatment*. London: King's Fund Centre, 1992: 1–48

5 Reynolds JV. Gut barrier function in the surgical patient. *Br J Surg* 1996: **83**, 1668–1669

6 Rombeau J, Sitges-Serra A. International Association for Surgical Metabolism and Nutrition. *World J Surg* 1999: **23** (6):

7 Wastell C, Nyhus L, Donahue PE. *Surgery of the Esophagus, Stomach and Small Intestine*, 5th edn. Boston: Little, Brown, 1994

16

Neuromuscular system

The motor system
    An overview of the motor unit
    The muscle action potential
    Muscle contraction
Neuromuscular-blocking drugs
    Monitoring of neuromuscular blockade
    Neuromuscular-blockers and nerve stimulator use
    Onset of neuromuscular blockade
    Pharmacodynamics
    Elimination of neuromuscular-blocking drugs
    Reversal of residual neuromuscular blockade
    Risks of neuromuscular-blocking drugs
Other drugs and ions which affect the neuromuscular
        system
    Aminoglycosides
    Calcium balance
    Magnesium balance
Diseases affecting the neuromuscular system in
        surgical and anaesthetic practice
    Poliomyelitis
    Botulism
    Tetanus
    Denervation injury

Myasthenia gravis
Myasthenic syndrome
Malignant hyperthermia
Pathways of transmission of painful stimulation
    Spinal cord pharmacology
    Descending pathways
Local anaesthetics
Opiates
    Actions of opiates
    Immediate hazards of opiate use
    Routes of opiate administration
Non-steroidal anti-inflammatory drugs
    Side effects
Miscellaneous analgesic agents
    Clonidine
    Ketamine
    Tramadol
Practical methods of pain relief in the surgical patient
    Local anaesthetic blocks
    Epidural analgesia
    Patient-controlled analgesia
    Miscellaneous methods of pain relief

C. J. R. Parker

Several neuromuscular topics are of interest to the surgeon and anaesthetist; these can broadly be divided into those involving the afferent system for transmission of painful stimuli and those involving efferent output to the muscles. The importance of the afferent system for treatment of postoperative pain is obvious but an understanding of the motor system is also essential to appreciate the production of muscle relaxation during surgery, as well as certain states of muscle weakness seen in surgical practice.

THE MOTOR SYSTEM

An overview of the motor unit

The motor unit is the basic component of the efferent neuromuscular system; it comprises the anterior horn cell in the spinal grey matter, its axon and the muscle fibres which it innervates. The lower motor neurones each give rise to a single axon which typically innervates a number of muscle fibres. The number of muscle fibres which comprise one motor unit is variable. In muscles which control posture and gross movement up to 2000 muscle fibres may be innervated by one neurone. The number is much smaller for those muscles which are required to produce very finely graded movements, such as the extraocular muscles.

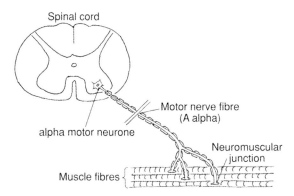

Figure 16.1 The organisation of the motor unit. The figure shows the motor neurone cell body lying in the anterior horn of the spinal grey matter, with its myelinated axon reaching the muscle fibres which it innervates at the neuromuscular junction.

Excitable tissue

Each of the structures in the motor unit, the motor neurone, its axon and the muscle fibre is excitable; that is, they are capable of transmitting a propagated action potential. As in all cells, the principal intracellular monovalent cation is potassium and the intracellular sodium concentration is much lower than that in the extracellular fluid. In their resting state, these tissues are selectively permeable to potassium, which diffuses down its concentration gradient to set up a resting membrane potential which opposes further potassium loss from the cell. The size of the resting membrane potential is given by the Nernst equation.

$$E = \frac{RT}{zF} \log\left(\frac{[K^+]_e}{[K^+]_i}\right)$$

Figure 16.2 The Nernst equation for potassium. The electrical potential difference across the membrane, E, which would exactly oppose the movement of the potassium ion down its concentration gradient, is given by the equation shown, where

R = the universal gas constant (joule mole^{-1} kelvin^{-1})
T = absolute temperature (kelvin)
z = valence of the ion concerned, in this case 1
F = the Faraday (coulombs per mole)
$[K^+]_e$ = the external (extracellular) potassium concentration (mMolar)
$[K^+]_i$ = the internal (cellular) potassium concentration (mMolar).

Table 16.1 The sodium (Na$^+$) and potassium (K$^+$) concentrations inside and outside the nerve axon

	Ion concentration (mM)	
	Intracellular	Extracellular
Na$^+$	15	140
K$^+$	140	5

The membrane of the excitable tissues also contains voltage-gated sodium channels. These are activated (opened) by depolarisation; opening of the sodium channels leads to depolarisation, because they cause membrane permeability to sodium to become greater than that to potassium and the membrane potential tends to a

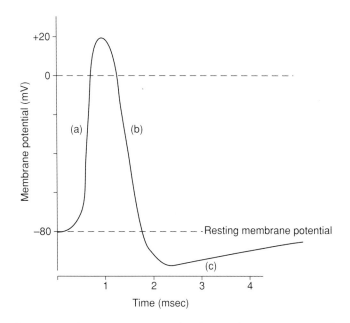

Figure 16.3 The nerve action potential is shown. There is a resting membrane potential of around 80 mV, negative internally. During phase (a), there is a rapid increase in sodium permeability due to the opening of voltage-gated sodium channels. In phase (b), the sodium channels become inactivated and voltage-gated potassium channels open. In phase (c), the axon is temporarily refractory to further stimulation.

value given by the Nernst equation for the sodium ion. The opening of the sodium channels which causes depolarisation thus leads to further opening of sodium channels; the effect is one of positive feedback. It is a feature of the sodium channels that they are rapidly inactivated; after a short open period they spontaneously close and for a short time are refractory to further depolarisation. Thus the depolarisation of the action potential is transient; repolarisation is further facilitated by opening of voltage-sensitive potassium channels.

The sodium channels are the site of action of local anaesthetic drugs (see below) and the inactivation of sodium channels by sustained depolarisation is thought to be involved in the action of the neuromuscular-blocking drug suxamethonium (see below).

Anterior horn cell

The anterior horn cell is located in the ventral horn of the spinal grey matter. It has several dendrites and gives rise to a single axon at the axon hillock. The resting membrane potential of the anterior horn cell is about 70 mV, negative internally. It receives synaptic inputs on both its dendrites and on the cell body; the inputs are both excitatory and inhibitory and arise from higher centres and from the segmental reflexes at the level of the spinal cord. The excitatory inputs cause a depolarising excitatory postsy-

Table 16.2 A classification of nerve fibres by their size and myelination, together with some of the main functions of the fibre types

	Myelination	Diameter (μm)	Function
A alpha	+	12–20	Motor to skeletal muscle
A beta	+	5–12	Touch sensation Proprioception
A gamma	+	3–6	Motor to muscle spindles
A delta	+	2–5	Fast pain sensation Temperature sensation
B	+	3	Preganglionic autonomic efferent
C	–	0.5–2	Pain Postganglionic autonomic efferent

naptic potential (EPSP), which results from an increase in sodium permeability. Inhibitory inputs produce a hyperpolarising response, the inhibitory postsynaptic potential (IPSP), owing to an increase in potassium or chloride ion permeability. The EPSPs and IPSPs are transmitted to the axon hillock by passive 'electrotonic' conduction; the overall activation of the cell is determined by the membrane potential at this site. The summation of sufficient EPSPs is followed by a suprathreshold depolarisation of the axon hillock and the generation of an action potential which is conducted along the axon to the muscle. The axons leave the spinal cord through the ventral root at their segmental level.

Motor nerve fibres

Motor nerve fibres are myelinated. The motor neurones principally innervate the muscle fibres which constitute the bulk of the muscle. These are large-diameter fibres (up to 20 μm diameter), known as A-alpha fibres. Their conduction velocity is around 100 m sec^{-1}. Some of the axons innervate the intrafusal fibres of the muscle spindles. These axons, though still myelinated, are of smaller diameter (up to 6 μm) and have a lower conduction velocity. They are known as A-gamma fibres. The A-gamma fibre innervation of the muscle spindle is thought to be important in adjusting the length-sensing mechanism of the muscle spindle to the length changes resulting from contraction of the surrounding muscle fibres.

The neuromuscular junction

The motor nerve fibres reach the muscle fibre at a specialised area, the motor endplate; this is adapted for the chemical transmission of excitation. Acetylcholine is released from the nerve terminal and interacts with nicotinic acetylcholine receptors in the postjunctional muscle fibre membrane which causes a depolarisation of the muscle fibre. The mammalian endplate is compact and occupies a length of around 25 μm; it is therefore a tiny fraction of the total muscle fibre length and in health, acetylcholine sensitivity is restricted to this region of the muscle membrane. In cer-

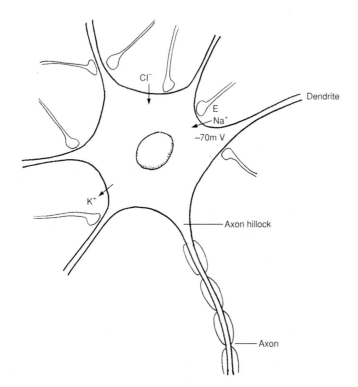

Figure 16.4 The motor neurone is illustrated. It receives inputs on both the cell body and the dendrites, which are both excitatory and inhibitory. The excitatory inputs increase sodium permeability to cause depolarisation; the inhibitory inputs cause hyperpolarisation by increasing potassium or chloride permeability. The axon arises at the axon hillock, where the action potential is generated if there is a sufficient depolarisation.

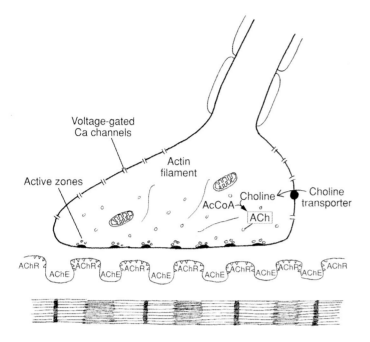

Figure 16.5 A diagram of the neuromuscular junction. Acetylcholine is synthesised in the nerve terminal and is concentrated into vesicles there. The vesicles are concentrated near the active release zones, opposite the ridges of the postjunctional membrane where there is a high concentration of nicotinic acetylcholine receptors (AChR). Vesicle release is triggered by calcium entry through voltage-gated calcium channels. Acetylcholinesterase (AChE) is located in the junctional cleft, in particular in folds of the postjunctional membrane.

tain conditions, notably following denervation injuries and burns, there is a proliferation of acetylcholine receptors along the length of the muscle fibre.

Acetylcholine is synthesized in the axoplasm of the nerve terminal by the enzyme choline acetyltransferase. This reaction requires choline, which is taken up into the nerve by active transport, and an acetyl group, derived from acetyl-coenzyme A, which is synthesised within the nerve terminal. The acetylcholine is taken up by active transport into vesicles, whose diameter is about 50 nm, from which it is released into the junctional cleft following the invasion of the nerve terminal by an action potential. Each vesicle contains about 10 000 molecules of acetylcholine.

Vesicle release is calcium dependent; the required calcium enters the nerve terminal through voltage-sensitive calcium channels in the axon membrane, following the depolarization induced by the action potential. These calcium channels are not sensitive to dihydropyridine-type calcium channel antagonists which are used to

$$CH_3-\overset{\overset{\displaystyle CH_3}{|}}{\underset{\underset{\displaystyle CH_3}{|}}{N^+}}-CH_2-CH_2-O-\overset{\overset{\displaystyle O}{\|}}{C}-CH_3$$

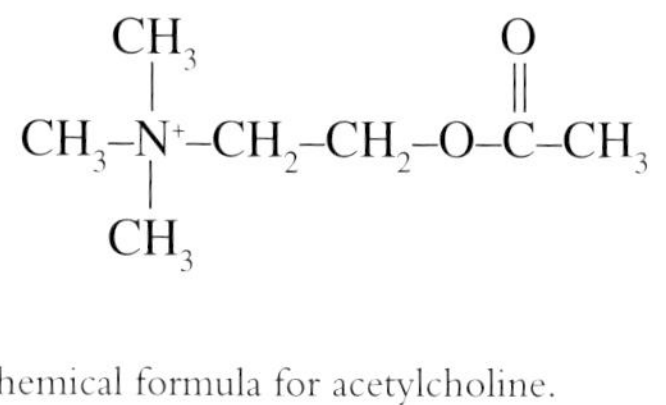

Figure 16.6 The chemical formula for acetylcholine.

treat angina and hypertension. Magnesium is capable of entering the axon terminal in competition with calcium but it is not active in activating acetylcholine release; thus it acts as an antagonist of calcium in the release process.

The release of acetylcholine vesicles occurs at specialised zones of the prejunctional nerve terminal, 'active zones', and involves the interaction of specialised proteins in the vesicle membrane with docking proteins in the axon plasma membrane. Acetylcholine storage, mobilisation and release are controlled by a series of proteins in the vesicle membrane; elucidation of their roles allows understanding of the action of certain toxins.

Random release of single vesicles occurs spontaneously and this gives rise to miniature endplate potentials. Invasion of the nerve terminal by an action potential causes about 100 vesicles to be released; thus about a million molecules of acetylcholine are released by each action potential. The junctional cleft is about 50 nm in width and release of acetylcholine is followed by rapid diffusion of the transmitter to the postjunctional membrane.

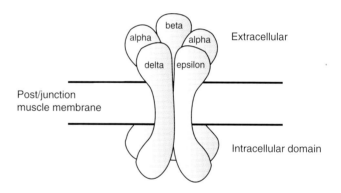

Figure 16.7 The nicotinic acetylcholine receptor. The receptor is a transmembrane protein, consisting of five subunits arranged around a central pore. Each subunit spans the membrane. Acetylcholine binds to the alpha subunits.

The nicotinic acetylcholine receptor is a very well-characterized transmembrane, ligand-gated ion channel. It comprises five subunits, arranged around a central pore. There are four types of subunit (alpha, beta, delta and epsilon); the receptor is composed of two alpha subunits and one each of the other types. The amino acid sequence of each of the five subunits is known and they have substantial sequences in common. The molecular weight of each subunit is between 40 000 and 70 000 daltons and in each subunit there are four sequences which span the membrane. The alpha subunit contains the binding site not only for acetylcholine but also for neuromuscular-blocking drugs (see below) and for the cobra venom alpha-bungarotoxin.

The receptors are very tightly packed, with a density of up to 20 000 per μm² of postjunctional membrane. When a molecule of acetylcholine binds to both of the two alpha subunits, there is a change in the conformation of the receptor leading to opening of the channel and conductance of cations. The selectivity of the ion channel for cations is determined by the charge of the amino acid residues close to the channel openings. *In vivo*, the most important ion involved is sodium, because the resting membrane potential is far away from the equilibrium potential for this ion; activation of the nicotinic acetylcholine receptors leads to a depolarisation, termed the endplate potential.

The dynamics of the ion channel have been illuminated using the patch clamp technique, in which a single ion channel is isolated in the tip of a pipette and the electrophysiological properties may be studied in detail. Each ion channel has a unit conductance and is either 'on' or 'off'. Transition between the 'on' and 'off' states is sharp; when open, a channel has a typical lifetime before closing which is variable but can be characterised from a statistical point of view, as the mean open time. For the mammalian acetylcholine receptor, this is several milliseconds.

Fate of acetylcholine

Acetylcholine binding with the receptor is reversible and unbound acetylcholine is rapidly hydrolysed by the enzyme acetylcholinesterase. This is located in the junctional cleft and in particular in the folds of the postjunctional membrane. The mechanism of action of the enzyme is understood and it is the site of action of anticholinesterase drugs (see below).

The active site of the enzyme has two components: there is an anionic site, which is negatively charged and forms a site of attachment for the quaternary ammonium group of acetylcholine, and the esteratic site, at which the hydrolysis of acetylcholine actually occurs. At the esteratic site, the hydroxyl side chain of a serine residue reacts with the ester group of acetylcholine, so that the enzyme is acetylated and the choline moiety is released. The acetylated enzyme dissociates rapidly by release of the acetate group, so as to regenerate the enzyme.

Choline derived from the hydrolysis of acetylcholine is taken up into the prejunctional nerve terminal by active transport and is used again in the synthesis of further acetylcholine.

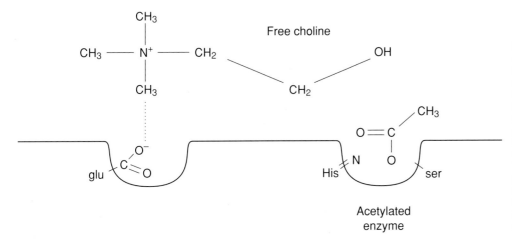

Figure 16.8 The active site of the enzyme acetylcholinesterase. There are two sites: the anionic and the esteratic. The anionic site attracts the positively charged choline moiety, the esteratic site catalyses the hydrolysis of the ester bond. In the upper panel acetylcholine is shown binding to the enzyme. In the lower panel, ester hydrolysis has occurred and the acetyl group remains bound to the enzyme whilst the choline group is free to dissociate. The acetylated enzyme is unstable and the acetyl group is freed rapidly. Carbamate esters like neostigmine react in a similar manner but the inactivated carbamylated enzyme is relatively stable; thus neostigmine acts as an inhibitor of this enzyme.

The endplate potential

The increase in endplate conductance to cations, with depolarisation of the endplate region, triggers the propagation of an action potential along the muscle fibre membrane. There is normally a 'margin of safety' of neuromuscular transmission which means that sufficient acetylcholine is released and sufficient acetylcholine receptors are activated to cause an endplate potential which is larger than that required to produce an action potential by a factor of about four. This ensures that each nerve action potential is reliably followed by a suprathreshold endplate depolarisation. The margin of safety determines some of the features of the neuromuscular-blocking drugs (see below); disorders of neuromuscular transmission are manifest only when the margin of safety is eroded.

The muscle action potential

The mechanism of the muscle fibre action potential is similar to that of the nerve action potential. The high speed of propagation of the action potential ensures that the whole of the muscle fibre is activated in a short period and so the whole fibre, which may be several centimetres long, is activated as a unit. The action potential invades the transverse tubular system or T-tubules, a series of invaginations of the muscle fibre membrane at each sarcomere.

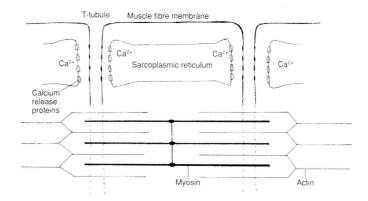

Figure 16.9 The transverse tubular system. This consists of a series of invaginations of the muscle fibre membrane and the tubules form a close relationship with the sarcoplasmic reticulum. Depolarisation in the T-tubule is transmitted to the calcium release proteins in the sarcoplasmic reticulum and leads to an increase in sarcoplasmic calcium ion concentration. Disorders of this mechanism are involved in the condition of malignant hyperpyrexia.

Calcium release

Muscle contraction is controlled by sarcoplasmic calcium concentration, normally very low, in the region of 10^{-4} mM. It is kept at this level by sequestration of calcium ions in the sarcoplasmic reticulum, a closed tubular system which forms a network surrounding each myofibril. Synchronised release of calcium from the sarcoplasmic reticulum occurs following the invasion of the transverse tubule (T-tubule) by the muscle action potential. The

T-tubule forms a very close association with the sarcoplasmic reticulum membrane and the appearance of the junction of a T-tubule with two adjacent systems of sarcoplasmic reticulum is known as a triad. Invasion of the T-tubule by the muscle fibre action potential causes a conformational change in a voltage-sensitive protein in the T-tubule membrane, which is transmitted to calcium release receptors (ryanodine receptors) in the adjacent membrane of the sarcoplasmic reticulum. The calcium release receptors are themselves calcium sensitive, leading to a rapid rise in calcium concentration in the muscle cell. The regulation of calcium release is of great importance in the condition of malignant hyperthermia (see below).

Muscle contraction

Muscle contraction involves repeated cyclical interaction between filaments of actin and myosin; in particular, there is repeated binding and unbinding of myosin filament heads to actin filaments. The process involves a conformational change in the myosin head with each cycle which results in contraction and the process is driven in one direction by the binding of ATP, its hydrolysis and subsequent unbinding of ADP.

Sarcoplasmic calcium ions control muscle contraction by binding to the C subunit of troponin-tropomyosin complex, a set of proteins attached to the actin filament, which control the access of myosin heads to the actin filaments. Calcium binding results in a conformational change in troponin, which exposes the actin filaments to the heads of the myosin filaments.

NEUROMUSCULAR-BLOCKING DRUGS

The most common cause of interruption of the normal function of the neuromuscular system in surgical practice is the use of neuromuscular-blocking drugs, which may be divided into depolarising and non-depolarising agents. The former has only one exemplar in common use, suxamethonium; the other drugs in everyday use (for example, atracurium, vecuronium, rocuronium and mivacurium) have a non-depolarising action. The distinction is based upon the fact that suxamethonium activates the nicotinic acetylcholine receptor, mimicking the action of acetylcholine, whereas the non-depolarising neuromuscular-blocking drugs are all competitive inhibitors of the action of acetylcholine at the nicotinic acetylcholine receptor and do not simulate it.

The non-depolarising neuromuscular-blocking drugs are relatively selective agents and thus have few side effects, though some of the older exemplars of this group such as tubocurarine had a propensity to release histamine from mast cells, resulting in hypotension and bronchospasm. Other agents, notably gallamine and pancuronium, have a tendency to block cardiac muscarinic acetylcholine receptors and hence cause a tachycardia.

Thus the principal effect of the non-depolarising neuromuscular-blocking drugs is paralysis of skeletal muscle. This includes the

Table 16.3 A comparison of some of the properties of suxamethonium and the non-depolarising neuromuscular-blocking drugs

	Suxamethonium	Non-depolarising neuromuscular-blocking drugs
Mode of action	Probably sodium channel inactivation	Competitive antagonism of acetylcholine
Initial stimulation	+	–
Fasciculation	+	–
Onset	Within 60 seconds	More than 60 seconds
Metabolism	Hydrolysis by plasma cholinesterase	Various, including: renal excretion, hepatic uptake, spontaneous degradation (atracurium), hydrolysis by plasma cholinesterase (mivacurium)
Recovery	Few minutes	Variable, most >30 min
Fade of train of four	Little	Substantial
Side effects	Many	Few
Malignant hyperthermia risk	+	–

muscles of respiration and the administration of a dose of a neuromuscular-blocking drug is followed by a cessation of respiration within about three minutes. It is essential to provide artificial positive pressure respiration, preferably through an endotracheal tube.

Indications for the use of a muscle relaxant drug in the operating theatre are as follows.

1. To facilitate surgery where this would otherwise be impeded by muscle tone; for example, surgery on the abdominal or thoracic cavity. Producing profound muscle relaxation without the use of a neuromuscular-blocking drug used to require deep anaesthesia, a technique which had adverse physiological consequences.

2. To facilitate the maintenance of physiological stability; for example, during neurosurgery, where the use of muscle relaxant drugs facilitates intermittent positive pressure ventilation to control arterial carbon dioxide tension and hence cerebral blood flow.

3. To facilitate anaesthesia in small children, where positive pressure ventilation is desirable to facilitate maintenance of lung volume above closing volume.

4. To facilitate endotracheal intubation where this is necessary for other reasons; for example, during head and neck surgery or eye surgery.

5. To limit the adverse effects of muscle contractions during the convulsions induced by electroconvulsive therapy. Without the use of a muscle relaxant drug, there would be a risk of fractures.

This group of drugs is also valuable in the intensive care unit. Though most patients receiving artificial ventilation in the intensive care unit are managed using sedative drugs only, the muscle relaxants are useful in patients with particularly uncompliant lungs, and to permit permissive hypercapnia in the management

of severe asthma; they also have a role in patients with raised intracranial pressure.

Monitoring of neuromuscular blockade

The action of the neuromuscular-blocking drugs used in the operating theatre is monitored by the anaesthetist to ensure that relaxation is adequate. The method depends upon the administration of a short electrical stimulus, transcutaneously to a convenient peripheral motor nerve. Often the ulnar nerve at the wrist, the posterior tibial nerve at the ankle or the facial nerve is used. The electrical stimulus should be less than the duration of a nerve action potential and a duration of 0.2 msec is usually chosen so that a single volley of nerve action potentials results. The stimulus should be strong enough to stimulate all the nerve fibres in the nerve ('supramaximal') which requires a current in the region of 50 mA.

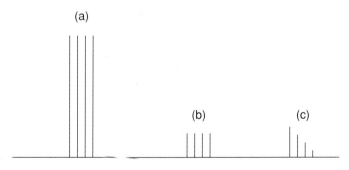

Figure 16.10 The train of four, used in neuromuscular monitoring; four supramaximal stimuli are applied to the motor nerve at 2 Hz. The twitch responses of the muscle are shown. The control response, obtained before the administration of a neuromuscular-blocking drug, is shown in (a), with four strong twitches. In (b), the response of a muscle partially paralysed with suxamethonium is shown; there are four weak but equal twitches. Panel (c) denotes the response of a muscle partially paralysed with a non-depolarising neuromuscular blocking drug; the responses are all smaller than the control but there is a progressive lessening of the responses to successive stimuli, known as fade.

It is usual to administer four stimuli at a rate of 2 Hz, a pattern known as the 'train of four'. Following the administration of a non-depolarising neuromuscular-blocking drug, the response to the train of four is characterised by 'fade'; that is, the height of the fourth response is much smaller than the first response in the series. Such a response is not normally seen following a single dose of suxamethonium.

Neuromuscular-blockers and nerve stimulator use

Occasionally it may be necessary for a surgeon to identify a nerve using a nerve stimulator; this is required, for example, during dissection of the parotid gland to identify the facial nerve. Since the stimulus is applied under direct vision to an exposed nerve, the current requirement is much less than in the case of a transcutaneous nerve stimulator and is around 1 mA. If it is planned to use a nerve stimulator, it is essential that the anaesthetist should not use a long-acting neuromuscular-blocking drug, which would mask the response to nerve stimulation.

Onset of neuromuscular blockade

On occasion it is necessary to achieve as rapid an onset of neuro-muscular-block as possible following the administration of the drug. An example of such a situation is where a patient presents with intestinal obstruction; to minimise the risk of aspiration of gastric contents, an endotracheal tube should be passed as soon as possible following the induction of anaesthesia. In these circumstances, suxamethonium is the drug of choice.

The non-depolarising neuromuscular-blocking drugs have a relatively slow onset of action and even drugs such as rocuronium, which have been introduced in recent years with a more rapid onset, are still a little slower than suxamethonium in producing complete paralysis. The basis for this slow onset is the margin of safety of neuromuscular transmission; the preponderance of acetylcholine receptors and release of more than enough acetyl-choline to provide a sufficient endplate potential means that nearly all the nicotinic acetylcholine receptors at the neuromuscular junction must be occupied by neuromuscular-blocking drug before paralysis occurs. Clearly it takes time for a sufficient quantity of the relaxant drug to diffuse into the junctional cleft. Recent developments have been aimed at producing a drug of low potency, which is necessarily given in larger amounts. The greater number of molecules given generates a greater concentration gradient to encourage diffusion into the cleft compared with a more potent agent. The greater concentration gradient results in a more rapid onset of neuromuscular-block.

Pharmacodynamics

The action of the non-depolarising neuromuscular-blocking drugs is closely related to their concentration in the plasma.

Indeed, the relationship between drug plasma concentration and the effect has perhaps been more thoroughly quantified than for any other class of drug. That does not mean that the degree of paralysis at any time is directly proportional to the plasma drug concentration; rather, it is related to a time-lagging function of the recent history of plasma drug concentration. The relationship has been formalised in terms of a model where an 'effect compartment' is related to the plasma concentration profile by a single rate constant k_{eo}. The effect of the drug is related to the drug concentration in the effect compartment by the Hill equation.

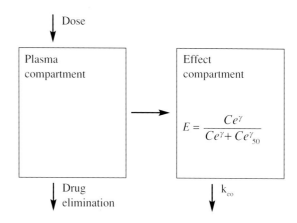

Figure 16.11 The effect compartment model for non-depolarising neuromuscular blocking drugs. The drugs are administered by injection into the plasma, from which they are also considered to be eliminated by processes such as renal or hepatic elimination. The effect of the drug is related to the concentration of drug in an 'effect compartment', Ce. The value of Ce depends upon the recent history of the plasma drug concentration. It will be a lagging function of it; the higher the value of the rate constant k_{eo}, the more closely the effect compartment concentration mirrors the plasma concentration profile. The effect (E) is a non-linear function of Ce. A Hill equation is usually used to describe the relationship. The parameter Ce_{50} is the concentration in the effect compartment which gives rise to a 50% block of neuromuscular transmission; the parameter gamma describes the sigmoidicity of the concentration–effect relationship.

Elimination of neuromuscular-blocking drugs

The termination of the action of the neuromuscular-blocking drugs depends upon their elimination from the body. In the case of suxamethonium, this is by a circulating enzyme, plasma cholinesterase. The non-depolarising neuromuscular-blocking drugs are eliminated by various means including renal excretion, which applies to all drugs to some extent but is predominant for gallamine, and hepatic uptake, which is important for certain aminosteroid drugs such as vecuronium. The non-depolarising neuromuscular-blocking drug mivacurium is metabolised by plasma cholinesterase, whilst atracurium undergoes spontaneous degradation under physiological conditions of pH and temperature.

Reversal of residual neuromuscular blockade

After the end of surgery and before adequate respiration can be reestablished, it is usually necessary to antagonise or 'reverse' the residual action of the non-depolarising neuromuscular-blocking drugs. This is done by the administration of an antagonist of acetylcholinesterase, the enzyme which destroys acetylcholine at the neuromuscular junction. To antagonise this enzyme increases the life of released acetylcholine and hence shifts the balance of competitive inhibition in favour of acetylcholine.

Two categories of anticholinesterase are in common clinical use.

● Drugs such as neostigmine act by reacting with the active site of the enzyme. They are carbamate esters and by reacting with the enzyme in an analogous manner to acetylcholine, they form a carbamylated enzyme complex, which is inactive. Unlike the acetylated enzyme, the carbamylated enzyme does not dissociate immediately but has a half-life of about 30 minutes. During this time the enzyme is inactive.

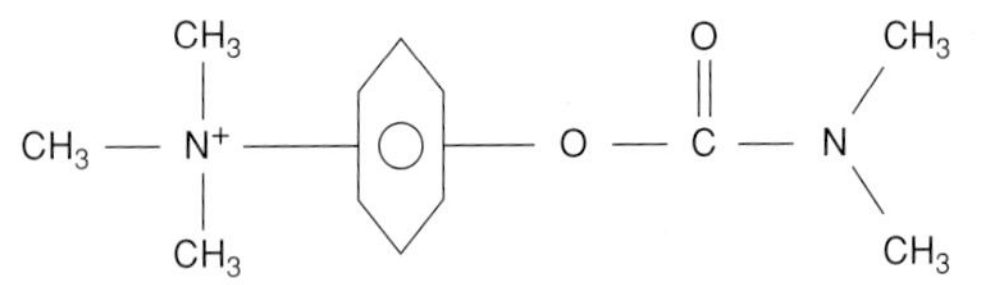

Figure 16.12 The chemical formula of neostigmine.

● The second category, exemplified by edrophonium, simply acts as a competitive antagonist of acetylcholine at the anionic site of the enzyme. It does not combine with the esteratic site; its attachment to the enzyme is shortlived and the drug has a short duration of action. It is used in the diagnosis of myasthenia gravis; a definite improvement in muscle power and fatiguability following the administration of a small intravenous dose of edrophonium strongly supports the diagnosis. Edrophonium has also been used to antagonise neuromuscular-block at the end of surgery but a much larger dose, around 0.5 mg kg^{-1} is then required. It is best suited to antagonism of relatively short-acting non-depolarising neuromuscular-blocking drugs.

The enzyme acetylcholinesterase is widely distributed, because acetylcholine is the neurotransmitter not only at the neuromuscular junction but also at the autonomic ganglia and at the parasympathetic postganglionic nerve endings. The administration of neostigmine by itself would therefore be followed not only by recovery of muscle power but also the effects of widespread activation of the muscarinic receptors in the parasympathetic nervous system. These include such undesirable effects as enhanced bronchial secretions, bronchial constriction, bradycardia and spasm of gastrointestinal smooth muscle. It is essential therefore when giving the anticholinesterase drug at the end of surgery to accompany it with an antimuscarinic drug such as atropine or glycopyrrolate.

When a neuromuscular-blocking drug has been used, it is important that the anaesthetist be sure that the muscle power has recovered to a level allowing the patient to breathe adequately and maintain airway patency, to cough and to swallow before the trachea is extubated and the patient discharged. This is facilitated by delaying pharmacological reversal until spontaneous recovery is

well under way. The adequacy of recovery of neuromuscular function can be assessed by asking the patient to raise the head from the pillow for five seconds.

Risks of neuromuscular-blocking drugs

The introduction of neuromuscular-blocking drugs into anaesthetic practice some 50 years ago was accompanied by the emergence of new hazards.

Disconnection

The most feared complication of the use of a neuromuscular-blocking drug is the total discontinuation of ventilation due to a technical mishap such as a disconnection of the anaesthetic breathing system from the endotracheal tube so that the patient is totally deprived of oxygen. This is a particular hazard during surgery on the head and neck, when the endotracheal tube is concealed under drapes and may be moved by the surgeon.

A prolonged period of hypoxia is eventually followed by cardiac arrest. The brain is more sensitive to hypoxia than is the heart, however, and it is particularly tragic that successful resuscitation is likely to be accompanied by permanent cerebral damage; typically, there is global cortical damage resulting in the patient suffering a persistent vegetative state.

Awareness

The pharmacological paralysis of the muscle means that the patient is no longer able to indicate his or her distress if the level of anaesthesia becomes insufficient to abolish consciousness. This may occur either due to mishap, for example where the anaesthetic vaporizer is empty, or where the anaesthetic is deliberately lightened to avoid the depressant effects of anaesthetic drugs, for example on the heart or, in the case of a patient undergoing caesarean section, the fetus. In any event, it can be a most unpleasant experience with long-term psychological sequelae.

Muscle weakness in intensive care unit

The use of neuromuscular-blocking drugs in the intensive care unit over a period of several days or weeks is sometimes followed by prolonged weakness. The origin of this condition is not completely clear. It may involve the presence of active metabolites of some of the drugs used or may be a manifestation of a peripheral neuropathy.

Anaphylaxis

Any drug with a quaternary ammonium group may directly cause release of histamine and other inflammatory mediators from mast cells. This may result in no more than a few wheals on the skin of the limb used for drug injection but rarely there may be a florid reaction with widespread flushing, hypotension and bronchospasm. The treatment of a severe reaction is to secure the airway, give oxygen, adrenaline and intravenous fluids. Secondary treatment will include intravenous steroids and perhaps antihistamines. It is impossible in the immediate aftermath of a reaction to distinguish between direct release of histamine, complement-mediated histamine release and true IgE-mediated anaphylaxis.

Blood samples taken at the time of the reaction and in the following 24 hours are assayed for mast cell tryptase; a rise in the level at the time of the attack confirms the nature of the reaction. Muscle relaxant drugs are often given at the start of anaesthesia together with an intravenous induction agent and an opiate. Drugs other than the muscle relaxant series can also provoke anaphylactic reactions and skin tests may be helpful in identifying the causative agent.

Any neuromuscular-blocking agent may be responsible but it was more likely with the now obsolete agents tubocurarine and alcuronium than with currently used agents. Suxamethonium is now probably the most common trigger of an anaphylactic reaction.

OTHER DRUGS AND IONS WHICH AFFECT THE NEUROMUSCULAR SYSTEM

Aminoglycosides

Although it is not often seen now, aminoglycoside antibiotics have been reported to cause failure of neuromuscular transmission, usually in the patient with peritonitis given intraperitoneal antibiotics as well as a neuromuscular-blocking drug. The modes of action in interfering with neuromuscular function include reduced calcium entry at the prejunctional nerve terminal and the paralysis is not reversed by neostigmine.

Calcium balance

Although calcium ions are intimately involved in both acetylcholine release and in excitation-contraction coupling, the clinical effects of hypocalcaemia on the neuromuscular system are dominated by muscular spasms, probably arising from an increase in nerve membrane excitability. A gentle tap over the facial nerve produces a twitch in the facial muscles; more importantly, there may be laryngospasm, a feature which can complicate the hypocalcaemia which may follow parathyroidectomy.

Magnesium balance

Magnesium is used clinically to control pre-eclamptic toxaemia. Magnesium is a competitor with calcium at the prejunctional nerve terminal; a progressive increase in the plasma concentration of magnesium is accompanied by increasing muscle weakness. Thus a therapeutic concentration is in the range 2–3 mM; the patellar tendon reflex is lost at levels in the range 3.5–5.0 mM and at higher levels there is danger of respiratory failure.

DISEASES AFFECTING THE NEUROMUSCULAR SYSTEM IN SURGICAL AND ANAESTHETIC PRACTICE

There are several medical conditions which can be understood in terms of interference with the physiology of the neuromuscular system, as outlined above.

Poliomyelitis

This viral disease affects the anterior horn cells of the spinal cord and motor nuclei of the cranial nerves and also neurones in the central nervous system concerned with control of the motor system, including the motor cortex and the cerebellum. There is necrosis of the anterior horn cells and degeneration of their axons. There is a consequent loss of muscle mass and muscle weakness. The remaining motor neurones will sprout new axon terminals to innervate the muscle fibres which have lost their innervation.

Botulism

Botulism is caused by an exotoxin produced by the bacterium *Clostridium botulinum* and it can be understood in terms of the action of the exotoxin at the neuromuscular junction. The exotoxin is an enzyme which cleaves a 25 000 dalton molecular weight protein found in the release zones of the nerve terminal membrane; its normal function is to bind a protein (synaptobrevin) in the membrane of the acetylcholine storage vesicle. The toxin thus interferes with acetylcholine release. Clinically the disease is characterized by diplopia, bulbar weakness and a progressive motor paralysis, which may involve respiratory muscles.

Tetanus

This disease is also caused by the exotoxin of a clostridium bacterium; the toxin acts centrally, both in the spinal cord and at higher centres, resulting in disinhibition of the muscular system and hence muscular spasms. Management requires the spasms to be controlled and in very severe cases this may require the patient to be pharmacologically paralysed with a non-depolarising neuromuscular-blocking drug and artificially ventilated for a prolonged period.

Denervation injury

Whatever the cause of the injury, where muscles are deprived of their normal motor innervation, the muscle responds characteristically by proliferation of acetylcholine receptors along the whole length of the muscle fibre membrane. The 'extrajunctional' receptors have a somewhat different molecular subunit composition from the normal junctional receptors but they retain their sensitivity to suxamethonium. Consequently, when a patient who has suffered a denervation injury is exposed to suxamethonium, there follows a massive opening of the proliferated receptors and potassium release from the muscle. The sudden and massive rise in plasma potassium concentration is likely to lead to a fatal cardiac arrest.

Myasthenia gravis

This disease is characterised by the onset of fatiguability and muscle weakness, often affecting initially the extraocular muscles, resulting in ptosis and diplopia. It can be understood as a failure of neuromuscular transmission and bears many similarities to a partial block with a non-depolarising neuromuscular-blocking drug. Often antibodies to the nicotinic acetylcholine receptor can be detected; the number of acetylcholine receptors is decreased. Treatment is with an anticholinesterase drug, usually pyridostigmine, to increase the availability of acetylcholine at the neuromuscular junction.

Such patients may present for surgery for thymectomy. They are exquisitely sensitive to non-depolarising neuromuscular-blocking drugs, which may, however, be required in reduced dosage. Management must take account of the need for anticholinesterase medication to be continued and postoperative monitoring of respiratory muscle function is essential.

Myasthenic syndrome

This condition is characterised by weakness and fatiguability usually of the pelvic girdle and limb musculature, often associated with a small cell carcinoma of the lung. It probably arises as a defect in the prejunctional calcium entry evoked by the nerve action potential. It does not respond to treatment with anticholinesterase drugs.

Malignant hyperthermia

This is a rare condition whose manifestation depends first upon an inherited predisposition and second upon exposure to a triggering agent. The predisposition is inherited in an autosomal dominant pattern; triggering agents include the depolarising neuromuscular-blocking drug suxamethonium and the volatile anaesthetic agents.

Although the condition may represent a group of genetically distinct defects, a common feature is a continuing rise in sarcoplasmic calcium levels. This leads to a continuing interaction of actin and myosin, with muscle rigidity and excessive utilisation of both energy and oxygen.

The development of the condition is marked by a rapid rise in body temperature, tachycardia and a rise in end-tidal carbon dioxide tension. These features reflect a massive hypermetabolic state and in a fully developed attack, the consequences of tissue damage become evident with myoglobinuria.

The condition is sufficiently rare that early diagnosis requires a high level of suspicion, together with routine monitoring of heart rate, end-tidal PCO_2 and body temperature. Early diagnosis and treatment are important because they minimise the metabolic disarray, end-organ damage and high risk of death which would otherwise result.

Treatment includes withdrawal of the triggering anaesthetic, the administration of dantrolene intravenously, cooling and intensive supportive care. Acidosis and hyperkalaemia are likely and in the fulminant attack renal failure may occur.

Diagnosis is confirmed, after the attack has subsided, by examination of the contracture of a muscle biopsy specimen in response to caffeine and halothane. In the United Kingdom, this test is carried out at the Malignant Hyperthermia Unit in Leeds.

PATHWAYS OF TRANSMISSION OF PAINFUL STIMULATION

The treatment of pain in the surgical patient demands a knowledge of the structure and function of the pathways involved in the transmission of painful stimuli.

A noxious stimulus activates the free nerve endings of peripheral afferent nociceptive fibres. These nerve endings lie free in the tissues and include both small myelinated (A-delta) fibres and unmyelinated (C) fibres. The A-delta fibres are between 2 and 5 μm in diameter and have a conduction velocity of 12–30 m sec^{-1}. The C fibres have a diameter of about 1 μm or less and have a conduction velocity an order of magnitude slower at 0.5–2 m sec^{-1}.

The act of damaging a tissue not only stimulates nociceptive primary afferent fibres but initiates an inflammatory response, with the release of a range of inflammatory mediators which have a bearing on the maintenance of painful stimulation. There are several classes of inflammatory mediator and they include such chemically diverse substances as eicosanoids (such as the prostaglandins and leukotrienes), oligopeptides (such as bradykinin) and polypeptides (such as the cytokines). Some are secreted from inflammatory cells, some arise from enzyme systems in plasma activated by tissue damage and others are released from primary afferent nerve terminals.

Some mediators stimulate primary afferent fibres and also lead to vasodilatation and oedema formation. There follows an ingress of inflammatory cells which synthesise cyclooxygenase at the site of the injury. The enzyme converts arachidonic acid, derived from cell membranes, to cyclic endoperoxides, which are converted to a variety of products including prostaglandins, thromboxane and prostacyclin. These products in turn contribute to the inflammatory response and intensify the algesic action of inflammatory peptides. The inhibition of cyclooxygenase by non-steroidal anti-

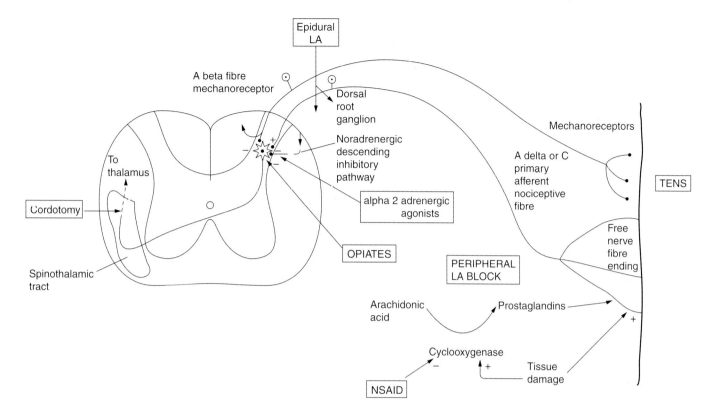

Figure 16.13 An outline of the peripheral and spinal pathway for transmission of painful stimuli, together with the sites of action of some therapeutic interventions. The primary afferent nociceptive fibres synapse with the second neurone in the pathway in the dorsal horn of the spinal grey matter. The second-order neurone projects centrally in the spinothalamic tract. Non-steroidal antiinflammatory drugs (NSAID) inhibit cyclooxygenase in the periphery, reducing the production of prostaglandins. Local anaesthetics (LA) may be applied to peripheral nerves or to the epidural space where they reach afferent fibres in the nerve roots. The dorsal horn of the spinal cord is a site of interaction of many factors and part of the action of the opiates is exerted here. There is a descending noradrenergic pathway and alpha-2 adrenergic agonists such as clonidine are thought to act on this system. Both opiates and clonidine may be given by the epidural route. Transcutaneous electrical nerve stimulation (TENS) is shown; this is thought to stimulate mechanoreceptors which modulate the transmission of painful stimuli through the dorsal horn. Section of the spinothalamic tract (cordotomy) has been used to provide temporary relief from pain due to advanced cancer in patients with a short life expectancy.

inflammatory drugs provides one mainstay of analgesic therapy (see below).

The primary afferent fibres enter the dorsal horn of the grey matter of the spinal cord, where they synapse with the next neurone whose axon crosses (decussates) to the opposite side of the cord and ascends to the thalamus in the spinothalamic tract. The spinothalamic tract is divided into anterior and lateral portions and is responsible for transmission of noxious stimuli as well as the sensations of temperature and deep pressure.

The anatomy and physiology of the synaptic arrangement in the dorsal horn of the spinal grey matter have been the subject of enormous interest in recent years. The dorsal horn is not simply a relay in the onward transmission of acute painful stimuli but is the site at which non-noxious stimuli, and higher centres acting through descending pathways, can modify the central transmission of painful stimulation. Furthermore, the pathway is not fixed but is itself modified by painful stimulation.

Spinal cord pharmacology

Pharmacological approaches to the dorsal horn have not only shed light on the mechanism for nociceptive transmission but also raised possibilities for new therapeutic interventions. There is evidence that the neurotransmission from the nociceptive primary afferent fibres involves release of both the amino acid glutamate and a peptide neurotransmitter. The action of glutamate at the postsynaptic NMDA receptor may be responsible for the phenomenon of 'wind-up'; that is, a volley of afferent stimuli in the nociceptive pathway results in an increasing response to subsequent stimuli. The putative peptide neurotransmitters include substance P and calcitonin gene-related peptide (CGRP) but the role of the peptides in neurotransmission is unclear.

Descending pathways

The dorsal horn receives input from descending pathways originating in brainstem nuclei. These include the locus caeruleus, which gives rise to a descending noradrenergic pathway, and the raphe nuclei, which give rise to descending fibres in which the neurotransmitter is serotonin or enkephalin. Activation of the descending pathways may reduce the central transmission of painful stimuli and forms a substrate for the analgesic action of alpha-2 adrenergic agonists (see below). The dorsal horn is rich in opiate receptors, which are predominantly of the mu type and are principally located on the nerve terminals of primary afferent C fibres. Activation of these presynaptic receptors diminishes release of the neurotransmitters glutamate and substance P.

The sites of action of several classes of drug which are useful in treatment of pain are shown in Figure 16.13 and are described in more detail below.

LOCAL ANAESTHETICS

The local anaesthetics comprise a group of drugs which were introduced into surgical practice following the discovery, over 100 years ago, of corneal analgesia from cocaine. Local anaesthetics have a common chemical structure, with an amine group joined to an aromatic group by a linking group. The local anaesthetics in current use are classified chemically as esters or amides, depending on the nature of this link.

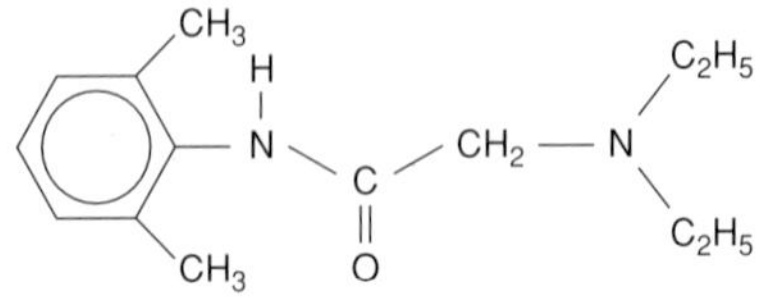

Figure 16.14 The chemical formula of lignocaine. There is an aromatic group which is joined to an amine group by a linking amide group.

The agents most commonly used today are all amides and this group includes lignocaine, bupivacaine, prilocaine and ropivacaine. They are all weak bases usually presented for clinical use as hydrochloride salts. They are ionised and water soluble; they exist *in vivo* in both ionised and unionised forms. The degree of ionisation depends upon the pH and upon the pKa of the local anaesthetic involved.

Local anaesthetics act by blocking the voltage-activated sodium channels which generate the nerve action potential (see above). They appear to reach the sodium channel from the axoplasmic side of the axon membrane or from within the membrane itself; in any case the local anaesthetic molecule which is deposited outside the nerve fibre must cross the lipid axon membrane before it can exert its action. Access to the site of action thus depends upon the existence of the molecule in the unionised form and hence upon the pKa of the drug.

(a) $B + H^+ \leftrightarrow BH^+$

(b) $pH = pKa + \log([B]/[BH^+])$

Figure 16.15 The ionisation of local anaesthetics. Local anaesthetics exist in ionised (BH+) and unionised (B) forms in equilibrium, as depicted in (a). The relative quantity of the two forms in a solution is determined by the hydrogen ion concentration and the pKa, which is the pH at which the ionised and unionised forms exist at an equal concentration. The relationship between pH, pKa and the ratio of the concentrations of the two species is given by the Henderson-Hasselbalch equation (b).

The pKa of bupivacaine is 8.1; this implies that at a pH of 7.4, the ionised form is preponderant over the unionised form by a factor of some 5:1. A small minority of the agent is unionised and onset is delayed. The pKa of lignocaine, at 7.7, is closer to physiological pH and so over 30% of the drug is present in the unionised form; the onset is therefore more rapid.

The potency of the local anaesthetic drugs is correlated with lipid solubility; thus the highly lipid-soluble bupivacaine is given in a lower dose than either lignocaine or prilocaine which are less lipophilic.

Table 16.4 Some of the contrasting properties of the commonly used amide local anaesthetics lignocaine and bupivacaine

	pKa	Onset speed	Potency
Lignocaine	7.7	Rapid	Moderate
Bupivacaine	8.1	Slow	High

The action of the local anaesthetic drugs is 'use dependent'. This means that a volley of action potentials in a partially anaesthetised nerve increases the extent of the block; the first action potential of a train may be propagated, whereas the subsequent action potentials will be blocked. The phenomenon is a result of the fact that local anaesthetics bind preferentially to sodium channels which are, or have recently been, activated. The action potential therefore increases the opportunity for the action of the local anaesthetic.

It is perhaps not surprising that the toxicity of local anaesthetics is exerted chiefly on those organs with a high concentration of excitable tissue, namely the brain and heart. The cerebral toxicity is manifest most seriously as convulsions, though there may be a premonitory phase of confusion and excitement. The cardiovascular toxicity includes a negative inotropic effect and cardiac arrhythmias. The cardiac toxicity of bupivacaine is prolonged and difficult to reverse and hence serious; it was responsible for fatality in patients undergoing intravenous regional anaesthesia and it is no longer recommended for that use.

The latest addition to the amide series of local anaesthetics is ropivacaine. Chemically this may be thought of as a modification of bupivacaine. First, the butyl (C_4H_9) side chain on the cyclic nitrogen of bupivacaine is replaced by a propyl (C_3H_7) group; second, the drug is presented as a single enantiomer, whereas bupivacaine is a racemic mixture of two optical isomers. The significance of this is that the cardiac toxicity is not equivalent for the two optical isomers and the cardiac toxic potential of ropivacaine is thought to be less than that of racemic bupivacaine.

OPIATES

The analgesic properties of the opiates have been known since ancient times; specific receptors were described in the early 1970s, shortly followed by the description of endogenous opioid ligands in 1975. Several opiate receptor subtypes have been proposed. The main groups are mu-receptors, delta-receptors and kappa-receptors. The mu-receptors mediate spinal and supraspinal analgesia, together with respiratory depression, euphoria, sedation and bradycardia. The kappa-receptor mediates part of the spinal analgesic action.

Chemically morphine is a T-shaped molecule, which combines with the opiate receptor in a stereo-specific manner. Opiates share certain common chemical features. There is an asymmetric carbon atom and this is separated from a tertiary ammonium group by two methylene groups, which are often part of a piperidine ring.

The clinically useful opiates can be classified into several groups.

- *Morphine* and its derivatives, such as codeine and diamorphine.

- *Phenylpiperidine* derivatives which include pethidine, fentanyl and alfentanil.

- *Methadone* derivatives. Methadone is well absorbed orally and it has a prolonged duration of action.

- *Thebaine* derivatives, such as buprenorphine.

Actions of opiates

Opiates remain a pillar of analgesic regimes. They have a diverse range of other effects apart from analgesia; these may be broadly classified to include acute side effects and those resulting from prolonged administration.

The acute side effects of opiates include:

- respiratory depression and cough suppression

- bradycardia

- sedation and euphoria

- smooth muscle spasm, resulting in constipation

- pupil constriction

- histamine release, causing bronchospasm and, particularly after large doses of morphine, hypotension.

Immediate hazards of opiate use

The most immediately threatening acute side effect of opiate use is respiratory depression. This is manifest clinically as a slowing of the respiratory rate rather than a diminution of tidal volume; the patient may take two or three deep breaths per minute. It is essential to give an opiate antagonist such as naloxone. This is given as an intravenous bolus dose initially and a swift clinical response confirms the original diagnosis of opiate intoxication. The duration of action of naloxone is less than that of many opiate agonists and the initial bolus dose will need to be followed by a continuous infusion of naloxone.

Routes of opiate administration

Intramuscular and intravenous routes

The opiate drugs have been traditionally given by intermittent intramuscular injection for postoperative pain relief. Thus morphine has often been prescribed for the adult patient in a dose of 10 mg IM repeated every three hours as needed. However, it is possible to apply the opiates by a variety of other routes; the administration of repeated small IV boluses is the basis of patient-controlled analgesia (see below).

Oral route

The use of oral morphine has a long tradition in the relief of pain in patients with advanced cancer; it is available as a slow-release preparation (MST) and the dose given by the oral route needs to take into account the poor oral bioavailability of morphine. This is due to its metabolism in the gut wall and in the liver, the so-called 'first-pass effect'; the systemic bioavailability is around 20–30% of the orally administered dose.

Epidural route

In recent years it has become common to administer opiates to the postoperative surgical patient by the epidural route. This is usually undertaken by continuous infusion together with a local anaesthetic drug. In order to reach its site of action in the dorsal grey matter of the spinal cord, the opiate must first diffuse across the dura mater, a relatively thick barrier. It is also advantageous to avoid rostral spread as far as the brainstem, which presumably occurs most readily from movement of the drug in cerebrospinal fluid. These aims are met by using a relatively lipophilic opiate drug; diamorphine and fentanyl are common choices.

Transcutaneous route

The potent and lipophilic opiate fentanyl has been formulated in transcutaneous patches which release the opiate at a steady rate of 25, 50, 75 or 100 µg/h for up to 72 hours. The patches differ in the exposed surface area, across which fentanyl will diffuse at a rate of 2.5 µg/h/cm² of patch. There is a lag of about two hours before systemic fentanyl absorption becomes significant and plasma fentanyl concentration reaches a plateau between six and 72 hours following application of the patch. Fentanyl patches have been used in both the immediate postoperative period, when they reduce morphine requirements, and in the treatment of chronic pain.

A difficult problem is posed by patients who present for surgery whilst receiving opiate drugs for a chronic painful condition. This may arise in patients with advanced cancer but also sometimes in patients with non-malignant conditions, such as chronic pancreatitis. In general, such patients need to continue to receive their existing opiate medication in order to achieve analgesia and to prevent the occurrence of a distressing withdrawal syndrome in the immediate postoperative period. The analgesic drug requirements to produce adequate pain relief in such patients may be very large.

NON-STEROIDAL ANTIINFLAMMATORY DRUGS

A full review of the non-steroidal antiinflammatory drugs is beyond the scope of this chapter. They are the mainstay of treatment of mild and moderate pain, when there is an element of tissue inflammation. They have a triad of actions:

- analgesic
- antiinflammatory
- antipyretic.

All three main actions of this group of drugs are explicable in terms of blockade of the enzyme cyclooxygenase. This enzyme initiates the conversion of the fatty acid, arachidonic acid, to a series of prostaglandins, thromboxane and prostacyclin.

The prostaglandins cause vasodilatation and increase capillary permeability in an area of inflammation; inhibition of prostaglandin synthesis will diminish that action. Furthermore, although the prostaglandins do not provoke pain in isolation they potentiate the algesic effects of inflammatory mediators such as bradykinin; hence inhibition of prostaglandin synthesis reduces pain. The antipyretic action is mediated centrally by interfering with the prostaglandin synthesis consequent upon the action of interleukin-1.

There are several classes of non-steroidal antiinflammatory drug depending upon their mechanism of inhibition of cyclooxygenase and upon their chemistry. Thus aspirin is an irreversible inhibitor of cyclooxygenase, acetylating the enzyme; ibuprofen is a competitive inhibitor and its action is reversible.

Prostaglandins are widespread throughout the body and have a multitude of physiological roles. The beneficial effects of non-steroidal antiinflammatory drugs are largely mediated through inhibition of cyclooxygenase at sites of inflammation. This enzyme is derived from inflammatory cells and its production is induced by the injury. This form of the enzyme is termed inducible cyclooxygenase or COX-2. Unfortunately, prostaglandins have numerous other functions and are synthesised continuously in the tissues by a somewhat different form of the enzyme, COX-1, which is expressed constitutively. The currently available non-steroidal antiinflammatory drugs are not selective and so they have adverse side effects which result from COX-1 inhibition. Drugs which selectively inhibit COX-2 have recently become available and can provide the analgesic and antiinflammatory effects without inhibiting COX-1, thus avoiding the complication of gastric ulceration.

Side effects

The adverse side effects of non-steroidal antiinflammatory drugs arising from inhibition of the enzyme COX-1 include the following.

- *Gastric ulceration.* This arises because prostaglandin synthesis in the stomach has a protective function in inhibiting acid secretion and enhancing mucus formation.

- *Renal failure.* In the renal circulation prostaglandins act as vasodilators; they counteract the vasoconstrictor actions of angiotensin and noradrenaline. Inhibition of renal prostaglandin synthesis in patients with an already diminished renal blood flow can worsen renal function and precipitate renal failure. This is a particular problem in the surgical patient with preexisting impairment of renal function, who may be dehydrated and hypotensive.

MISCELLANEOUS ANALGESIC AGENTS

Clonidine

This drug is an agonist at the alpha-2 adrenoreceptor. Although principally developed as an antihypertensive agent, it has been applied as an adjunct in analgesic therapy. It has been used both systemically, where it can reduce morphine requirements for postoperative pain relief, and intrathecally as part of the anaesthetic technique, where it prolongs the period of postoperative analgesia following a spinal local anaesthetic block. It is presumed to act on the descending adrenergic pathways which modulate nociceptive transmission through the dorsal horn of the spinal grey matter, though not all studies have found a greater effect when the drug is given by the epidural route than systemically.

Ketamine

This anaesthetic induction agent has been available for almost 30 years but has not achieved widespread use because of the dysphoric reactions that accompany recovery. It is, however, unique amongst intravenous anaesthetic agents in that it is strongly analgesic; it is used in subanaesthetic doses in patients undergoing painful interventions such as the change of burns dressings or the application of regional local anaesthetic blocks to patients with limb fractures. It is known to act on several chemical receptor systems including the NMDA subtype of glutamate receptor. Its activity is the sum of the actions of two optical isomers, one of which is responsible for most of the dysphoric reactions. In the future, a single isomer preparation might find a more widespread application than the racemic mixture.

Tramadol

This agent, released in the United Kingdom about five years ago, has been available in continental Europe for many years. It is an interesting drug, with several actions including a weak agonist action at the opiate mu-receptor and inhibition of the uptake of both noradrenaline and serotonin. It thus affects both the opiate and monoamine systems in the dorsal horn of the spinal cord. It is a racemic mixture of two optical isomers, which each account for different aspects of its action. It has an O-desmethyl metabolite which is an opiate agonist. It is hoped that it will find a place as an analgesic for moderate pain without the abuse potential of pure opiates.

PRACTICAL METHODS OF PAIN RELIEF IN THE SURGICAL PATIENT

Local anaesthetic blocks

In many operations on the periphery, it is possible to provide analgesia for several hours by the use of a local anaesthetic block. Examples are the block of discrete peripheral nerves such as the femoral and sciatic nerves for lower limb surgery and block of the brachial plexus.

Epidural analgesia

Epidural analgesia is achieved by injecting a dose of local anaesthetic solution into the epidural space. The epidural space is filled with fatty tissue and blood vessels and is crossed by segmental nerve roots; it is at this site that local anaesthetics exert their action. It is now usual to insert a catheter into the epidural space and infuse analgesic drugs for the first postoperative days. Many anaesthetists supplement the local anaesthetic with an opiate or even use an opiate as the sole agent in epidural analgesia.

Hazards of epidural analgesia

The insertion of an epidural catheter carries certain inevitable risks, regardless of the agents which will be used. The most feared hazards are the formation of an epidural abscess and the development of a haematoma of the vertebral canal.

As regards the risk of an epidural abscess, the presence of skin sepsis is a contraindication to the performance of an epidural block. The epidural catheter is inserted using a full aseptic technique. Note is taken of postoperative back pain and tenderness and the development of pyrexia in a patient with an epidural catheter *in situ* should raise suspicion of this possibility.

Like epidural abscess, vertebral haematoma following neuraxial block is very rare. Nevertheless, epidural block should be avoided in patients who suffer from bleeding disorders or are taking anticoagulant medication. The place of epidural block in patients who are treated with prophylactic subcutaneous heparin is controversial. The problem has been traditionally considered to be a minor one but there has been a series of reports following the combination of an epidural block and the prophylactic use of the low molecular weight heparin. The development of a haematoma may be associated with catheter removal as well as insertion.

The epidural space is limited by the dura, normally a tough membrane. It is possible to puncture the dura mater inadvertently during the performance of an epidural block. This is recognised by the escape of cerebrospinal fluid (CSF). This is referred to as a 'dural tap'; it is important to recognise the event. The persistent escape of CSF through the hole created in the dura leads to loss of CSF volume and often to a severe headache. Treatments include simple analgesics, caffeine, maintenance of good hydration and epidural infusion of crystalloid after siting an epidural catheter at an adjacent level. In severe cases, a volume of the patient's own blood is injected into the epidural space under strictly aseptic conditions; this is referred to as a 'blood patch', and it often provides dramatic relief.

The application of local anaesthetic to the epidural space is intended to block the afferent nociceptive fibres. Unfortunately, local anaesthetic agents are not specific and block both afferent and efferent nerve fibres. Amongst the efferent nerve fibres are two important groups which pose a serious hazard to physiological stability if they are blocked. First, the sympathetic nervous system emerges from the spinal cord between the levels of T1–L2 as preganglionic white rami. An epidural block providing analgesia at the mid-thoracic level will block the sympathetic outflow to some extent and hence diminish the resting sympathetic tone responsible for maintenance of a normal arterial blood pressure. Second, the innervation of the intercostal and accessory abdominal muscles of respiration may be affected by the local analgesic agent. The diaphragm, being innervated from the cervical cord (C3–5), is affected only by a very high epidural block.

In the event that the epidural catheter becomes displaced to lie in the subarachnoid space or if a dose of local anaesthetic appropriate to the epidural route is given intrathecally after a dural tap, then a very profound and extensive block of all spinal nerves, somatic and autonomic, will occur. This situation is referred to as a 'total spinal' block; there is profound hypotension and cessation of respiration. It is necessary rapidly to institute artificial respiration and support the systemic arterial blood pressure with intravenous fluids and vasopressor drugs.

The application of an opiate to the epidural space carries the risk of cephalad spread of the opiate in the CSF (see above). The consequence is respiratory depression which may be profound; the respiratory depression may also be delayed for some hours after the dose of opiate was given.

The above considerations explain the necessity to monitor both arterial blood pressure and respiratory rate regularly in the postoperative patient receiving epidural analgesia.

Patient-controlled analgesia

One of the problems with the intermittent administration of intramuscular bolus doses of opiates for postoperative pain relief is that opiate requirements vary enormously between individuals and traditional dosing regimes take this variability into account only to a limited degree. The idea of patient-controlled analgesia is to allow the patient to administer a small intravenous dose of a potent opiate, often morphine. The patient can adjust the dose of opiate to his or her requirements. The control is exerted by means of pushing a button. The patient is prevented from obtaining a large and dangerous dose in response to a rapid sequence of button pushes by a 'lockout'; the delivery of a dose is followed by a period of time, often five minutes, in which a further demand is ignored.

Often the dose of morphine received from a patient-controlled device is larger than would have been possible using a regime based upon the administration of a 10 mg dose every three hours.

Miscellaneous methods of pain relief

The following two techniques are mentioned to illustrate some of the anatomical and physiological principles outlined above.

Transcutaneous electrical nerve stimulation (TENS)

In this method, non-painful electrical stimuli are applied to the skin of the painful part through carbonised rubber electrodes; this often provides relief from the painful stimulus. The parameters of stimulus strength and frequency can be varied by the patient according to the response. It is thought to act because according to the gate theory of pain, non-nociceptive stimuli inhibit the central transmission of painful stimuli arising at the same segmental level. Although it has been applied to postoperative pain this method is perhaps most used for chronic painful conditions.

Cordotomy

The principle of this method is to apply a lesion to the spinothalamic tract above the level of the painful lesion. It can be done percutaneously under radiological control. Problems with the technique are first, that it may lead to unwanted damage to descending motor tracts. If a bilateral lesion is made in the cervical region this can lead to respiratory difficulties, though this is uncommon with a unilateral lesion. Second, although the initial result is frequently a success, the recurrence of pain despite the lesion is usual over the course of the following year. It is therefore best confined to patients suffering pain from malignant disease, where life expectancy is short.

FURTHER READING

1   Alberts B, Bray D, Lewis J, Raff M, Roberts K, Watson JD. Membrane transport of small molecules and the ionic basis of membrane excitability. In *The Molecular Biology of the Cell*, 3rd edn. New York: Garland, 1994; 507–549

2   Bowman WC. Prejunctional mechanisms involved in neuromuscular transmission. In: Booij LHDJ, ed. *Neuromuscular Transmission*. London: BMJ Books, 1996; 1–27

3   Checketts MR, Wildsmith JAW. Central nerve block and thromboprophylaxis – is there a problem? *Br J Anaesthesia* 1999; **82**: 164–167

4   Lambert DG, ed. Recent advances in opioid pharmacology. *Br J Anaesthesia* 1998; **81**: 1–84

5   Neher E, Sakmann B. The patch clamp technique. *Sci Am* 1992; **266** (3): 28–35

6   Wall PD. Inflammatory and neurogenic pain: new molecules, new mechanisms. *Br J Anaesthesia* 1995; **75**: 123–124

17

Endocrine emergencies

Introduction – endocrine loops
Thyrotoxicosis
    Thyroid hormones in the diagnosis of
        hyperthyroidism
    Hypocalcaemia following thyroid surgery
Hypercalcaemia
Hypertensive crisis
    Hypertensive emergency
    Hypertensive encephalopathy
Phaeochromocytoma
Conn's syndrome
Adrenal insufficiency
    Acute adrenal insufficiency: adrenal crisis

Devasenan Devendra, Terence J. Wilkin

INTRODUCTION – ENDOCRINE LOOPS

The long-prevailing view that endocrine organs are 'glands' and that their secretions are 'chemical messengers' is unduly simplistic and needs revision. Endocrine loops have evolved to provide biological control which is vital to the maintenance of health. They are ubiquitous in nature and maintain homeostasis as much in microbes as in man. Control loops are designed to constrain a function within a predetermined limit and failure to do so results in the symptoms and signs we associate with disease. The endocrine loops are one category of control system, whose function is to constrain the concentrations of substances in the circulation such as hormones, glucose and ions. Endocrine control is exerted over long distances but adjacent cells may control each other (paracrine) and each cell contains within it micro (autocrine) feedback loops which exercise the same kind of constraint over intracellular functions.

The endocrine control loop, like all control loops, comprises two components: a comparator, which compares the level of substance being controlled with the set (optimum) point, and a generator, which secretes the substance to be controlled. Examples of such control loops are pituitary-thyroid, pituitary-adrenal, islet-liver/muscle and parathyroid-kidney/bone. Where the set point has a biological rhythm (nycthermal, circadian or menstrual), the setting system lies in the hypothalamus, anatomically distant from the loop. Where the set point is potentially constant throughout life (e.g. calcium, glucose and sodium concentrations), the set point is incorporated within the comparator cells, although functionally it still lies outside the loop (e.g. parathyroid glands, islet beta cells and juxtaglomerular apparatus).

Disturbances in the set point are uncommon and, for the purposes of clinical perspective, endocrine disease can be reduced to disorders of either the comparator or the generator. Functionally, the disorder may be one of deficiency or one of excess. Excess is commonly due to autonomous adenomas, where function is unrestrained and inappropriate. Surgeons are seldom involved in the management of endocrine deficiencies and are more likely to be asked to remove autonomous tissue or carcinomas.

The nature of feedback control makes functional diagnoses straightforward, in theory at least. The administration of the substance controlled by the loop (cortisol, for example) will normally 'switch off' a healthy control loop by negative feedback to the comparator (pituitary). Its failure to do so suggests autonomy, either of the comparator or of the generator. It is worth reflecting that an upward shift in set point, while uncommon, may raise the output of the loop to pathological levels without (because the loop itself remains healthy) abrogating the feedback response to administered hormone. The fact that in many cases of pituitary-driven Cushing's disease it is possible to suppress ACTH production with high-dose dexamethasone (8 mg) but not with a low dose (1 mg) suggests that this condition originates as a rare example of disturbance in set point. If the hypercortisolaemia results from an adrenal tumour, which is always autonomous, there is no suppression with dexamethasone.

Where endocrine deficiency is suspected, stimulation tests of the gland in question are logical and appropriate. Failure of the adrenal cortex in Addison's disease is confined by failure of the serum cortisol to rise after stimulation of the adrenal cortex with synthetic ACTH (Synacthen). Failure of the pituitary gonadotrophic sector is demonstrated by its failure to release LH and FSH after injection of the hypothalamic hormone GnRH.

Endocrine diagnosis may be difficult clinically because deficiencies develop slowly and often involve many different systems. Endocrinology may be the last speciality to see the patient with hypothyroidism who has baffled the gastroenterologist (constipation), cardiologist (tamponade), dermatologist (dry skin), rheumatologist (bursitis) and even psychiatrist (personality change).

Endocrine control is central to all functions of the body and clinical endocrinology now extends well beyond thyroid disease to encompass bone disorders, gastrointestinal disease, hypertension, infertility and psychiatry. It is predictable that endocrine disturbance should underlie ill health since disease, by definition, reflects a loss of homeostatic control. This chapter deals with some of the classic endocrine disorders which can lead to surgical emergencies. They are rare but can be life threatening and their recognition is important because in most instances they can be readily reversed.

THYROTOXICOSIS

The thyroid gland is derived from the first and second pharyngeal pouches and descends during ontogeny down the thyroglossal tract to lie just below the level of the cricoid cartilage. Its surgical anatomy is well described elsewhere (*Fundamentals of Surgical Practice*, Chapter 14). Of the thyroid hormones, thyroxine (T_4) is a relatively inactive prohormone, converted in the peripheral tissues to the active hormone triiodothyronine (T_3).

The thyroid hormones exert two principal actions. The first is to increase oxygen consumption in selected tissues, thereby increasing metabolic rate. The second is to sensitise tissues bearing sympathetic adrenoceptors to sympathomimetic amines such as adrenaline. A raised metabolism stimulates appetite, catabolises fat stores, causes heat intolerance and increases in sweating and respiratory rate. The rise in sensitivity to sympathomimetic amines leads to tachycardia, palpitations, lid retraction, tremor, sense of anxiety, agitation and nausea.

The principal causes of hyperthyroidism are listed in Box 17.1. Hyperthyroidism is the generic term and thyrotoxicosis is conventionally reserved for the hyperthyroidism resulting from Graves' disease. The peripheral signs of thyroid eye disease, pretibial myxoedema and finger clubbing which sometimes accompany hyperthyroidism are all autoimmune and associated *only* with Graves' disease, which is due to TSH receptor-stimulating autoantibodies.

Box 17.1 Principal causes of hyperthyroidism

Graves' disease	Autoimmune – TSH receptor antibodies
Multinodular toxic goitre Single toxic nodule	Autonomous nodule(s)
Subacute thyroiditis	Postviral, de Quervain's
Self-administered thyroxine	Thyrotoxicosis factitia

Thyroid hormones in the diagnosis of hyperthyroidism

The tissues respond only to free thyroid hormone, which represents a small fraction of the total circulating hormone. Most laboratories will nowadays measure the free hormone level. Although serum T_4 is traditionally measured, the reasons are historical rather than biological. Indeed, T_4 is a prohormone and relatively less potent than T_3. T_3 is the cause of hyperthyroidism, although T_4 is usually raised at the same time. There are, however, well-recognised instances where the T_3 alone is elevated and measurement of the T_4 would be misleading. Some laboratories will now use serum TSH as a screening assay for hyperthyroidism, as it is highly sensitive to mild excesses of thyroid hormone. Nevertheless, the serum TSH may remain suppressed long after thyroid function has been restored following hyperthyroidism, so that, like all other thyroid function tests, TSH has its limitations. The serum T_3 is typically greatly elevated in thyrotoxic crisis.

Surgery is sometimes used for the treatment of Graves' hyperthyroidism, particularly when a large goitre is present. The autoantibodies responsible for stimulating the thyroid in Graves' disease frequently disappear after subtotal thyroidectomy and it is assumed that antigens released from the thyroid during the operation tolerise or paralyse the immune system. Surgery is not appropriate in the management of other causes of hyperthyroidism. In the case of single or multiple toxic nodules due to functional thyroid adenomas (single toxic nodule and multinodular toxic goitre), the non-autonomous thyroid tissue remains healthy but inactive, since pituitary TSH is switched off by the hyperthyroid nodules. Subtotal thyroidectomy in this situation is not only likely to miss some of the active nodules but will also remove much of the healthy tissue. Radioiodine, which is taken up only by active thyroid tissue, self-targets the active adenoma(s) and can frequently lead to a cure, with restoration of normal thyroid function once the adenomas cease to function.

Thyroid storm or crisis is a potentially fatal disorder which is now rare in developed countries. Graves' disease is usually the cause. It occurs where patients with poorly controlled and aggressive hyperthyroidism are exposed to a stressful and often catabolic state such as infection, trauma or surgery. The clinical presentation is one of fever, profuse sweating, agitation, nausea or vomiting, congestive cardiac failure due to a thyrotoxic cardiomyopathy, often psychotic behavioural change and ultimately hypotension,

coma and death. The onset is frequently acute and death may ensue within hours. Immediate management is crucial.

Treatment aims to support the heart, replenish fluid as appropriate (the patient may be in congestive failure), reduce thyroid hormone levels as fast as possible and normalise core body temperature. Propranolol is given by mouth, initially 80 mg every six hours, to protect the heart from excess sympathomimetic action and to block the peripheral conversion of T_4 to T_3. Iodide (Lugol's iodine 15 mg every four hours by mouth) is an effective means of blocking thyroid secretion (which it achieves by mechanically distending the thyroid follicles). Carbimazole, 40–60 mg daily, is given to block further synthesis of thyroid hormone. A saline/dextrose drip should be set up but the use of fluid replacement and beta-blockers must be judged according to cardiac status. Temperature can be normalised by the use of antipyretics (e.g. aspirin) and ice packs around the body.

Hypocalcaemia following thyroid surgery

Although seldom an emergency, there is considerable misunderstanding about the mechanisms of hypocalcaemia following thyroid surgery and its management.

Hyperthyroidism is not infrequently accompanied by thyrotoxic osteomalacia, in which the serum calcium and bone isoenzyme of alkaline phosphatase may be elevated. It was once thought that the early hypocalcaemia following thyroid surgery was due to the effect of 'hungry bones', in which previously osteomalacic bones, relieved of the hyperthyroid state, took back from the circulation the calcium they had previously lost. However, it was shown long ago that the frequency of hypocalcaemia and tetany following thyroid surgery is no different following surgery for euthyroid goitre than for Graves' hyperthyroidism and that accordingly the fall in calcium is more likely due to the release of calcitonin at the time of surgery. Cases of permanent parathyroid damage following thyroid surgery require lifelong treatment.

Serum calcium levels are regulated by a control loop incorporating the parathyroid glands and bone, the generator, which in adult life stores many kilograms of calcium. It is important to understand that there is no shortage of available calcium in the hypocalcaemia which follows thyroid surgery. Postthyroidectomy hypocalcaemia due to calcitonin release temporarily inhibits the action of PTH on the release of calcium from bone. Calcium infusion over a period of 24 or 48 hours may be all that is required to maintain circulating calcium levels. If the hypocalcaemia is the result of parathyroid damage, the cause is once again not a deficiency of calcium but rather a fall in its concentration due to loss of loop function through damage to the 'comparator' function. Treatment with calcium is inappropriate under these circumstances, which should be managed with high-dose vitamin D as a substitute for parathyroid hormone. The difference between calcium deficiency (virtually impossible in view of bone stores) and downregulation of its control through parathyroid damage is crucial in understanding the need for vitamin D rather than long-term calcium.

HYPERCALCAEMIA

The serum calcium levels in health are maintained within tight limits by a negative feedback control loop no different in principle from the system which controls thyroid hormone levels. As with thyroid hormones, much of the serum calcium is protein bound (in this case about 60%, by serum albumin) and only the free calcium in its ionised state is metabolically active. Accordingly, it is appropriate to adjust the total serum calcium according to the serum albumin by an increment of 0.02 mmol per litre for every gram per litre of albumin below 40 g/l. This is important, as many of the malignancies in which hypercalcaemia occurs are associated with low albumin. The factors controlling serum calcium are depicted in Figure 17.1. The point of key importance is that serum calcium levels are controlled by PTH, which is analogous to TSH in the thyroid system. PTH acts mostly on bone, where it stimulates bone turnover, though bone resorption rather more than its formation. Its effects on the kidney are largely phosphaturic, where it controls the conversion of inactive 1-OH-D3 to the active 1, 25-$(OH)_2$ D3. It is the PTH-activated dihydroxy vitamin D which regulates intestinal absorption of calcium, not the PTH itself. Most cholecalciferol (vitamin D3) in humans is produced by the action of sunlight on the skin and little is derived from food.

Most cases of hypocalcaemia are due to parathyroid hormone insufficiency, either through autoimmune destruction of the parathyroid glands or their damage following neck surgery. However, vitamin D deficiency, particularly in the institutionalised elderly deprived of sunlight, is an increasingly important cause of hypocalcaemia. The common causes of hypercalcaemia are listed in Box 17.2 according to clinical circumstance. While incidental hypercalcaemia due to spontaneous adenomas of the parathyroid glands is common, it is seldom severe. Hypervitaminosis D is uncommon and is readily diagnosed by higher serum vitamin D levels in the presence of high serum calcium and suppressed parathyroid hormone level.

The causes of hypercalcaemia in hospitalised patients are most frequently associated with malignancy. The levels of serum calcium are often very high, above 3.0 mmol/l, and the cause of significant morbidity. The serum PTH is suppressed and the phosphate often normal (unlike primary hyperparathyroidism where the raised PTH levels are phosphaturic). The hypercalcaemia of malignancy may be due to the infiltration of bone by metastases but there are many cases of hypercalcaemia in malignancy where there is no evidence of bone metastasis. Typically squamous carcinomas or tumours of the genitourinary tract, these tumours secrete not PTH but a PTH-like hormone referred to as parathyroid hormone-related protein (PTHrP). PTHrP is encoded on chromosome 12 and PTH on chromosome 11. It is believed that these two chromosomes are derived phylogenetically from a single chromosome, which would account for the close sequence homology of PTH and its related protein. Unlike PTH, PTHrP *reduces* conversion of cholecalciferol to dihydroxy vitamin D. It stimulates bone resorption but not bone formation, accentuating the degree of hypercalcaemia. PTHrP is identical in sequence with PTH over the first 13 amino acid residues from the N-terminal but differs thereafter. This sequence homology has allowed the development of a two-site immunoassay in which one antibody recognises the mutually identical sequence, while the second distinguishes the subsequent sequence differences. Using this assay, PTHrP was found to be elevated some 10-fold in the majority of patients with hypercalcaemia and solid tumours. PTHrP is suppressed in hyperparathyroidism.

The clinical features of hypercalcaemia are listed in Box 17.3. They can be explained by the metabolic effects of calcium on many different systems and the diuretic effects caused by imposing an osmotic load on the renal tubules. Patients with hypercalcaemia of malignancy can become stuporose and severely hypovolaemic. Urgent treatment is needed under these circumstances.

Symptomatic hypercalcaemia of malignancy can be improved or cured by lessening or removing the tumour load. Symptomatic treatment is otherwise directed at maintaining hydration and at reducing bone resorption. Where primary hyperparathyroidism is discovered incidentally, the situation is rarely critical and a considered decision for or against neck exploration and parathyroid removal can be made. In symptomatic cases, volume expansion with isotonic saline improves the general condition of the patient and most particularly provides the increase in glomerular filtration which allows greater urinary calcium excretion. Unlike glucose, another common cause of osmotic diuresis, calcium has a low molecular weight and is osmotically efficient, so that fluid intake may have to be considerable in order to achieve any significant

---

Box 17.2 Causes of hypercalcaemia, in order of frequency

Symptomatic/ hospitalised patients	Asymptomatic/ ambulatory patients
Overt malignancy	Primary hyperparathyroidism
Primary hyperparathyroidism	Drugs (thiazides, lithium,
Renal failure (2° hyperpara-	vitamin D)
thyroidism)	Occult malignancies
Thyrotoxicosis	Familial hypocalcaemic
Granulomatous disease	hypercalcaemia
Phaeochromocytoma	Multiple endocrine neoplasia
Multiple endocrine neoplasia	
Hypoadrenalism	

Box 17.3 Symptoms of hypercalcaemia

Fatigue
Weakness
Personality change
Arthralgia
Headache
Polyuria/polydipsia
Bone pain
Constipation

net gain in circulating volume. For this reason, also, the hypocalcaemic effect of fluids is modest and only perhaps 20% of patients will become normocalcaemic with fluid replacement alone.

Loop diuretics are traditionally advised in malignant hypercalcaemia because they reduce calcium reabsorption but their effects are limited and they should be used only when hydration is completed. Again, corticosteroids have been traditionally advocated to lower calcium levels but results are inconsistent and they are nowadays little used. Steroids probably act best by reducing the load of haematogenous tumours and by raising resistance to the action of dihydroxy vitamin D on calcium absorption from the gut. However, as steroids have little effect in reducing the mass of solid tumours and as dihydroxy vitamin D levels are already reduced in the presence of PTHrP, steroids are of little value in these circumstances.

Pharmacological doses of calcitonin given by injection can produce a rapid reduction of serum calcium within 2–4 hours, although the duration of action is short and 'escape' is common. It is given intramuscularly as short-term therapy and will achieve normocalcaemia during the first 48 hours or so of treatment in some 30% of patients.

Mythromycin is an antitumour therapy which has a rapid and profound antiresorptive effect on bone. It is effective in most cases of hypercalcaemia of malignancy at a dose of 15–25 µg per kilogram as an infusion, with a peak effect at around 48 hours. It lasts for rather longer than calcitonin but can be severely toxic in the longer term. It is little used nowadays.

One of the most effective longer term therapies in malignant hypercalcaemia is the family of bisphosphonates. The bisphosphonates (etidronate, clodronate, pamidronate, alendronate and risedronate) are all poorly absorbed orally but attach tightly to hydroxyapatite crystals on bone and reduce its resorption rate. Their half-life in the body is probably as long as the bone to which they attach. The most rapid action is obtained by intravenous infusion and both clodronate and disodium pamidronate are effective in more than 60% of patients. A single dose infusion of between 15 and 60 mg pamidronate is effective within 4–10 days and the effect may last many weeks. Oral bisphosphonates may be sufficient to maintain normocalcaemia, once achieved.

HYPERTENSIVE CRISIS

Hypertension is the presence of an elevated blood pressure that places patients at increased risk of target organ damage in several vascular beds including the heart, retina, kidneys and the brain. Hypertensive crisis is the turning point in the course of hypertension when immediate management of elevated blood pressure plays a decisive role in the eventual outcome and is arbitrarily defined as a diastolic blood pressure above 120 mmHg.

Hypertensive crises are classified as *hypertensive emergencies* in the presence of end-organ damage or as *hypertensive urgency* in the absence of end-organ damage. The title malignant hypertension is synonymous with hypertensive emergency and has largely been replaced.

Hypertensive crisis (see Box 17.4) is most commonly seen in patients who are chronically hypertensive. Important predisposing causes include failure to take the prescribed medication or inadequately prescribed medication. Hypertensive crisis is believed to be due to an abrupt increase in systemic vascular resistance due to a rise in the circulating levels of noradrenaline, angiotensin II or antinatriuretic hormone. As a consequence of the severely elevated blood pressure, arteriolar fibrinoid necrosis occurs, causing endothelial damage, platelet and fibrin deposition and loss of autoregulatory function, resulting in end-organ ischaemia. In the kidney, besides fibrinoid necrosis, the classic onion-skin lesions of hyperplastic arteriolitis may be seen on histology. End-organ damage includes congestive heart failure, aortic dissection or neurological dysfunction.

Box 17.4 Causes of hypertensive crisis

Sudden increase in blood pressure in chronic hypertensive patients
Renovascular disease
Parenchymal renal disease
Scleroderma and other connective tissue diseases
Pregnancy induced hypertension
Phaeochromocytoma
Head injury
Withdrawal of anti-hypertensive treatments
Autonomic instability in patients with spinal cord injuries
Ingestion of drugs (cocaine, amphetamines, tricyclic antidepressants)

The history, examination and investigations are directed towards determining the presence of end-organ damage in order to distinguish a case of hypertensive emergency from hypertensive urgency. Important investigations include an electrocardiogram, chest radiograph, urinalysis, full blood count and the serum urea and electrolyte levels.

Evidence of chest pain (myocardial infarction, aortic dissection), dyspnoea (pulmonary oedema) and neurological changes (cerebrovascular accident) in the history, retinopathy (see Figure 17.1) or increase in urea and creatinine will help to distinguish hypertensive emergency from hypertensive urgency.

As soon as a hypertensive emergency is diagnosed, the patient should be monitored electrocardiographically, intravenous access established and an arterial line inserted to confirm the diagnosis and monitor progress with therapy. The goal of therapy is a reduction in systemic vascular resistance. Beta-adrenergic receptor antagonists are generally avoided since they result in a reduction in cardiac output. However, they are useful in cases of myocardial infarction and aortic dissection.

Hypertensive emergency

The goal in therapy in a hypertensive emergency is to lower the mean arterial pressure by approximately 25%, to reduce the dias-

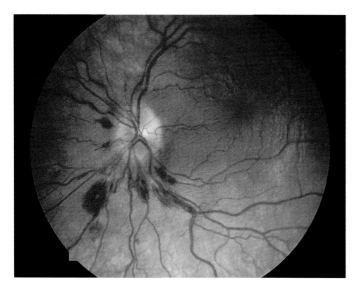

Figure 17.1 Hypertensive retinopathy: optic disc blurring, flame shaped haemorrhages and tortous blood vessels.

tolic blood pressure to 100 mmHg. This must be done carefully and, depending on the circumstances, may take a period of several minutes to several hours. An overzealous reduction in blood pressure to hypotensive levels should be avoided as it will provoke end-organ ischaemia.

Sodium nitroprusside is the drug of choice for the treatment of hypertensive emergencies but levels must be monitored in view of the risk of thiocyanate and cyanide toxicity. Intravenous labetalol is also frequently used. If intravenous access cannot be obtained sublingual nifedipine can be effective in producing an immediate reduction in blood pressure.

Most patients who have a hypertensive crisis are volume depleted, possibly due to pressure-related diuresis, and thus will require fluid resuscitation. In cases of volume depletion as evidenced by a decrease in central venous pressure or pulmonary capillary wedge pressure, an increase in blood urea and marked postural hypotension, fluid replacement with isotonic saline solution may improve renal function. The use of diuretics and fluid restriction should be reserved for patients who are clinically overloaded.

Hypertensive encephalopathy

Hypertensive encephalopathy is believed to be caused by cerebral oedema resulting from failure of autoregulation of cerebral blood flow. The symptoms include headache, nausea, vomiting, visual disturbances, confusion and weakness. The signs include disorientation, focal neurological signs, seizures, retinopathy, nystagmus and asymmetric reflexes. The diagnosis is made by exclusion once stroke, subarachnoid haemorrhage, mass lesions, seizure disorders, vasculitis and encephalitis have been ruled out. Sodium nitroprusside is the agent of choice in the treatment of this disorder.

PHAEOCHROMOCYTOMA

Phaeochromocytomas are responsible for only 0.1–0.2% of hypertensive patients. There are certain distinctive manifestations; most patients experience the sudden onset of headaches, sweating, palpitations and nervousness. The presence of these spells should aid in distinguishing the very few who need laboratory investigation from the larger population who have essential hypertension. Ambulatory blood pressure monitoring is very useful in detecting patients with these spells who are not consistently hypertensive.

There are conditions that simulate phaeochromocytoma (see Box 17.5) due to excess secretion of catecholamines. This is particularly seen in patients with essential hypertension who have further rises in blood pressure and episodes of tachycardia which are thought to be triggered by emotion. This form of pseudophaeochromocytoma is associated with high plasma levels of dopamine.

The 24-hour urine collection for the measurement of noradrenaline and adrenaline is very sensitive and specific in the detection of these tumours. Provocative pharmacological tests are rarely needed and may be reserved for patients who have familial multiple endocrine neoplasia 2 syndrome, who are more likely to have bilateral phaeochromocytoma which is usually quiescent. If the results of abdominal imaging are negative, scintigraphic localization with ^{123}I-MIBG can be considered.

The treatment of choice in the situation of a hypertensive crisis is intravenous phentolamine. Beta-adrenergic receptor antagonists should only be used after alpha-adrenergic receptor blockade since the unopposed beta-receptor antagonist may exacerbate the hypertension. Most patients who are not in an emergency hypertensive

---

Box 17.5 Differential diagnosis of phaeochromocytoma

Cardiovascular disorders
Labile hypertension
Paroxysmal tachycardia
Angina
Hypertensive crisis
Rebound hypertension from cessation of anti-hypertensive medication

Endocrinological disorders
Menopausal symptoms
Diabetes mellitus
Hypoglycaemia
Carcinoid syndrome
Thyrotoxicosis
Mastocytosis

Psychoneurological disorders
Anxiety
Migraine
Porphyria
Lead poisoning
Brain tumour
Stroke

---

crisis should be commenced on the mixed alpha 1 and 2 blocker phenoxybenzamine. The starting dose is 5–10 mg orally which should be titrated upwards until satisfactory blood pressure control is achieved. Twenty-four hours after starting phenoxybenzamine, a beta-blocker such as propranolol 40 mg tds should be started.

Surgical removal should be undertaken after the institution of appropriate pharmacological blockade. With proper preoperative preparation and careful anaesthesia, the majority of patients are fairly easily managed. During the surgical procedure there should be continuous monitoring of arterial pressure, central venous pressure and electrocardiographic changes. Pulmonary capillary wedge pressure is essential in patients with preexisting cardiac disease. Hypotension during the procedure usually relates to fluid loss and responds better to fluid replacement rather than vasoconstrictors. Postoperatively, a transient episode of hypertension may occur due to fluid shifts and autonomic instability. This often responds to diuretic therapy. Urinary measurements for catecholamines should be repeated approximately a week after the operation.

CONN'S SYNDROME (PRIMARY HYPERALDOSTERONISM)

Aldosterone, the most important mineralocorticoid steroid produced by the zona glomerulosa of the adrenal gland, plays an important role in sodium homeostasis. It acts on the distal nephron, exchanging sodium for potassium and hydrogen ions. Excess production leads to sodium retention and the loss of potassium. Hypokalaemia is an important pointer to the possibility of mineralocorticoid excess and is usually associated with a metabolic alkalosis.

Conn's syndrome, an aldosterone-secreting adenoma of the adrenal cortex causing hypertension and spontaneous hypokalaemic alkalosis, is responsible for less than 1% of cases of hypertension. It typically occurs in symptomatic, young to middle-aged patients and is slightly more common in females. Hypertensive crisis unusually occurs in this condition. Idiopathic bilateral hyperplasia of the adrenal cortex is a cause of primary aldosteronism but hypokalaemia is less pronounced.

The diagnosis is suggested by persistent hypokalaemia in a non-oedematous patient on a normal sodium intake who is not receiving potassium-wasting diuretics (e.g. thiazide diuretics, frusemide). In patients with hypovolaemia or renal vascular disease, the reduced perfusion to the kidneys will result in increased renin production, leading to secondary hyperaldosteronism. The main difference between primary and secondary hyperaldosteronism is therefore in the plasma renin level; a low renin level suggests the diagnosis of primary aldosteronism.

Primary aldosteronism due to an adenoma is detected by CT scan and usually treated by surgical excision. Only 50% of patients are normotensive after an adrenalectomy and older patients are more likely to be hypertensive postoperatively. However, in some cases, patients can be managed successfully by medical management. Spironolactone is effective in controlling hypertension and hypokalaemia but is limited by its side effect profile which includes decreased libido, erectile dysfunction and gynaecomastia. When idiopathic hyperplasia of the adrenal cortex is suspected, surgery is indicated only when significant symptomatic hypokalaemia cannot be controlled by medical therapy.

ADRENAL INSUFFICIENCY

The adrenal cortex produces three major classes of hormones. Aldosterone, the major mineral corticoid, is produced by the zona glomerulosa and maintains electrolyte balance and normal plasma volume. Cortisol, the major glucocorticoid, is produced by the zona fasciculata and is one of the main modulators of the stress response. The adrenal androgens are produced in the zona fasciculata and zona reticularis. Their physiological role is relatively unknown but in both sexes they stimulate axillary and pubic hair growth.

In primary adrenal insufficiency, the glands are themselves the site of a destructive process or enzyme deficiency and the causes are shown in Box 17.6. Secondary adrenal insufficiency results from the lack of adrenocorticotrophin (ACTH) hormone. This is most often the result of chronic suppression of the hypothalamus-pituitary-adrenal axis by administration of glucocorticoids (iatrogenic Cushing's syndrome) but can occur as a result of pituitary disease or surgery. Aldosterone is not ACTH dependent, so that mineral corticoid activity tends to remain intact in secondary adrenal insufficiency. Tertiary adrenal insufficiency is caused by loss of hypothalamic production or delivery of corticotrophin-releasing hormone (CRH).

Box 17.6 Causes of primary and secondary adrenal insufficiency	
Primary adrenal insufficiency	Secondary adrenal insufficiency
Autoimmune adrenalitis	Pituitary tumour
Tuberculosis	Craniopharyngioma
Metastatic carcinoma	Pituitary surgery or radiation
Fungal infections	Empty sella syndrome
Opportunistic infections in AIDS patients	Postpartum pituitary necrosis
Adrenal haemorrhage	Long term glucocorticoid treatment

Acute adrenal insufficiency: adrenal crisis

Adrenal crisis is a medical emergency that manifests as hypovolaemic shock. It may be precipitated by infection, trauma, blood loss or poor compliance with steroid treatment. Adrenal insufficiency may present with malaise, weakness, anorexia, vomiting and diarrhoea. Laboratory results that may indicate an acute adrenal insufficiency include hyponatraemia, hyperkalaemia, acidosis, hypoglycaemia, normocytic anaemia, lymphocytosis and eosinophilia.

The initial goal of treatment is to restore blood pressure by fluid replacement and to treat the underlying cause of the crisis. A recommended treatment for adrenal crisis is outlined below.

1. IV cannula, measurement of electrolytes, glucose, and cortisol and plasma ACTH.

2. Infuse 2–3 litres of 0.9% saline as quickly as possible. Monitor fluid overload in the elderly with central venous pressure monitoring.

3. Inject 100 mg hydrocortisone initially and every six hours thereafter.

4. Treat the underlying precipitating cause (infection, blood loss).

5. Continue IV infusion of 0.9% saline at a lower rate for the next 24–48 hours.

6. If the patient is not known to have Addison's disease, perform a short Synacthen test.

7. Convert to oral steroid replacement if the patient is free of gastrointestinal symptoms and euvolaemic.

8. Begin mineralocorticoid replacement with fludrocortisone (in primary adrenal disorder) when saline infusion is stopped.

All patients with adrenal insufficiency should carry a steroid therapy card and recommendations for treatment in emergency situations. Vials of hydrocortisone should be stored in the patient's home so that in the event of vomiting, the patient may self-inject steroids without delay. These patients should also wear some type of warning bracelet or necklace, such as those issued by MedicAlert.

FURTHER READING

1 Calhoun DA, Oparil S. Treatment of hypertensive crisis. *N Engl J Med* 1990; **323**: 1177–1183

2 Oelkers W. Adrenal insufficiency. *N Engl J Med* 1996; **335**: 1206–1212

3 Wilson JD, Foster DW, eds. *Williams Textbook of Endocrinology*. Philadelphia: WB Saunders, 1992

Section 3

Surgical Pathology

18

General concepts

Disease types
Definitions of common pathological conditions
  Malignant
  Benign
  In situ
  Borderline
  Dysplasia
  Differentiation
  Tumour grade
Disease staging
  TNM classification

Disease classification
  International Classification of Diseases (ICD)
Epidemiology
  Incidence
  Prevalence
  Screening
  Death certification
  Mortality data

Paul Newman

Surgical pathology is, as the name implies, the study of pathological processes as they apply to the practice of surgery or, as succinctly put by L V Ackerman in the preface to his classic *Surgical Pathology* textbook, it is 'the pathology of the living'. From a surgical standpoint, this traditionally was taken to mean predominantly gross or macroscopic pathology where appearances learned from museum pots are translated to findings in patients on the operating table. From a pathologist's standpoint, surgical pathology is the examination of tissue specimens to provide clinically relevant information in respect of diagnosis, extent and severity of disease, completeness of surgical removal and sometimes the underlying disease aetiology.

Over time, the surgical concept has changed somewhat. With the development of increasingly sophisticated imaging, the need for a snap macroscopic diagnosis during a 'completely blind' exploratory laparotomy is reduced (a good thing, as museum pots may be quite different from pathology seen 'in life'). Within pathology, ever-increasing endoscopic procedures are producing smaller specimens for histological examination and histological samples are being replaced by cytological specimens for diagnosis. Immunohistochemical and molecular biological techniques are enabling extra information to be extracted from these smaller diagnostic samples while the development of 'minimum datasets' requires accurate description and measurement of many parameters from cancer resection specimens. These developments in practice require a close working relationship between surgeon and pathologist and each must understand the language of the other.

In this introductory chapter to the surgical pathology section, some of the basic terminology and concepts are discussed, together with an overview of disease classification, epidemiology and a short section on aspects of death.

It must also be realised that despite being regarded as the gold standard of diagnosis, histopathological diagnosis is as much an art as a science. A diagnosis is based primarily on human interpretation of a visual image and is therefore dependent on the knowledge, experience and judgement of the observer (the pathologist). Observation may produce a differential diagnosis and special stains may help in making a choice between these diagnoses but the interpretation of such stains is crucial as few of themselves give a clearcut answer and knowledge of the clinical situation pertaining to the case may be vital.

A histopathological report is an opinion rather than absolute fact and many factors (such as the clinical features of a case) may weigh heavily in forming that opinion. Pathologists and surgeons should not feel threatened if diagnoses or interpretations are questioned by the other in the light of further developments. In this respect, a good clinical history given to the pathologist is often of far more value than any number of special stains.

DISEASE TYPES

The spectrum of human disease is so wide that some form of categorization is required to put any sort of order into one's thinking on how patients or organ systems are affected by disease. There is no real right or wrong way to do this but all doctors should develop a system that allows a logical progression through the range of diseases that may apply in any circumstance.

One system that is fairly flexible is a modification of the old 'surgical sieve'. This aims to subclassify disease on a broadly aetiological basis, initially into very large categories and subsequently further subdividing these into narrower and narrower bands, in a manner similar to a family tree.

Conditions are initially divided into congenital or acquired. The congenital conditions are usually few (except in paediatric practice) and can further be divided into structural or functional (e.g. tetralogy of Fallot or thyroid dyshormonogenesis). The acquired conditions might be subdivided into metabolic, neoplastic, inflammatory, degenerative or traumatic. These can in turn be further split up. For instance, 'inflammatory' might encompass autoimmune, infective and toxic; 'infective' can be further split into bacterial, fungal, viral, protozoal, etc. (Figure 18.1). Each of these categories could possibly be further divided by specific organism.

It is therefore obvious that such a system can be made as simple or as complex as you wish. It should not be followed slavishly but is a useful starting point. As disease is frequently multifactorial, there will always be conditions that do not easily fit into artificial categories. Is cholecystitis due to gallstones 'inflammatory', 'metabolic' or even 'traumatic'?

A similar approach can be used in a more focused manner when thinking about how a symptom may be caused by disease. Try using 'vomiting' at the top of the tree in place of 'diseases of the stomach'.

However, the most significant separation of disease types which must be made by surgeons and pathologists working together (and frequently now in collaboration with radiologists and molecular biologists) is the separation of neoplastic from non-neoplastic conditions and the separation of malignant neoplasms from benign ones. Each of these groups is then further divided into specific tumour types (Figure 18.2). Much of the emphasis on surgical pathology is placed in this area although it is often not as challenging histologically as is subdividing inflammatory conditions. In the next few sections, aspects of the nomenclature and classification of neoplastic conditions are discussed and more details are given in Chapter 19.

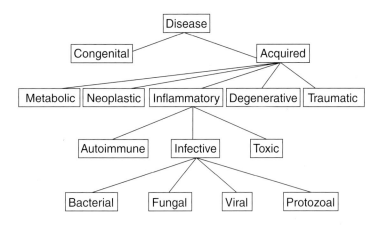

Figure 18.1 Classifying diseases.

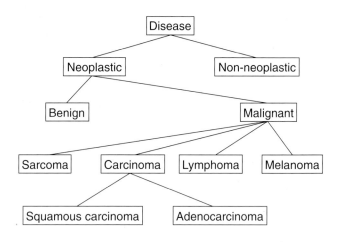

Figure 18.2 Neoplastic or non-neoplastic classification.

DEFINITIONS OF COMMON PATHOLOGICAL TERMS

Malignant

A malignant tumour is one that, if left untreated, has the potential to produce distant metastases (by blood, lymphatic or transcoelomic spread) and thereby cause the death of the patient. That is not to say that all malignant tumours will metastasize. For example, high-grade gliomas of the brain almost never spread outside the central nervous system (unless they have been previously operated upon) but they may seed within the central nervous system. They are nevertheless in all other criteria fully malignant. Nor is it true to say that all tumours producing metastases will invariably lead to the death of the patient, even if left untreated. Some tumours which produce metastases readily in local lymph nodes may have a very indolent clinical course. The classic example is papillary carcinoma of the thyroid which may be present in the lymph nodes of the neck for many years without progression, its presence being confirmed at autopsy performed in relation to some other condition. The behaviour in such cases is so indolent that for years there was debate as to whether the tissue in the nodes represented tumour or 'lateral aberrant thyroid'.

The importance of designating a tumour as malignant is that it will invade locally and have the *potential* (even if unlikely) to produce metastases. Even basal cell carcinomas, which usually cause destruction by local infiltration, may on rare occasions metastasise. It is the prime role of the surgical pathologist when presented with a biopsy from a tumour to attempt to determine whether the tumour is malignant. This is sometimes far from easy, especially on small biopsies, and on occasion may not be possible. For further discussions on the histological differences between benign and malignant tumours, see Chapter 19.

Benign

A benign tumour as opposed to a malignant tumour is one that does not have the potential to produce distant metastases. The importance of this is that it implies that if a benign tumour is completely excised locally, the patient will be cured. If the lesion is incompletely excised, the residual tumour tissue may continue to proliferate and there may be local recurrence, which should perhaps more accurately be called persistence. It is this local recurrence or persistence that partly determines a benign tumour's clinical effects.

A pathologically benign tumour is not necessarily a clinically benign one. An ameloblastoma in the jaw may not metastasize but if untreated it can attain such a size that the patient cannot feed and dies of starvation or the airway is obstructed and the patient is asphyxiated. This is fortunately now very rare and therefore not generally remembered in regions with well-developed health-care systems but tragically still occurs where access to surgery is limited, as in parts of Africa. Benign tumours may also cause death due to haemorrhage, as from hepatic adenomas, or from the effects of hormones or other biologically active substances produced by the tumour, as in pheochromocytoma.

In situ

In situ is the term used to describe a cellular proliferation (nearly always epithelial but occasionally melanocytic) which has a fully developed cytologically malignant phenotype but in which the tumour cells have not breached the basement membrane by which they are bounded. If a tumour is truly *in situ*, it does not produce metastases and therefore complete local excision will be curative. However, it is sometimes not possible to be absolutely certain on light microscopy whether a lesion really is *in situ* and it must not be forgotten that histological diagnosis is based on examination of samples of a lesion. It may therefore be that a small area of invasive tumour has not been sampled during the diagnostic process. In some locations such as the breast or bladder, carcinoma *in situ* may be more difficult to treat, due to widely spread clinically inapparent disease, than is a localised established invasive malignant tumour.

Borderline

Borderline is a term used by pathologists in relation to some tumours and not infrequently leads to misunderstanding. The term was originally used in the field of ovarian pathology for tumours which had some but not all the features of malignancy. Most had a biologically benign course but some were associated with disease progression and ultimately death. It was not possible pathologically to accurately predict which tumours would behave in a clinically benign or malignant fashion and so the concept of a borderline tumour was devised. In ovarian pathology, these tumours have a defined and reproducible histological pattern and are not diagnoses made by 'borderline pathologists' who cannot make up their minds! The diagnosis is made on the appearance of the primary tumour only and the presence or absence of deposits in the peritoneum has no bearing on the diagnosis of borderline tumour. Such tumours have also been referred to as 'carcinomas of low malignant potential' or 'atypically proliferating tumours'.

'Borderline' subsequently became a term rather loosely used in other areas of surgical pathology but strict definitions were not always applied and there was much less interobserver agreement than in the field of ovarian tumours. The term was generally used (as in ovarian tumours) where a lesion had some features of malignancy but where the histological features were not a good predictor of biological behaviour. It is not surprising that histological findings cannot always predict behaviour. Carcinogenesis is a multistep process and until the fully malignant phenotype has developed, it may not be possible to say how far down the road to malignancy a tumour has come.

Trends are changing and pathologists are perhaps now more open (or are surgeons more willing to accept?) that in some cases they cannot make a definite decision between benign and malignant. Such lesions are now sometimes given the label 'of uncertain malignant potential'. This obviously may lead to difficulties in treatment planning and close dialogue between surgeon, oncologist and pathologist with explanation to and involvement of the patient is essential to agree any further requirement for therapy.

Dysplasia

This is a term that has caused misunderstanding in the past, largely due to varying application of the same word. Literally, dysplasia means 'abnormal growth'. Traditionally, it was applied to abnormally formed organs often in relation to congenital abnormalities such as renal or pulmonary dysplasia, but also to abnormalities that developed later (e.g. mammary dysplasia). Within pathology, cytological and histological dysplasia referred to the microscopic morphological abnormality seen in preneoplastic or neoplastic states. The prefixes 'histological' and 'cytological' have been lost in many routine settings and unless otherwise specified, dysplasia now generally refers to neoplastic or preneoplastic cellular abnormalities. For further discussion of dysplasia, see Chapter 19.

Differentiation

Differentiation is a histological feature used to indicate the degree to which a tumour resembles the presumed 'tissue of origin' from which it arose. The term is only applied to malignant tumours, mainly carcinomas, and is one of the factors used to determine tumour grade. The closer to the normal histological structure the tumour elements are, the better the degree of differentiation. Tumours are usually described as well, moderately or poorly differentiated, with the moderately differentiated group traditionally represented by the middle 50% of tumours, the upper and lower quartiles being designated well and poorly differentiated respectively. This is obviously a subjective assessment but there is in general fairly good agreement between observers.

In adenocarcinomas, differentiation refers to the extent of tubule or gland formation and in squamous carcinoma, to the degree of keratinisation. Some adjustment for the degree of nuclear pleomorphism may be made but this is more formally performed in tumour grading.

The degree of differentiation has some effect on prognosis but is not as important as stage or the subsequent calculated grade.

In colorectal carcinoma, the well and moderately differentiated tumours may be grouped together as 'usual differentiation'.

Tumour grade

The development of the concept of tumour grade is an attempt to more accurately stratify prognosis on the basis of the histological parameters of a malignant tumour than is possible using differentiation alone. Criteria for grading are closely defined but kept as simple as possible to retain reproducibility between observers. Criteria vary between tumours but in general include differentiation, mitotic count and nuclear pleomorphism. With some tumours, the different parameters are given numerical values and the total of these values gives the overall grade. An example of this is the Elston modification of the Bloom and Richardson grading system for breast carcinoma, as used in the National Health

Box 18.1 Modified Bloom and Richardson grading system for breast carcinoma

		Score
Tubule formation	Majority of tumour (greater than 75%)	1
	Moderate amount (10–75%)	2
	Little or none (less than 10%)	3
Nuclear pleomorphism	Regular, uniform	1
	Larger with variation	2
	Marked variation	3
Mitoses	Mitoses per 10 high-power fields:	
	0–5	1
	6–10	2
	>11	3

The exact number of mitoses per field varies slightly depending on the size of the visual field of the microscope used.

Grade 1 = total score 3–5
Grade 2 = total score 6–7
Grade 3 = total score 8–9

Box 18.2 Dukes' staging for colerectal carcinoma

Stage
A   Tumour is confined to the bowel wall
B   Tumour penetrates through the serosa
C   Tumour involves regional lymph nodes
D   Distant metastases present

Service breast screening programme (Box 18.1). In general, the poorer the differentiation, the greater the mitotic count and the more pleomorphic the tumour cell nuclei are, the higher the tumour grade and the poorer the prognosis.

Confusion may arise in areas of oncology where more than one grading system exists. In one grading system for transitional cell carcinomas of the bladder, there are four grades, whereas another has three. This is another instance where dialogue between surgeon, pathologist and oncologist is vital to ensure that all are using the same system.

In the field of soft tissue sarcomas and lymphomas, tumours are usually referred to as of high or low grade depending on nuclear pleomorphism, mitoses and necrosis.

DISEASE STAGING

Diseases present at different stages of their natural history so to enable treatment to be planned appropriately, a meaningful prognosis to be given to the patient or to allow statistical comparison between different treatments, a disease must be staged for that patient.

To be effective, a staging system should be easy to use and should reliably stratify differences in prognosis between groups. Although some chronic inflammatory conditions such as hepatitis and sarcoidosis are staged, most staging relates to malignant disease where the stage is given by assessing the extent of the primary tumour, the extent of regional lymph node metastases and the presence or absence of distant metastases.

Staging is of two types: clinical, which is determined by physical examination of the patient (including operative findings and imaging), and pathological, which is only possible after histological examination of resected tissue. It might be thought that pathological staging would always upgrade a patient from the clinical stage by the finding of microscopic metastases in lymph nodes. However, this is not always the case and sometimes clinically enlarged lymph nodes are found on light microscopy to be reactive rather than harbouring metastatic tumour. It must not be forgotten that not all apparent 'tumours' seen at surgery are in fact metastases (particularly small subcapsular lesions in the liver) and biopsy of such lesions is advisable.

In terms of ease of use, the Dukes' staging system for colorectal carcinoma (a pathological staging system) probably comes closest to the ideal (Box 18.2). All that is required is knowledge of whether the tumour is confined to the bowel wall (stage A), through the serosa (stage B) or metastatic to lymph nodes (stage C). Stage D for distant (usually hepatic) metastases was added later. This system, however, does not include data on prognostically important information such as invasion of a major vein, tumour perforation or the involvement of the radial resection line.

When tumours are in more complex anatomical locations, staging of the primary tumour can be more difficult. To address this problem, the TNM system was devised.

TNM classification

The TNM system was designed by the International Union against Cancer (UICC) in the 1950s in an attempt to produce an internationally acceptable system of tumour staging. It is based on the assessment of the primary tumour (T), regional lymph node metastases (N) and distant metastases (M). If a feature cannot be assessed, the code is given a suffix 'X' (TX, NX, MX). Codes derived from pathological examination are indicated by a prefix 'p' (pT, pN, pM).

For each primary tumour, criteria are laid down based on size or local structures infiltrated by the tumour to assign the lesion into one of four T categories. This may be very simple, as in carcinomas of the colon or the thyroid (Box 18.3). It may be extremely complex, as in the case of the larynx where the organ is separated into three anatomical sites and eight subsites; the T code is dependent on the involvement of varying numbers of these (Box 18.4). In all cases, *in situ* tumours are designated Tis.

Box 18.3 T stage for carcinoma of thyroid

TX Primary tumour cannot be assessed

T0 No evidence of primary tumour

T1 Tumour 1 cm or less in greatest dimension, limited to the thyroid

T2 Tumour more than 1 cm but not more than 4 cm in greatest dimension, limited to the thyroid

T3 Tumour more than 4 cm in greatest dimension, limited to the thyroid

T4 Tumour of any size extending beyond the thyroid capsule

Box 18.4 T codes for carcinoma of the larynx

Anatomical sites and subsites

1. Supraglottis
   i) Suprahyoid epiglottis [including tip, lingual (anterior) and laryngeal surfaces] } Epilarynx (including marginal zone)
   ii) Aryepiglottic fold, laryngeal aspect
   iii) Arytenoid
   iv) Infrahyoid epiglottis } Supraglottis excluding epilarynx
   v) Ventricular bands (false cords)

2. Glottis
   i) Vocal cords
   ii) Anterior commissure
   iii) Posterior commissure

3. Subglottis

T codes (clinical classification)

Primary tumour

TX Primary tumour cannot be assessed

T0 No evidence of primary tumour

Tis Carcinoma *in situ*

Supraglottis

T1 Tumour limited to one subsite of supraglottis with normal vocal cord mobility

T2 Tumour invades mucosa of more than one adjacent subsite of supraglottis or glottis or region outside the supraglottis (e.g. mucosa of base of tongue, vallecula, medial wall of piriform sinus) without fixation of the larynx

T3 Tumour limited to larynx with vocal cord fixation and/or invades post-cricoid area and/or preepiglottic tissues

T4 Tumour invades through thyroid cartilage and/or extends into soft tissues of the neck, thyroid and/or oesophagus

Glottis

T1 Tumour limited to vocal cord(s) (may involve anterior or posterior commissures) with normal mobility

    T1a Tumour limited to one vocal cord

    T1b Tumour involves both vocal cords

T2 Tumour extends to supraglottis and/or subglottis and/or with impaired vocal cord mobility

T3 Tumour limited to the larynx with vocal cord fixation

T4 Tumour invades through thyroid cartilage and/or extends to other tissues beyond the larynx, e.g. to trachea, soft tissues of the neck, thyroid, pharynx

Subglottis

T1 Tumour limited to subglottis

T2 Tumour extends to vocal cord(s) with normal or impaired mobility

T3 Tumour limited to larynx with vocal cord fixation

T4 Tumour invades through cricoid or thyroid cartilage and/or extends to other tissues beyond the larynx, e.g. trachea, soft tissues of the neck, thyroid, oesophagus

---

Assessment of regional lymph nodes is frequently simple. With some tumours the nodes are either involved (N1) or not involved (N0). Degrees of nodal involvement may be further specified (N2 and N3) and with some tumours such as the breast, there are very detailed and complex criteria for pathological lymph node assessment (Box 18.5).

Distant metastases are designated as either present (M1) or absent (M0).

The TNM is a very detailed system but with 24 possible divisions when using the basic four T, three N and two M codes, it is unwieldy for day-to-day patient management and for all but the largest clinical trials. TNM categories are therefore usually grouped into four stage groupings or stages. These simplify matters but again the stages may be subdivided (Box 18.6).

DISEASE CLASSIFICATION

To enable meaningful communication between doctors, it is vital that all parties mean the same thing by the same term. Even within one country, this can be a problem but when international communication and collaboration are required, the possibility of significant misunderstanding is markedly raised. To avert this, the World Health Organisation (WHO) produced two major standard sources of reference. The first is a series of books giving the standard histological diagnostic features of all major tumours in each organ system, with reference photomicrographs. The second is a standardised list of diseases, the International Classification of Diseases (ICD), which is used in the development of data storing and archiving systems around the world.

International Classification of Diseases (ICD)

The ICD was initially established as a means of standardising causes of death (see later) but since 1948 it has also included causes of morbidity. It has become increasingly more complex and is now really the preserve of statisticians and epidemiologists. The current ICD classification (ICD10) is no longer merely an 'International Classification of Diseases' but is now the 'International Statistical Classification of Diseases and Related Health Problems'. Thankfully, the letters ICD have been retained!

In view of its complexity, more focused versions of ICD are produced to facilitate work in specific areas. For most surgeons, the most relevant is most probably the ICD-O (ICD for Oncology) but classifications for ophthalmology, dentistry and stomatology are also produced. A linked classification is SNOMED (Systemised Nomenclature of Medicine) produced

---

Box 18.5 N codes for carcinoma of the breast

pNX Regional lymph nodes cannot be assessed (not removed for study or previously removed)

pN0 No regional lymph node metastasis

pN1 Metastasis to movable ipsilateral axillary node(s)

    pN1a Only micrometastasis (none larger than 0.2 cm)

    pN1b Metastasis to lymph node(s), any larger than 0.2 cm

        pN1bi Metastasis to one to three lymph nodes, any more than 0.2 cm and all less than 2.0 cm in greatest dimension

        pN1bii Metastasis to four or more lymph nodes, any more than 0.2 cm and all less than 2.0 cm in greatest dimension

        pN1biii Extension of tumour beyond the capsule of a lymph node metastasis less than 2.0 cm in greatest dimension

        pN1biv Metastasis to a lymph node 2.0 cm or more in greatest dimension

pN2 Metastasis to ipsilateral axillary lymph nodes that are fixed to one another or to other structures

pN3 Metastasis to ipsilateral internal mammary lymph node(s)

Box 18.6 TNM stage grouping for carcinoma of the breast

Stage 0	Tis	N0	M0
Stage I	T1	N0	M0
Stage IIA	T0	N1	M0
	T1	N1	M0
	T2	N0	M0
Stage IIB	T2	N1	M0
	T3	N0	M0
Stage IIIA	T0	N2	M0
	T1	N2	M0
	T2	N2	M0
	T3	N1, N2	M0
Stage IIIB	T4	Any N	M0
	Any T	N3	M0
Stage IV	Any T	Any N	M1

---

by the College of American Pathologists which is used by most histopathology departments to classify their archived cases. It is directly comparable with ICD-O and, like ICD-O, is based on a combination of topography and morphology codes. The topography code indicates the site of the body affected and the morphology code indicates the disease process.

EPIDEMIOLOGY

Epidemiology is the study of patterns of disease within a population. It has grown from the tabulation of death rates from specific infectious diseases in the 18th and 19th centuries to a highly complex statistical discipline which is fundamental to health-care planning. It is not appropriate in a chapter on surgical pathology to examine the topic in any depth as there are several clear and readable texts devoted specifically to it. However, there are aspects of epidemiology which are important in surgical practice. In one respect, standardised staging of malignant disease, as described above, allowing grouping of patients and comparison of cases, is a form of epidemiology. Some other factors that should be considered are standardisation of disease nomenclature, the concepts of incidence and prevalence of disease (which provide the rationale for screening programmes) and also the collection and analysis of mortality data.

Incidence

The incidence of a disease is the number of *new* cases of that disease that arise within a population at risk during a specified period of time. The incidence rate can therefore vary with differing populations and with differing periods of time. Analysis of changing incidence may provide evidence of increasing or decreasing risk factors within a population or the effectiveness of preventive treatment. Analysis of incidence within differing populations may show a particular population that is at higher risk of developing a particular disease and this may allow screening to be targeted at that population.

Note that the incidence relates to an 'at-risk' population. Those who are not at risk of developing a disease, either because they already have it at the start of the period in question or because they could not be affected (testicular cancer does not occur in women!), are excluded from the population under study.

Prevalence

The prevalence of a disease is the total number of cases of that disease within a population at any particular time. This can be represented as a snapshot of a population at a defined moment (point prevalence) or taken over a period of time (period prevalence). Prevalence in a population is determined by the number of new cases developing (the incidence) and the rate of recovery or death from the disease in question.

The first round of a screening programme will have a higher rate for the detection of abnormalities than subsequent rounds due to the prevalence of subclinical disease within the population. The detection rate of later rounds is determined by the rate of new cases developing, that is, the incidence.

Screening

Screening is the quest for disease or disease precursors in apparently healthy individuals before symptoms or signs of the disease become manifest. It is very different from usual medical practice where a patient consults the doctor due to a perceived medical problem.

The rationale for screening is that if a disease process can be detected in its early preclinical phase, it is more amenable to cure with less damage to the patient than if detected later. In the field of screening for cancer, the aim is to detect the disease before development of the fully malignant phenotype, i.e. while the disease is still *in situ* or at least before it has metastasised.

While this concept may appear self-explanatory and of obvious benefit to the population, there are several factors that need to be assessed in connection with screening before a screening programme is established.

1. Those being screened are, in their own opinion, well and the majority will not have the disease for which they are being screened. The screening process should do no harm physically or emotionally to those who come for screening.
2. The natural history of the disease process is known and sufficiently predictable to make early treatment worthwhile and likely to be successful.
3. If a disease is found, a treatment that is acceptable to the patient is available.
4. The level of disease in the population is such that it justifies the high cost of a screening programme.

In a cash-limited health service, the last point is basically a political decision but if the first three points cannot be answered in the affirmative, it is unlikely that public money would now be made available for the establishment of a new screening programme.

Features of a screening test

To be effective, a screening programme needs a high uptake rate from those being screened (particularly from any identified high-risk groups). The test itself should be simple, minimally invasive and acceptable to those being screened. It should be a good discriminator between the individuals who have disease or are likely to develop it and those who do not, so that those who do not have disease are not subject to unnecessary treatment which may be both physically and emotionally harming. There is also an expectation from the public that a test will reliably detect the disease when present. Failure to do so may also be perceived as harm.

The features of a test which determine how suitable it is for screening are its sensitivity and specificity and its positive and negative predictive values. The sensitivity is the probability that the test will be positive if the disease is truly present. The specificity is the probability that the test will be negative if the disease is truly absent.

The sensitivity and specificity of a test can only be determined if those who have been screened are followed up and their outcomes correlated with the test results. This will enable false-positive and false-negative rates to be calculated and thus determine the predictive values of the test. The positive predictive value is the probability that if the screening test is positive, the individual will truly have disease while the negative predictive value is the probability that if the screening test is negative, the individual is truly disease free (Table 18.1).

Table 18.1 Test characteristics

	Disease status		
	Present	Absent	Total
Test positive	a	b	a + b
Test negative	c	d	c + d
Total	a + c	b + d	

Test specificity = d/b+d
Test sensitivity = a/a+c
Positive predictive value = a/a+b
Negative predictive value = d/c+d

Screening in Britain is a politically emotive issue and some of the perceived problems with the screening programmes result from lack of awareness of the balance that must be struck between sensitivity and specificity to enable the programme to benefit the population at large without causing harm to individuals within that population from overtreatment.

Death certification

The earliest attempts at epidemiological study were concerned with tabulating causes of death and can be traced back to 1632, when John Graunt published his 'Observations' based on the weekly London Bills of Mortality, in which he divided deaths into one of 63 categories. In the 18th century, deaths in Edinburgh were correlated by William Cullen. It was not, however, until 1836 when the Registration Act was passed in England and Wales that more widespread data became available. In the following year, the General Register of England and Wales was established, enabling William Farr, who is regarded by some as the father of modern epidemiology, to produce weekly returns of deaths in London. These returns proved their worth when they were used by John Snow in tracing an outbreak of cholera to the public water pump in Broad Street some 20 years before the germ theory of disease had been expounded.

In 1853, the first International Statistical Conference was held in Brussels and commissioned Farr and Marc d'Espine of Geneva to devise a classification of causes of death. This was adopted at the next meeting in 1855 and modified in 1893 by Bertillion as the 'International List of Causes of Death'. The list was to be reviewed every 10 years. In 1898, the American Public Health

Association recommended that the Bertillion system as used in Europe be adopted in the Americas and so the International Classification of Diseases (ICD) was established. In 1920, responsibility for the Classification became shared between the International Statistical Institute and the Health Organisation of the League of Nations. In 1946, responsibility for the classification passed to the WHO. It was not until 1948 in the sixth revision of the ICD that non-fatal conditions were included in the Classification.

Early death certificates were usually not completed by doctors. Following the establishment of the General Register Office in London, however, it was realised that many bizarre causes of death were being recorded and to try and prevent this (and to allay fears of undetected homicide) the Births and Deaths Registration Act of 1874 made it mandatory for an attending physician to sign a certificate as to the cause of death.

The death certificate

To ensure comparability, the ICD system requires a death certificate (more correctly called the medical certificate of cause of death) to be completed in a standard manner which separates the underlying cause leading to death (Part 1) from other factors which are not related to the underlying cause but which have contributed to death (Part 2). The underlying cause is defined as:

> a) the disease or injury which initiated the train of morbid events leading directly to death, or b) the circumstances of the accident or violence which produced the fatal injury.

The standard form of death certificate allows further information to be given showing how the underlying cause lead to death. For example, a carcinoma of the colon could lead to death in several ways. It might lead to intestinal obstruction with vomiting, aspiration and pneumonia in which case the cause of death would read:

> 1a) aspiration pneumonia, due to
>
> 1b) intestinal obstruction, due to
>
> 1c) carcinoma of the colon.

The tumour might perforate, in which case the cause of death could read:

> 1a) faecal peritonitis, due to
>
> 1b) intestinal perforation, due to
>
> 1c) carcinoma of the colon

or it may become widely disseminated, leading to a generalised deterioration with many organ systems failing due to sheer tumour load in which case an appropriate cause of death might read:

> 1a) disseminated carcinoma of the colon.

In all cases, the primary underlying cause of death is carcinoma of the colon and this should be the last condition recorded in Part 1 (remember: 'The bottom line is the bottom line').

Part 2 is only for conditions that have contributed to death and is not to be used for other conditions that a patient may have suffered from at the time of death but which did not have any significant bearing on death. For example, if an elderly patient has a fall and sustains a fractured neck of femur leading to immobility and a terminal bronchopneumonia, the circumstance that produced the fatal injury is the fall and this should be recorded under Part 1. However, if that patient is known to have marked osteoporosis, this obviously makes the likelihood of a fracture following a fall much higher. The osteoporosis was not itself the cause of the fall but it almost certainly played a significant part in the train of events leading to death and should therefore be included under Part 2. If, however, instead of osteoporosis, the patient had a stage 1 carcinoma of the breast, this would obviously play no part in the train of events and should not be included under Part 2. Sometimes, however, particularly in elderly patients where multiple pathologies are present, it can be difficult to decide which is the primary or underlying cause of death and which other conditions have merely contributed.

It must be remembered that the 'failures' (that is, cardiac failure, respiratory failure, renal failure, hepatic failure) are not *causes* of death. They are *modes* of death and as such, they should not be given as the underlying cause of death. The underlying cause in such cases of death due to organ failure is the underlying disease process that led to the failure. For instance, 'cardiac failure' is commonly due to coronary artery atheroma but may be due to valvular disease or even acute hypovolaemia due to a stab wound. It is therefore imperative that the underlying cause is stated. Registrars of Births and Deaths are instructed by the Home Office not to accept certificates for registration where only a mode of death has been given.

Mortality data

Valuable information for health-care planning can be gained by analysis of mortality data (causes and rates of death) but when data are compared between populations it is important to compare like with like. Mortality rates are therefore quoted as crude, specific or standardised rates.

A crude death rate is the rate that refers to an entire population.

$$\frac{\text{All deaths}}{\text{Total population at mid year}}$$

A specific death rate refers to deaths in a specific group within a population (usually either an age range or specified gender); for example:

$$\frac{\text{Deaths in people aged 25--35}}{\text{Number in population aged 25--35 at mid year}}$$

A standardised death rate removes bias from a population due to differences in age profile or other confounding variables. Using a non-standardised rate to compare populations can produce unexpected and entirely misleading results. Age is the most important factor in determining the death rate in almost every population. If one population has a larger percentage of old people than another, it will usually have a higher crude death rate. This effect of age can be very startling. If a third world population is compared with one from an affluent society with a well-developed health-care system, the third world population will usually have the lower crude mortality rate even though it has a higher age-specific mortality in all age ranges. This is because its increased age-specific mortality in a generally younger population does not make up for the sheer number of older people in the wealthier population.

To more meaningfully compare two populations, a standardised mortality rate can be used which makes allowance for the age distribution of the population by one of two means: direct standardisation and indirect standardisation.

In direct standardisation, the age-specific death rates calculated for the study population are applied to the age profile of a known standard population (often the national average) and the totals in death per thousand population are compared.

In indirect standardisation, it is the age-specific death rates of the standard population that are applied to the test population to produce the 'expected' death rate for that test population. The expected rate can then be compared with the actual measured or 'observed' rate within the population to produce the standardised mortality ratio (SMR).

$$SMR = \frac{\text{observed number of deaths}}{\text{expected number of deaths}} \times 100$$

Comparing mortality rates between populations by the indirect method is not always valid. Strictly, the SMR should only be used to compare one population with the standard population but sometimes the SMRs of several populations are compared. Provided that the age distributions of the different populations are similar, comparisons are valid, but if the age populations are significantly different (say, comparing a garrison town with a retirement area), they are not.

Box 18.7 WHO definitions of deaths in the first year of life

Neonatal death	A liveborn infant that dies within 28 days
Early neonatal death	A liveborn infant that dies within seven days
Late neonatal death	A liveborn infant that dies after seven days but within 28 days
Stillbirth	A foetus that dies before birth but after a presumed 24 weeks of gestation
Perinatal death	A combination of stillbirths and early neonatal deaths
Postneonatal death	Deaths from one month to one year of age
Infant deaths	Deaths under one year of age

The reason why the indirect method of standardisation is so widely used is that it is easier to calculate than the direct method: only the total number of deaths in a population and the age structure of that population are required (rather than requiring calculation of the age-specific death rates for the population).

In addition to studying whole-population mortality, a general measure of the overall health of a population can be obtained by assessing deaths in early life. These deaths have been separated into strictly defined groups depending on the age of the infant at death. Some categories include stillbirths, others do not. The definitions are given in Box 18.7.

FURTHER READING

1 McGee J O'D, Isaacson PG, Wright NA. *Oxford Textbook of Pathology.* Oxford: Oxford University Press, 1992

2 Cotran RS, Kumar V, Collins T. *Robbins Pathologic Basis of Disease*, 6th edn. Philadelphia: WB Saunders, 1999

3 Rosai J. *Ackerman's Surgical Pathology*, 8th edn. St Louis: Mosby, 1996

4 Farmer R, Miller D, Lewannon R. *Lecture Notes on Epidemiology and Public Health Medicine*, 4th edn. Oxford: Blackwell Scientific Publications, 1996

19

Cell growth, differentiation and degeneration

Cell growth
  Cell cycle
Cellular adaptation
  Hypertrophy
  Hyperplasia
  Hypoplasia
  Atrophy
  Metaplasia
  Dysplasia
Neoplasia
  Aetiology
  Environmental factors
  Intrinsic factors
  Genetic basis of cancer
  Tumour classification
Cellular accumulations

Fatty change
  Calcification
  Hyaline change
Amyloid
  Composition
  Pathogenesis
  Classification
  Systemic amyloidosis
  Localised amyloid deposits
  Diagnosis
Ageing

Frances McCormick

In mammals, growth and cellular differentiation begin in embryonic life and continue to the point of death. Throughout life complex genetic, hormonal and environmental factors affect both the whole organism as well as its individual cells. The cells respond to the physical and chemical alterations of their microenvironment in an attempt to maintain tissue and organ viability. This may lead to changes in cell proliferation and/or cell differentiation and function. Changes in differentiation may lead to abnormal morphological variants which may seriously compromise cell function. Alternatively, disordered cell proliferation may produce either a reversible non-neoplastic, controlled proliferation or an irreversible neoplastic, uncontrolled proliferation.

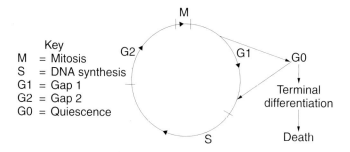

Figure 19.1 The cell cycle.

CELL GROWTH

Mammalian cells may be subdivided into three main classes. For a given stimulus, the cellular response depends upon the growth potential and class of the particular stimulated cell.

Labile cells are in a constant state of renewal, replacing those lost to terminal differentiation. They include the epidermal cells of the skin, the epithelial lining of the gastrointestinal tract and cells of the haemopoietic system. These tissues contain stem cells that divide continuously through asymmetrical division. After each division one daughter cell becomes a stem cell whilst the other follows the irreversible route to terminal differentiation. When stem cells produce progeny that differentiate into only one cell type they are called *unipotent,* whilst those generating more than one cell type are called *pluripotent.*

Stable cells are found in tissues that normally renew slowly. These cells are capable of entering into the cell cycle and rapidly dividing in response to damage. Tissues containing stable cells include glandular organs such as liver, kidney and pancreas as well as mesenchyme.

Permanent cells are terminally differentiated and usually cannot re-enter the cell cycle. Typically, they have lost the ability to divide by birth or shortly after. Neurones and cardiac muscle are thought to be incapable of dividing. Smooth muscle has definite regenerative capacity. That of skeletal muscle is small; the transformation of satellite cells within the endomysial sheaths enables a limited degree of regeneration.

Cell cycle

Cellular proliferation of both labile and stable cells is rigorously controlled through the cell cycle to maintain appropriate cell numbers. The cell cycle is defined as the time interval between two successive mitoses and it is divided into four phases, of varying duration (Figure 19.1). Immediately following cell division, the cell enters the G1 (gap 1) cycling phase. This is the most variable phase and in labile, rapidly dividing cells, it is extremely short. This is followed by the S or synthesis phase, during which time the DNA of the nucleus replicates. The next phase, G2 (gap

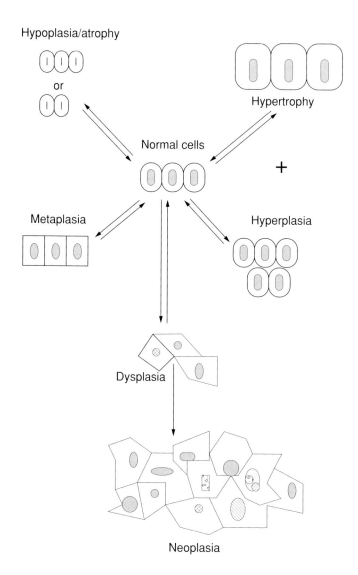

Figure 19.2 Cellular adaptation.

2), is short and precedes the beginning of mitosis, the M phase. Following mitosis, some cells leave the cell cycle and enter a resting phase, G0, from which they can reenter the cell cycle. Others, however, terminally differentiate and lose the ability to divide further.

An increase in cell production may occur either by shortening the cell cycle or by recruiting those cells in G0 back into the cell cycle.

CELLULAR ADAPTATION

In order to survive, cells must continuously adapt to their changing microenvironment and react to stress or increased demands (Figure 19.2). These alterations may occur in either physiological or pathological circumstances. Cellular adaptation is a reversible change, which attempts to prevent cell injury. Removal of the stimulus may enable the cell to return to its original state. However, prolonged stimulation may lead to irreversible change, ultimately leading to cell injury, cell death or genomic transformation and neoplasia (Figure 19.3).

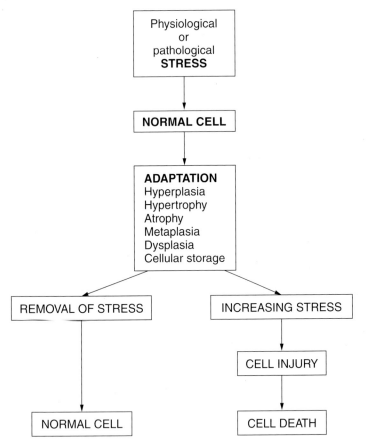

Figure 19.3 Cellular adaptation to stress.

Hypertrophy

This is the enlargement of individual cells with an increase in structural components, including DNA. There is an associated increase in cellular functional capacity. Although the tissue or organ may increase in size, the total cell population remains constant. This reversible process may be either physiological or pathological and is caused by either increased functional demand or hormonal stimulation. Pure hypertrophy (not associated with hyperplasia) occurs only in muscle.

Physiological hypertrophy is seen during pregnancy when increased hormonal stimulation causes hypertrophy of the myometrium of the gravid uterus. Similarly, repeated exercise through increased functional demand causes skeletal muscle hypertrophy.

Pathological hypertrophy is seen in several common settings. Obstruction of a hollow muscular viscus leads to smooth muscle hypertrophy of the muscle coat. In elderly men, benign enlargement of the prostate gland causes bladder outflow obstruction, producing hypertrophy of the detrusor muscle of the urinary bladder. Cardiac muscle hypertrophy of the heart is seen when there is pressure or volume overload (Figure 19.4). This is commonly seen in systemic hypertension where there is increased cardiac workload. The cardiac muscle hypertrophy reaches a limit beyond which the compensatory mechanism breaks down. This eventually leads to myocyte injury, with chamber dilatation and eventual heart failure.

In certain circumstances there is *individual organelle hypertrophy*, rather than enlargement of the whole cell. Classically, this is seen in patients treated with barbiturates. Barbiturates are metabolised in the smooth endoplasmic reticulum of hepatocytes. The resultant hypertrophy of the smooth endoplasmic reticulum leads to increased tolerance to this drug.

It is important to remember that some tissues are unable to respond to stimuli that would cause hypertrophy in other tissues.

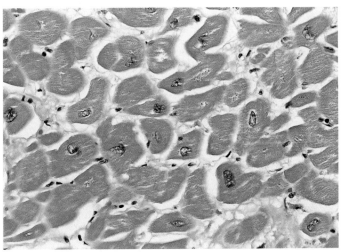

Figure 19.4 Hypertrophied cardiac myocytes with enlarged hyperchromatic nuclei.

Alas, neurones fail to undergo hypertrophy no matter how hard we think!

Hyperplasia

This is an increase in the total number of cells within a tissue or organ and may be associated with an increase in organ or tissue size as well as increased functional activity. Different adult tissues show variation in their capacity for hyperplastic growth. Epithelia and hepatocytes respond readily whilst neurones, cardiac and skeletal muscle have essentially no capacity. Limited capacity for hyperplastic growth is seen in smooth muscle, bone and cartilage.

Whilst they are two distinct processes, hyperplasia may be coupled with hypertrophy. This is a reversible process with both physiological and pathological causes.

Physiological hyperplasia is seen at puberty in both sexes with enlargement of the gonads and the secondary sexual organs. Female breast enlargement may also be seen during pregnancy and lactation when there are increased levels of circulating oestrogen and progesterone.

Compensatory hyperplasia is a form of physiological hyperplasia seen when there is enlargement of the remaining one of paired organs or within the remains of a single organ. After a nephrectomy the remaining kidney may increase its mass by 80–90% of normal by hyperplasia and hypertrophy of the remaining nephrons.

The term *pathological hyperplasia* is used when there is unwanted and/or unnecessary hyperplasia. Many examples are caused by excessive hormonal or growth factor stimulation.

- Endometrial gland hyperplasia is caused by an imbalance of oestrogen and progesterone and results in menorrhagia. It typically occurs in perimenopausal women and in younger women with persistent anovulatory cycles. Simple hyperplasia with an increase in glands and stroma is not preneoplastic. However, atypical hyperplasia may progress to endometrial carcinoma.

- In men defective androgen metabolism in the prostate gland leads to benign prostatic hyperplasia. The hyperplasia of the epithelial and connective tissue components leads to nodular enlargement of the prostate gland (Figure 19.5) with resultant urinary outflow obstruction.

- In individuals who live at high altitude, where the air has a low oxygen concentration, an increase in erythropoietin levels leads to hyperplasia of erythrocyte precursors in the bone marrow with a resulting increase in circulating red blood cells which is an example of secondary polycythaemia.

- Persistent trauma to epithelium may lead to hyperplasia and this is seen in the skin of the foot when the mechanical trauma of ill-fitting shoes leads to the development of calluses and corns.

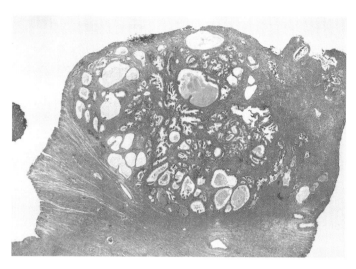

Figure 19.5 A hyperplastic predominantly glandular nodule seen in benign prostatic hyperplasia.

Hypoplasia

This is a reduction in the number of cells in a tissue or organ and may be either a developmental (congenital) abnormality or acquired after a period of normal growth. The affected organ is smaller than normal and may be dysfunctional.

Congenital hypoplasia is usually present at birth.

- In DiGeorge syndrome failure of development of the third and fourth pharyngeal pouches leads to hypoplasia of the thymus gland and T cell deficiency.

- In cryptorchidism the maldescended or undescended testis undergoes hypoplasia and at puberty there is failure of normal spermatogenesis. If both testes are affected the individual will be sterile.

Acquired hypoplasia is seen after prolonged parenteral feeding or surgical bypass intervention leading to hypoplasia of the intestinal mucosa.

Agenesis is the severest form and is the complete failure of a tissue or organ to develop. Unilateral renal agenesis is an uncommon anomaly that is compatible with life and is associated with compensatory hyperplasia and hypertrophy of the solitary developed kidney. Bilateral agenesis is incompatible with survival.

Aplasia is a term applied when there is sudden cessation of development with minimal regeneration. Aplastic anaemia is the term applied to pancytopaenia caused by either failure or suppression of the multipotent myeloid stem cells of the bone marrow to release the differentiated cell lines. The commonest causes are exposure to drugs and chemicals and whole-body irradiation.

Atrophy

This is a reversible response where the individual cell reduces its mass of functional cytoplasm but is still capable of survival. The total number of cells may remain constant or decrease. The overall size of the organ involved may be reduced. The resultant shrinkage in cell volume minimises the cell's energy requirement, with loss of cell differentiation. This is caused by the repression of the differentiation genes whilst retaining the expression of the 'housekeeping' genes that maintain cellular integrity. The causes of atrophy may be physiological or pathological.

Involution is used synonymously with *physiological atrophy* and is seen in the foetus, infant and in later life. Embryonic structures, such as the ductus arteriosus, branchial clefts and notochord, atrophy during foetal development. The thymus gland atrophies at puberty whilst the uterus decreases in size after parturition.

Pathological atrophy may be either localised or generalised.

- Reduced functional activity (disuse atrophy). Prolonged bedrest leads to skeletal muscle atrophy and muscle weakness. Astronauts experiencing prolonged reduced gravitational force experience skeletal muscular atrophy and also decalcification of bones.

- Loss of innervation (neuropathic atrophy). Traumatic paraplegia or neurological diseases causing destruction of the motor neurones cause atrophy of the denervated skeletal muscle.

- Reduced blood supply. Chronic reduction of the blood supply to an organ, typically through partial occlusion of the main arterial supply or poor collateral circulation in a completely occluded blood vessel, causes atrophy.

- Ageing. This typically affects tissues composed of permanent cells.

- Diminished nutrition. This may be seen in starvation or in the cachexia of malignant disease. The body's carbohydrate and fat stores are used up first. Later proteins from skeletal muscle are metabolised. Those of the heart and brain are the last to be used.

- Loss of hormonal stimulation. The secondary sexual organs atrophy after the menopause. Adrenocortical atrophy affecting the glucocorticoid zones follows withdrawal of ACTH stimulation, for example in hypopituitarism or corticosteroid therapy.

Other types of atrophy include *postradiation atrophy* which is caused by genetic damage which interferes with mitosis. *Pressure atrophy* of an organ is seen when either an internal or external tumour compresses an organ and interferes with the function and/or the blood supply.

Atrophy may progress to irreversible injury and ultimately cell death.

Metaplasia

Metaplasia comes from the Greek word *metaplasis* which means a moulding afresh and it is the condition where one differentiated cell type changes to another. This is usually caused by persistent injury, either from chronic irritation or chronic inflammation which stimulates tissue growth. Metaplasia can occur in either epithelia or connective tissue. It is a reversible adaptive response but it is not harmless as it results in loss of specialist function.

Cancer is recognised to occur in certain metaplastic tissues. However, it is uncertain whether a particular form of metaplasia predisposes to cancer or whether it is caused by the underlying chronic tissue damage.

Epithelial metaplasia

Squamous metaplasia is the transformation of glandular epithelium to stratified squamous epithelium. Any site may be affected, one of the commonest examples involves the bronchial ciliated respiratory epithelium in smokers. Loss of specialised ciliary function leads to mucus accumulation, with predisposition to recurrent chest infections and pneumonia. Also, the squamous metaplasia may progress through grades of dysplasia to *in situ* and then to invasive squamous cell carcinoma. Squamous metaplasia is also seen in other mucus membranes including those of the endocervix (Figure 19.6), nose, salivary ducts and urinary bladder.

Vitamin A deficiency is a recognised contributory factor to epithelial metaplasia in both respiratory and transitional epithelia.

Glandular metaplasia is the conversion of squamous epithelium to glandular mucosa or alternatively, the conversion of one specialised glandular epithelium to another.

- Repeated gastrooesophageal reflux affects the distal oesophagus, with glandular columnar epithelium replacing the normal squamous epithelium. When intestinal-type mucosa lines the

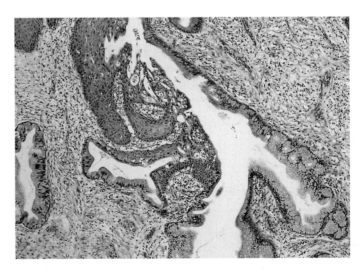

Figure 19.6 An endocervical crypt with focal squamous metaplasia.

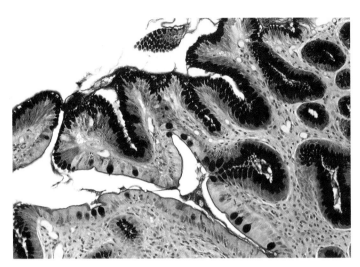

Figure 19.7 Focal complete intestinal metaplasia arising within gastric mucosa.

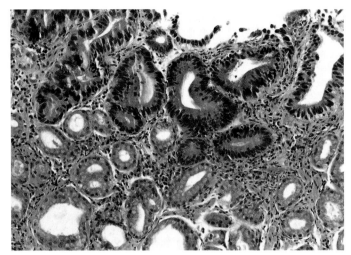

Figure 19.8 Glandular dysplasia arising in normal mucosa showing nuclear hyperchromasia and loss of polarity.

distal oesophagus above the oesophagogastric junction, it is described as Barrett's oesophagus.

● In chronic gastritis or gastric ulceration, acid-secreting oxyntic gastric mucosa is replaced by mucin-producing complete or incomplete intestinal epithelium. In the complete form (Figure 19.7), fully formed small intestinal crypts and villi are present. In incomplete metaplasia there is a variable degree of intestinalisation but fully formed villi are sparse and there is no evidence of Paneth cells.

The endocervical epithelium may convert from mucin secreting glandular mucosa to squamous mucosa, for example under the influence of oestrogens or the human papilloma virus. Such squamous metaplasia precedes the squamous dysplasia of CIN.

Connective tissue metaplasia

Osseous metaplasia is seen in soft tissue following dystrophic calcification. Marrow showing normal haemopoietic differentiation may develop within the metaplastic bone. Cartilaginous metaplasia may be seen when there is undue mobility in healing bones.

Dysplasia

This is a premalignant, reversible condition that is characterised by disorderly epithelial cell growth with an associated compromise in function. There is both cellular and organisational atypia. The constituent cells show nuclear pleomorphism with hyperchromasia, increased mitotic activity and an atypical growth pattern showing architectural disorder (Figure 19.8).

Dysplasia may occur in hyperplastic or metaplastic epithelium but may be seen in any tissue under chronic stress. Dysplastic cells are thought to have a survival advantage over non-dysplastic cells, as

they are more resistant to injury because of poor cellular differentiation and loss of specialist function. This enhances their survival and helps to maintain the integrity of the tissue or organ.

Dysplastic cells share many morphological features with neoplastic cells and dysplasia is a recognised preneoplastic condition that is considered to be part of the multistep evolution of cancer. In many tissues the presence of dysplasia is graded and considered to be a form of intraepithelial neoplasia, as in the cervix and prostate gland. When dysplasia is severe and involves the full thickness of the epithelium, the lesion is considered to represent a preinvasive neoplastic state and is called carcinoma *in situ*. This lesion is treated aggressively in an attempt to prevent invasive malignancy.

Thus, although dysplasia is considered a reversible process, the persistence of noxious stimuli may cause the cellular abnormalities to become increasingly atypical, ultimately leading to malignant transformation of the dysplastic cell into a cancer cell.

NEOPLASIA

Neoplasia literally means new growth and the resultant lesion is a neoplasm.

Cell proliferation is intricately coupled with and inversely related to its ability to differentiate. The tumour cell population is thought to arise from divisions of a single cell that has acquired an accumulation of damage to its genome. Potentially, all cell types within the human body may give rise to neoplasia, at any stage along the differentiation pathway between stem cell and the fully differentiated state. Therefore, both the morphological appearance and the characteristics of neoplasia may differ between organs.

Aetiology

Studies in human populations have indicated possible factors implicated in cancer aetiology. However, it is usually impossible to determine the specific cause of a particular cancer. Generally, the causes of cancer may be subdivided into:

1. factors extrinsic to the patient (environmental factors)

2. factors intrinsic to the patient that include genetic, physiological and pathological factors, e.g. hormonal balance, immune status.

It is important to realise that these factors do not operate independently; owing to the complexity of carcinogenesis, one particular neoplasm may have a number of different causes whilst conversely, a single causal factor may be responsible for several different types of tumour.

Environmental factors

The incidence and mortality for specific cancers vary dramatically around the world; for example, the death rate for carcinoma of the stomach is eight times higher in Japan than in Western Europe. It is thought that most of the geographical differences are due to environmental factors rather than racial differences.

Carcinogens are active mutagens with the ability to cause DNA damage and there is a positive correlation between carcinogens and cancer induction. Typically, cigarette smoking is recognised as a causative factor in the development of carcinoma of the lung; however, it is also implicated in the aetiology of cancer of the mouth, larynx, oesophagus, bladder, pancreas and cervix.

An environmental agent may not act alone and its effect may be modified by the genetic make-up of the individual, as illustrated by those with fair complexions who are more susceptible to sun-induced skin cancers.

The interaction of environmental factors may have a synergistic effect on tumour development; for example, cigarette smoking and asbestos exposure have an additive effect in the development of lung cancer. This is the commonest malignant tumour developing in those with asbestosis, outnumbering the more typically accepted single-factor association of asbestos exposure and mesothelioma.

Intrinsic factors

Age

Most carcinomas tend to occur in older individuals with the peak mortality from cancer in the 55–74 age group. However, a smaller peak incidence occurs in children under the age of 15 years, when approximately 10% of deaths are due to cancer, most commonly acute leukaemia and central nervous system neoplasms.

Heredity

For many types of cancer a hereditary predisposition as well as exposure to environmental factors appears to be implicated in tumour development. Up to 10% of all human tumours are thought to involve heredity. These are subdivided into three groups.

Inherited cancer syndromes

This is indicated by a strong family history of uncommon cancers. There is an autosomal dominant pattern of inheritance whereby inheritance of a single mutant gene greatly increases the risk of developing a cancer. Familial adenomatous polyposis causes the development of numerous adenomatous colorectal polyps that ultimately progress to colorectal adenocarcinoma.

Familial cancers

Familial clustering of malignant neoplasms is evident with an early age of onset. These cancers may be multiple and/or bilateral. In certain cancers the inherited predisposition may not be obvious whilst others are linked to the inheritance of mutant genes. BRCA-1 and BRCA-2 genes are linked to familial breast and ovarian cancers.

Defective DNA repair

Patients with the inherited disorder xeroderma pigmentosum are at an increased risk of developing sun-induced skin cancers. Ultraviolet light exposure causes damage to the DNA which is not adequately repaired due to the defective DNA repair system. This enables the development of multiple skin cancers, basal cell and squamous carcinoma and malignant melanoma.

Genetic basis of cancer

Sequential acquisition of non-lethal somatic mutations in the cellular genome leads to the development of cancer. The conversion of a normal cell to a malignant one never occurs in a single step and cannot be attributed to the mutation of a single gene. Thus, tumour development is associated with an accumulation of mutations leading to the progression of the malignant phenotype. A multifactorial range of genetic changes therefore determines the behaviour and severity of any cancer. The rate-limiting steps depend on the tumour cell type, its requirements for growth factors and its ability to escape the host immune response.

A detailed explanation of the acquisition of the malignant phenotype is beyond the scope of this chapter. Nevertheless, the following is a brief outline of the main factors leading to malignant transformation.

Oncogenes

Protooncogenes are cellular genes that promote normal growth and differentiation. Oncogenes are the oncogenic form of cellular protooncogenes created by:

- point mutations
- gene amplification
- chromosomal rearrangements.

Oncogenes act by encoding components of the signal transduction cascade and the cell cycle regulatory pathway. Normally, cells receive signals to proliferate via growth factors that bind receptors located on the cytoplasmic or nuclear membrane. Signal transmission causes the activation of proliferation factors thereby producing a net growth response. Oncogenes are often altered so that proliferative signals are jammed in the 'on' position. Activated oncogenes are thought to be dominantly acting and even a single copy is sufficient to drive the cell to malignancy.

KRAS is one member of a family of three human RAS genes that are protooncogenes. They encode small guanosine triphosphatase (GTP) binding proteins that are involved in signal transduction through tyrosine kinase receptors, such as the epidermal growth factor (EGF) receptor. They participate in signalling for a variety of cellular functions including cellular differentiation, cell cycle progression, cytoskeletal organisation and protein transport and secretion. Up to 20% of all human tumours contain mutated RAS genes. KRAS mutations are the commonest genetic event described in pancreatic carcinoma.

Tumour suppressor genes

These are genes that negatively regulate cell proliferation and, by inference, promote cell differentiation. Loss of these genes leads to tumour development.

This type of gene was discovered through studying the rare retinoblastoma tumour, a paediatric tumour that shows both sporadic and familial occurrences. The familial predisposition is transmitted as an autosomal dominant trait. Knudson suggested the 'two-hit hypothesis' of oncogenesis. In hereditary cases one recessive genetic mutation in the retinoblastoma (Rb) gene is inherited and is present in all somatic cells, whilst the second abnormality is acquired. A heterozygous child inherits a recessive mutation to one allele of the Rb gene. This predisposes to neoplasia and these individuals may go on to develop a cancer if the mutation is made homozygous by damage to the remaining intact allele. The loss of both copies of any tumour suppressor gene at a critical time leads to tumour formation by enabling inappropriate expression of proliferative genes. In the sporadic cases both mutations are acquired and are seen only in the retinal cells.

Several tumour suppressor genes have been isolated:

- p53 gene
- retinoblastoma (Rb) gene

- gene deleted in cancer cells from patients with neurofibromatosis (NF)
- gene deleted in colon cancer (DCC).

Mutation to p53 is so common that it may represent the commonest mutation in all human cancers. It is estimated that approximately 50% of human tumours contain mutations of this gene. In the Li-Fraumeni syndrome, a heritable mutation in p53 is thought to predispose to a range of malignancies, including breast cancer, osteosarcoma, rhabdomyosarcoma, retinoblastoma and ovarian cancer.

Apoptosis regulation

Genes that induce or prevent programmed cell death are implicated in tumour development. By inhibiting apoptosis, damaged cells persist and accumulate. The anti-apoptotic gene bcl-2 is seen in 85% of follicle centre cell lymphoma. The regulation of apoptosis involves not only the interaction of bcl-2 but also p53 and the protooncogene c-myc.

DNA repair

DNA is constantly being damaged. Normal cells either repair the non-lethal DNA damage or undergo apoptosis if the damage is irreparable. The inability of a cell to maintain the integrity of the genome leads to an increased risk of developing cancer. As already discussed, in xeroderma pigmentosum there is an increased risk of sun-induced malignancies. A family of DNA mismatch repair genes (hMSH2, hMLH1, hPMS1 and hPMS2) is recognised to be defective both in hereditary non-polyposis colon cancer and in some types of sporadic cancer. Abnormalities of these genes allow ubiquitous somatic mutations or replication errors to accumulate throughout the genome, producing widespread alterations of the simple repeat sequences. This is called microsatellite instability (MSI) and is seen in several tumours including colorectal and gastric tumours.

Growth factors

There is excessive expression of several growth factor receptor-ligand families which participate in aberrant autocrine and paracrine pathways, so contributing to tumour cell growth. Some of these changes also occur in benign conditions, suggesting that overexpression of these receptor-ligand systems in itself is not sufficient to produce malignant transformation but in combination with other genetic abnormalities may lead to a distinct growth advantage. Examples include the epidermal growth factor family of receptors and ligands and the fibroblast growth factor family; the latter is deranged in prostate cancer.

Host immune response

Little is understood about the genes that control the reaction of cancer cells with the host immune system. Studies have shown that cancer cells express tumour antigens and these can form the basis of an antitumour immune reaction. The significance of this is illustrated by the rare phenomenon of spontaneous regression of cancers that cannot be attributed to treatment. The concept of immune surveillance may partially explain the observed age-related incidence of cancers and the increased incidence of cancer in the immunosuppressed.

Tumour development probably represents the failure of the host immune system to control the growth of transformed cells. Possibly the acquisition of genetic mutations in the development of the malignant phenotype enables the malignant cells to evade the host immune system. It is of importance that the tumours seen in immunosuppression are usually of viral association, e.g. squamous carcinoma of anogenital origin and skin and HPV; lymphoma and EBV; Kaposi's sarcoma and herpes hominis.

Metastases genes

Other genetic components of tumour progression are thought to be as important as oncogenes and tumour suppressor genes. Whilst the localised tumour mass may pose little direct threat to the individual, the most life-threatening feature of cancer is its ability to spread individual cells to distant regions where they initiate secondary tumours. Not all tumour cells have the same capacity to metastasise from within the same tumour population. For tumour cells to become metastatic they have to acquire several properties and most of these are under genetic control. Reduced expression of the nm23 gene in a melanoma cell line is associated with the malignant phenotype of these cells whilst increased expression seems to suppress the malignant phenotype.

Tumour classification

Tumours may be classified in several ways based on their morphological, histological and behavioural characteristics.

When tumours are classified according to their constituent cells they can be subdivided into three main groups:

- tumours of epithelial origin

- tumours of connective tissue origin

- other tumours.

The names ascribed to tumours tend to reflect their tissue of origin and their behavioural pattern (Table 19.1). Benign neoplasms of surface epithelia are called papillomas, whilst those showing glandular differentiation are called adenomas and, if cystic, are called cystadenomas. Malignant epithelial neoplasms are all called carcinomas; a malignant glandular tumour is called an adenocarcinoma (Figure 19.9). In connective tissues, the benign tumours are called after the tissue of origin with the addition of the suffix -oma, such as a leiomyoma, which is a benign tumour of smooth muscle cells. Malignant connective tissue tumours are called sarcomas, such as a leiomyosarcoma which is a malignant tumour of smooth muscle cells. Lymphomas are tumours arising from solid lymphoid tissue, whilst leukaemias are tumours derived from the haemopoietic elements where malignant cells circulate in blood. Embryonic tissue, present during development but absent in adult life, may also give rise to neoplasms. These tumours tend to occur in infancy and childhood.

Neoplasms may also arise from germ cells and these commonly occur in the ovary and testis. As germ cells are totipotent they may differentiate into any tissue of the body and are called teratomas. Neuroendocrine tumours are derived from cells of the neuroendocrine system and are essentially epithelial in nature, i.e. they behave as carcinomas.

Differentiation

Tumour assessment also includes neoplastic cell differentiation which is judged according to the degree of similarity between the

Table 19.1 Classification of tumours

Tissue of origin	Benign	Malignant
Epithelium		
Squamous	Squamous papilloma	Squamous cell carcinoma
Transitional	Transitional cell papilloma	Transitional cell carcinoma
Glandular	Adenoma	Adenocarcinoma
Connective tissue		
Fibrous tissue	Fibroma	Fibrosarcoma
Fat	Lipoma	Liposarcoma
Bone	Osteoma	Osteosarcoma
Cartilage	Chondroma	Chondrosarcoma
Lymphatics	Lymphangioma	Lymphangiosarcoma
Blood vessels	Haemangioma	Angiosarcoma
Smooth muscle	Leiomyoma	Leiomyosarcoma
Others		
Haemopoietic cells		Leukaemias
Lymphoid tissue		Malignant lymphoma
Totipotent cells	Mature teratoma	Immature teratoma
(in gonads)		Malignant teratoma

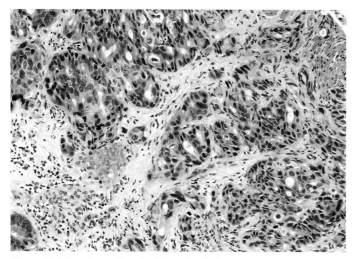

Figure 19.9 Invasive moderately differentiated adenocarcinoma.

neoplastic cell and the normal cell. Well-differentiated tumours closely resemble their normal counterparts. At the other end of the spectrum the cells are unspecialised and primitive and are called poorly differentiated or undifferentiated. The middle of the spectrum includes cells showing degrees of specialisation and these cells are described as moderately differentiated. The degree of differentiation of a tumour tends to correlate with the growth rate of tumours. Rapidly growing cells tend to be poorly differentiated whilst slowly growing tumours tend to be well differentiated.

Benign versus malignant

Neoplasms may be described as either benign or malignant and this can be determined from either tumour morphology and/or their clinical behaviour. Usually benign tumours can be easily differentiated from malignant tumours on morphology alone (Table 19.2).

In benign neoplasms the constituent cells closely resemble the parent tissue and so are well differentiated. They tend to be localised, expansile, cohesive masses that grow slowly. They are non-infiltrative and the surrounding tissues may develop pressure atrophy whilst the remaining compressed connective tissue forms a capsule, though not all benign tumours are

encapsulated. Benign tumours rarely show evidence of haemorrhage or necrosis. There are few mitotic figures and those present are normal.

In comparison, malignant neoplasms are generally unencapsulated with infiltrative growth into adjacent normal tissues. Speed of growth is variable but generally more rapid than the benign equivalent. The constituent malignant cells may show a full range of morphology from well differentiated to poorly differentiated. Typically, malignant cells show a variety of morphological features that include nuclear pleomorphism, variation in nuclear size and shape, and when this is extreme the cells are described as anaplastic and show no obvious evidence of differentiation. Nuclear hyperchromasia is caused by an excess of DNA and the nuclei tend to be disproportionately larger than the cytoplasm with an increased nuclear to cytoplasmic ratio. The chromatin is often coarsely clumped and is distributed along the nuclear membrane. There may be prominent nucleoli, indicating high synthetic activity. High proliferative activity is reflected by the increased number of mitotic figures and many are atypical, producing tripolar or multipolar forms. The tumour stimulates the growth of new blood vessels from the original vascular bed to support it; this is called angioneogenesis. However, when tumours grow quickly they tend to outstrip their blood supply and undergo central ischaemic necrosis.

Some tumours show intermediate malignancy. This term is applied to morphologically malignant-appearing tumours that are locally invasive but have little or no tendency to metastasise. Examples of such tumours are basal cell carcinomas and carcinoids.

Metastases

Another feature of malignant neoplasms is the ability to metastasise. This is the capacity to spread to and grow at sites distant from the primary lesion and these metastases are called secondary tumours. The ability to metastasise is due to the invasiveness of the neoplasm. While in general there is some correlation between the size of the primary tumours and the incidence of metastases, regrettably there may be widespread metastases with small or clinically undetectable primary tumours.

Table 19.2 Benign tumour versus malignant tumour	
Benign tumour	**Malignant tumour**
Well-differentiated cells, resembling cell of origin	Loss of cell differentiation
Well circumscribed	Ill-defined and infiltrative
Few mitoses, normal forms	Many mitoses with abnormal forms
Uniform cells	Cellular pleomorphism
No necrosis	Necrosis

Direct infiltration

Malignant tumours directly invade the surrounding tissues. They also spread along the lines of least resistance, such as the perineural sheath.

Haematogenous spread

This pathway is common for sarcomas but is also seen in carcinomas. Arteries are less readily penetrated than veins because of their thicker walls. Venous invasion leads to metastases that follow the venous flow. Liver and lungs are the most frequently involved organs.

Lymphatic spread

This is the commonest means of distant dissemination for carcinomas. The pattern of lymph node involvement follows the normal routes of drainage. Regional lymph node involvement may act as a barrier to further tumour dissemination.

Transcoelomic spread

Tumour cells spread directly across the coelomic spaces. The peritoneal and pleural cavities are most commonly affected but other sites, including pericardial and subarachnoid cavities, may also be involved.

It should be noted that the distinction between haematogenous and lymphatic invasion is not precise because there are numerous intercommunications between the vascular and lymphatic systems.

The release of tumour cells into lymphatic or blood circulation does not result in a uniform distribution of metastases. The distribution is irregular and partly related to the site and type of the primary tumour. Certain organs such as liver, lung, bone, lymph nodes and adrenal gland are frequently the sites of metastases, whilst others such as kidney or muscle are rarely involved.

CELLULAR ACCUMULATIONS

This is a normal process in multicellular organisms. Fat, glycogen, vitamins and minerals are commonly stored for use at another time. However, materials can accumulate in abnormal amounts either within the cytoplasm or the nucleus of a cell by several means.

- Normal cellular constituents may accumulate in excess when there is a normal rate of production but a decrease in catabolism.

- An unusual substance may be produced as a product of abnormal metabolism. For example, lack of a particular enzyme within a specific metabolic pathway encourages the develop-

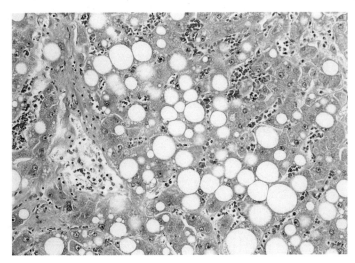

Figure 19.10 Fatty change (macrosteatosis) within hepatocytes.

ment of an alternative pathway, with the formation of atypical metabolites which then accumulate.

- An exogenous substance may accumulate when the cell lacks the metabolic capacity to deal with it or an inability to transport it to other sites. Carbon inhaled into the lung parenchyma accumulates in alveolar macrophages.

These accumulations may be harmless or toxic to the cell and may ultimately lead to cell death.

Fatty change

This is an abnormal *reversible* accumulation of neutral fat within parenchymal cells. It may be seen in several organs, including cardiac muscle and kidney, but is most often seen in the liver (Figure 19.10). An absolute increase in intracellular lipid causes the formation of fat vacuoles within the cytoplasm.

Pathogenesis

Normally, lipids are transported to the liver from both adipose tissue and the gastrointestinal tract (from dietary fat). Lipids released from adipose tissue are transported only as free fatty acids; however, dietary lipids are transported as either chylomicrons (a mixture of triglyceride, phospholipid and protein) or as free fatty acids. The liver can also synthesise free fatty acids.

On entering the liver, most free fatty acids are esterified to triglycerides, though some are converted into cholesterol or phospholipids or oxidised to ketone bodies. The triglyceride is then excreted by the liver by being complexed with specific apoproteins to form lipoproteins.

Fatty change develops from an excess accumulation of triglycerides and this can happen at any stage along the complex pathway of fat metabolism. There are three main causes:

- increased delivery of fatty acids to the liver

- reduced catabolism or increased formation of fatty acids within the liver

- reduced hepatic secretion.

An increase in free fatty acid transport to the liver is seen during starvation. Adipose tissue is broken down and the released fatty acids are transported to the liver. Increased endogenous fatty acid synthesis or reduced fatty acid breakdown leads to an increase in triglyceride formation. Accelerated conjugation of fatty acids to triglycerides is seen in alcoholic poisoning.

Alcohol is the commonest cause of fatty liver in industrialised nations. It is a hepatotoxin that deranges hepatocyte metabolism, altering the pathway of fat metabolism at several different loci.

The significance of fatty change depends on the cause and severity of the accumulation. When mild, there may be no alteration in cellular function though more severe accumulations may impair function or result in cell death with consequent inflammation, as in alcoholic hepatitis.

Calcification

Calcium deposition is normally seen in the formation of bone from cartilage. When calcium salts are deposited in tissues other than osteoid or tooth enamel it is described as *heterotopic calcification*. It is often associated with the deposition of smaller quantities of other mineral salts including iron and magnesium. Calcification develops as a two-stage process of initiation and propagation. Initiation occurs either in extracellular membrane-bound vesicles that have budded off from cells or within the intracellular mitochondria. Then propagation occurs with enlargement of the deposits.

Dystrophic calcification is the localised deposition of calcium salts in dead or degenerate tissue and it occurs in normal calcium and phosphate serum levels (Figure 19.11). The calcium deposition is seen in dead and injured cells that cannot maintain a steep calcium gradient across the cell membrane and the minerals are derived from the interstitial fluid or from the circulation. The deposits may be either intracellular or extracellular. Cells originally forming a papillary architecture may be converted to lamellated calcified structures called psammoma bodies. Depending upon the site, dystrophic calcification may have no functional consequence. However, where it develops in crucial sites, such as the mitral or aortic valves, it can cause impediment to blood flow due to narrowed valvular orifices and rigid valve leaflets and cause cardiac impairment.

Metastatic calcification tends to occur when there is a derangement of calcium metabolism producing hypercalcaemia. This may occur in hyperparathyroidism or in high plasma phosphate levels as seen in chronic renal failure. The deposits tend to be laid down

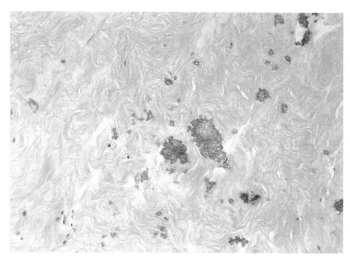

Figure 19.11 Basophilic dystrophic calcification within fibrous scar tissue.

in normal tissues and can occur widely throughout the body. Generally there is no clinical dysfunction, though massive deposition may ultimately compromise function.

Another form of pathological calcification is the formation of calcium carbonate calculi, which may be seen in the gallbladder, renal pelvis, urinary bladder and pancreatic ductal system.

Hyaline change

This is a histological term that describes the intracellular or extracellular change that produces a homogeneous, glassy, pink appearance to tissue seen on histological haematoxylin and eosin (H&E) sections. A multitude of different mechanisms and materials can produce this change, only some of which are recognised. The intracellular material Mallory's hyaline, seen in the hepatocytes of alcoholics, consists of aggregates of prekeratin intermedi-

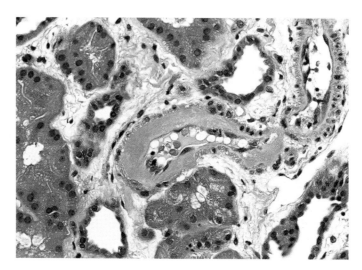

Figure 19.12 Hyalinisation of a renal arteriole showing glassy amorphous eosinophilic thickening of the vessel wall.

ate filaments. Viral inclusions may be associated with intracytoplasmic or intranuclear hyaline inclusions. Extracellular hyaline is seen in the hyaline found in renal arterioles in hypertension and diabetes mellitus (Figure 19.12) and is derived from basement membrane.

AMYLOID

This is a misleading name given to the deposition of an extracellular proteinaceous material (Figure 19.13). Amyloid is not a solitary disease as both the nature and the cause of amyloid deposits vary widely. Amyloid deposition may produce a variety of effects. Typically, the deposits are laid down between parenchymal cells and their blood supply, causing the cells to be isolated. The amyloid causes either a direct toxic effect or else a deleterious reduction in cellular nutrition and oxygenation. This ultimately causes atrophy of the affected cells leading to impaired mechanical function. Affected blood vessel walls are fragile and prone to bleeding, with resultant haemorrhage. Deposition in the glomerular basement membrane results in increased permeability, proteinuria and potentially the nephrotic syndrome.

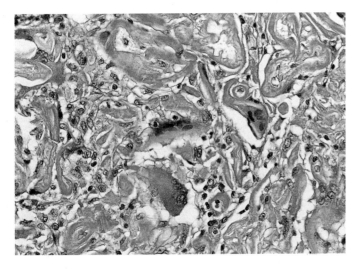

Figure 19.13 Deposits of amorphous eosinophilic amyloid which has elicited a multinucleated giant cell reaction.

Composition

Amyloid has two main components: a protein component, which makes up 90% of the amyloid, and a glycoprotein component which makes up the remaining 10%.

Protein component

The protein component is mainly a fibrillary protein whose amino acid composition varies with the underlying disease. However, in spite of their chemical differences, these protein fibrils are folded so that they share common ultrastructural and phys-

ical properties. The aggregated fibrils are between 7.5 and 10 nm long and are rigid, non-branching fibrils that form a beta-pleated sheet, giving amyloid its characteristic histological and chemical properties. These fibrils are insoluble and resistant to digestion.

In human disease two common chemically distinct classes have been identified. *Amyloid light chain (AL) type* is composed of partial or complete immunoglobulin light chains, usually lambda light chains. This is usually associated with plasma cell dyscrasias such as multiple myeloma. The malignant cells produce an abnormal monoclonal immunoglobulin that appears as an M band on serum electrophoresis. In multiple myeloma there is an excess of light chains that passes into the urine and is called Bence-Jones protein.

Amyloid-associated (AA) type amyloid is derived from a unique protein produced in the liver. It is found in cases where there is chronic inflammatory disease, such as rheumatoid arthritis, tuberculosis or rarely Crohn's disease. The fibrils are derived from a precursor protein serum amyloid-associated protein, that circulates in association with a subclass of lipoproteins. It is found in all normal individuals but its level increases with age and is elevated in chronic disease.

Other biologically distinct forms of amyloid are as follows.

Transthyretin

This is a normal serum protein that binds and transports thyroxine and retinol. A mutant form of this protein is deposited in the neuropathic forms of heredofamilial amyloidosis. These diseases are generally inherited as autosomal dominant traits and include familial amyloid polyneuropathy and familial Mediterranean fever. It is also found in senile systemic amyloid which is associated with ageing.

Beta amyloid protein

This is found in the cerebral plaques and blood vessel walls in Alzheimer's disease and is derived from a transmembrane glycoprotein called amyloid precursor protein (APP). In transmissible spongiform encephalopathies including Creutzfeldt-Jacob disease and new variant Creutzfeldt-Jacob disease as well as kuru, plaques similar to senile plaques are seen. It has been shown that the amyloid within these plaques is composed of prion protein (PrP).

Beta-2 microglobulin

This is found in chronic renal failure patients on long-term haemodialysis. It is a component of the major histocompatibility complex class 1 molecules and a normal serum protein. The protein accumulates because it is not removed by conventional dialysis membranes. Sites of deposition are often periarticular and include tendon sheaths, giving rise to carpal tunnel syndrome.

Hormone precursors

The hormone precursors procalcitonin and proinsulin have also been found as localised amyloid in endocrine glands.

Glycoprotein component

The second constituent forming approximately 10% of amyloid is composed of *amyloid P component*. This is a pentagonal glycoprotein that is present in all forms of amyloid. It is derived from a normal circulating serum protein, serum amyloid P (SAP).

Other components

Apolipoprotein E (apoE) is another component and this is a normal constituent of high-density lipoproteins.

Pathogenesis

All forms of amyloid are derived from soluble precursor proteins but form insoluble proteinaceous aggregates through proteolytic degradation. The physiological function of the amyloid precursor protein determines the localisation of the specific form of amyloid. Several factors are thought to work in concert including quantitative or qualitative increases in the precursor proteins coupled with defective or deficient proteolysis.

Classification

Classification of amyloid is unsatisfactory with classifications depending on the tissue distribution and the presence or absence of an identifiable predisposing condition.

Systemic amyloidosis

Amyloid is described as primary when associated with plasma cell dyscrasia or secondary when there is an underlying chronic inflammatory condition. Hereditary amyloidosis has several distinctive patterns of organ involvement.

Kidney involvement is a major feature and is the main cause of death followed by cardiac death. All the systemic forms of amyloidosis have a poor prognosis, though AA amyloidosis has a more protracted course than AL amyloidosis. Treatment of the underlying disease may occasionally lead to resorption of amyloid but this is a rare occurrence.

Localised amyloid deposits

These typically occur in the endocrine glands, the heart and the skin. Amyloid deposits are common in the islets of Langerhans in diabetes mellitus and islet cell tumours such as insulinomas.

Amyloid derived from calcitonin is deposited in the stroma of medullary carcinoma of the thyroid. Amyloid is frequently seen in the heart of the elderly and is derived from transthyretin. However, in isolated atrial amyloidosis the amyloid fibrils contain immunoreactive human atrial natriuretic peptide. Sometimes a localised mass of amyloid develops, examples being the lung and larynx. The amyloid is usually of AL type. These localised forms are unrelated to systemic deposition.

Diagnosis

Gingival, rectal and abdominal fat biopsies may be used to demonstrate the presence of amyloid for diagnosis. Using molecular biology, it is possible to identify genetic abnormalities common in the heredofamilial forms.

AGEING

Senescence is the finite capacity of normal human cells to divide in cell culture. A limited lifespan with death occurring after approximately 60 divisions is a fundamental characteristic of normal mammalian diploid cells in culture. However, this does tend to vary in magnitude between species and cell type. Though the senescence of cells in culture is different from the senescence of organisms in the environment, it may help to explain why life is finite. Studies have shown that the proliferative potential of cells in culture correlates inversely with the age of the donor in a range of normal human tissues. Hence cell senescence may be implicated in the pathogenesis of the normal ageing process. Possibly the accumulation of senescent cells contributes to the development of age-related disease.

Senescence is associated with a wide range of changes within both the cytoplasm and nucleus of the cell. Studies using fibroblasts have shown an increase in cell size as well as an increase in nuclear size. Lysosomes become enlarged with increased lysosomal enzyme activity. Although the mitochondrial mass increases, respiratory efficiency decreases. The cellular cytoskeleton becomes more rigid and there is irreversible growth arrest. Whilst the kinetics of senescence appears to vary between cell types, any stress that triggers a cell population to proliferate has been shown to alter the proportion of growing and senescent cells.

There are two main theories of senescence.

1. The random error hypothesis explains senescence as the passive accumulation of damage to cellular constituents.

2. Programmed senescence regards ageing as an active predetermined process related to the decrease in chromosomal telomeres.

This latter theory has increasingly been accepted as the probable mechanism of senescence.

The limited lifespan of human somatic cells is associated with the steady loss of nucleotides from the telomeres at the end of each chromosome. Telomeres are a sequence of six nucleotides, TTAGGG, that are repeated from a few hundred to a thousand times. They enable the replication of the ends of the chromosomes and are thought to be essential in maintaining chromosomal integrity by preventing exonuclease activity. With each cell division there is a loss of telomeres and in human diseases where there is premature ageing, such as ataxia-telangiectasia and Down's syndrome, there appears to be an increase in the rate of telomere shortening. This eventually results in damage and loss of chromosomes, enabling the development of senescence and eventual cell death.

The lifespan of the cell appears to depend upon the original length of the telomere balanced against the number of cell divisions. Germ cells possess a telomerase enzyme that is capable of synthesising DNA by reverse transcriptase. This enables the maintenance of the original length of the telomeres and so enables them to divide continuously. Malignant cells also contain this enzyme which is thought to be associated with the immortality of malignant cells.

FURTHER READING

1   Cotran RS, Kumar V, Collins T. *Robbins' Pathologic Basis of Disease*, 6th edn. Philadelphia: WB Saunders, 1999

2   Faragher RGA, Lipling D. Detection and significance of senescent cells in tissue. In: Lowe DG, Underwood JCE, eds. *Recent Advances in Histopathology*. Edinburgh: Churchill Livingstone, 1999: 173

3   Lewin B. *Genes V*. Oxford: Oxford University Press, 1994

4   Rubin E, Farber JL. Cell injury. In: Rubin E, Farber JL, eds. *Pathology*, 3rd edn. Philadelphia: Lippincott-Raven, 1999: 1, 154

20

Handling of specimens

General rules for biopsy procedures
Frozen sections
  Uses
  Disadvantages
Fixation and transport
  Fixatives
  Volume
  Container
  Speed of fixation
Aspiration cytology
  Uses
  Methods

Advantages
Disadvantages
Complications
Exfoliative cytology
Microbiological specimens
  Pus, swabs, exudate and tissue
  Sputum
  Blood
  Urine

Hannah Monaghan

GENERAL RULES FOR BIOPSY PROCEDURES

1. It is essential that the patient's name, date of birth, his/her ward or department and consultant are identified. Otherwise the results may go astray. Likewise the requesting doctor must be identified so that they can be contacted for further information and urgent results.

2. It is also essential that a comprehensive clinical history be submitted with each specimen. The content must depend ultimately on judgement in the individual case but apparently unrelated facts may prove of significance. The more obvious aspects such as previous diagnosis of malignancy, previous radiotherapy and/or radiomimetic chemotherapy, drug history, serological findings and associated diseases should be provided.

3. In a large lesion, multiple biopsies are desirable in order to assess variation throughout the lesion. Also clips or stitches should be attached to aid orientation of the specimen when specific resection margins need to be assessed, e.g. breast lumps.

4. By definition, assessment of depth of invasion requires receipt of subepithelial tissues, e.g. in staging an invasive carcinoma.

5. In ulcerated lesions, the more informative tissue is likely to derive from the edges of the lesion. Samples from the ulcerated, junctional and apparently normal tissues are preferable. All specimens should be submitted for examination.

6. Unless arrangements for frozen section examination have been made, the specimen should be placed in fixative with as little delay and interference as possible.

7. Several methods of obtaining tissue are available: endoscope, laser, etc. The latter produces the least satisfactory result due to heat damage and distortion of tissue and consequent lack of cellular detail and imperfect staining.

FROZEN SECTIONS

The only benefit of frozen sections is speed. Hence their use should be restricted to intraoperative decisions, the result of the frozen section determining management. Techniques used include liquid nitrogen, CO, shows, and heat exchange plate.

Uses

- The examination of lymph nodes for metastatic spread of carcinoma. If positive, the chance of curative surgery is reduced and this may limit the extent of surgery.

- The identification of liver metastases. In a Whipple's procedure, if positive, this would negate cure and hence a more limited palliative procedure would be undertaken.

- The identification of an unexpected finding at surgery, e.g. a localised lesion in the omentum during abdominal surgery. This may simulate malignancy but in fact be caused by an inflammatory reaction, e.g. to foreign material (following previous surgery), fat necrosis, etc. All these lesions will look macroscopically like pale nodules mimicking tumour.

- The assessment of adequacy of excision, e.g. examination of resection margins in a tumour of the larynx. It would clearly be unwise for the surgeon to attempt reconstruction of tissue which involves residual tumour or dysplasia at the margins.

- The identification of a parathyroid adenoma which, when removed, will cure the patient's hyperparathyroidism and hypercalcaemia.

- The diagnosis of a localised swelling in the thyroid gland. If this is a neoplasm, its nature (benign or malignant) and if malignant, type of carcinoma (papillary or follicular) will determine the nature of the appropriate surgery.

- Distinction of benign from malignant breast lesions.

Disadvantages

- Selection of representative area. In a large lesion only one or two small areas can be examined and these may not be representative.

- The cytological features are slightly different from those of a paraffin section and the interpretation of these features may prove difficult and preclude a definite diagnosis being offered, e.g. lymphoma. If possible, some tissue should be reserved in formalin and paraffin section in addition to the requirement to process the actual frozen section specimen.

- Malorientation, e.g. skin lesions. This may prevent accurate assessment of depth of the lesion.

- Technical difficulty, e.g. adipose tissue, bone.

- Infective risk, e.g. TB, hepatitis B or C, HIV, etc.

FIXATION AND TRANSPORT

Sometimes it is better to receive tissues in an unfixed state, e.g. for inflation of lung tissue in order to recreate the lung spaces, rendering the tissue nearer to its functioning state prior to its removal from the body.

Some immunohistochemical and histochemical methods are technically easier and more accurate when performed on unfixed tissue. This relates to the glycogen content of cells as revealed by PAS staining and the expression of CD molecules on certain lymphocytes, especially those of the T series. Also receptor profile/concentration, cytogenetics, e.g. on a Ewing's tumour, cell culture and microbiological culture can be performed on unfixed tissue. However, if a clinician is faced with the choice of delayed fixation with a prolonged period prior to freezing or immediate fixation, the latter should be chosen since most histochemical and immunohistochemical methods can be performed on fixed tissue.

Fixation can be carried out at room temperature. Tissue should not be frozen once it has been placed in the fixative solution, as ice crystal distortion will occur.

Fixatives

1. 10% buffered formalin (best).
   - Cheap.
   - Compatible with special stains.
   - Tissue can stay in it for long periods without deteriorating.
   - Shrinkage of tissue is minimal.
   - Preservation is satisfactory without refrigeration.

2. Zenker's fixative.
   - Expensive.
   - Contains mercury and therefore needs careful disposal.
   - Care with fixation times and washing procedures to remove mercury precipitates.

3. Bouins' fixative.
   - Desirable for testicular biopsies.

4. Carnoy's fixative.
   - This mixture contains chloroform so whilst it fixes tissues, it dissolves most of the fat, which is useful in the identification of lymph nodes in radical dissection specimens.

5. Universal fixative.
   - Suitable for both light and electron microscopy examination.
   - 4% commercial paraformaldehyde and 1% glutaraldehyde in a neutral buffer.

Volume

Ten times the volume of the tissue.

Container

This should have an opening large enough to allow tissue to be removed easily after hardening with fixative. The fixative should surround the specimen on all sides, e.g. the top of a specimen should be covered with absorbent material if exposed. Likewise, if the bottom of the container is in close contact with the specimen then absorbent material should be placed between the specimen and the container wall.

Speed of fixation

Approximately 1 mm/hour so a fixation time of several hours is needed for most specimens. This can be speeded up by the use of a commercial microwave oven (this induces an almost instantaneous fixation by controlled heating at 63–65°C) or by fixing the specimen in a large beaker containing fixative kept at 60°C and in continuous motion by the action of a heater-rotor.

ASPIRATION CYTOLOGY

Uses

A variety of materials may be subject to cytological examination: fluids, surface scrapings, endoscopic washings and brushings and material obtained by fine needle aspiration (FNA).

FNA has been particularly useful in the management of the following diseases.

Breast lumps

Fine needle aspiration cytology has a sensitivity of 87% and specificity and a positive predictive value of almost 100%. This has transformed the management of breast lumps. Breast aspirates are given one of the following scores which, along with the clinical and radiological scores, allow definitive management to be determined prior to surgery.

C1 Inadequate/insufficient cellular material
C2 Definitely benign
C3 Atypical, probably benign
C4 Atypical, probably malignant
C5 Definitely malignant

This technique avoids the need for immediate and sometimes stressful intraoperative decisions based on frozen section assessment.

Solitary thyroid nodules

Aspiration cytology is also used extensively in the preoperative assessment of solitary thyroid nodules. Published results claim a sensitivity and specificity of over 90% and most papillary carcinomas and other types of malignancy can be identified with ease. The main difficulty lies in the differentiation between a minimally invasive follicular carcinoma and a follicular adenoma, as the diagnosis is dependent upon capsular and vascular invasion. Most thyroid aspirates are described in one of the following three ways.

1. Probably benign nodule, when the material is composed largely of colloid, histiocytes and a few normal-looking follicular cells. This will be an indication for a conservative approach unless the clinical data suggest otherwise.

2. Follicular neoplasm, when cellularity is higher than that found in the usual hyperplastic nodule but the nuclear features of papillary carcinoma are absent. The diagnosis of Hurthle cell neoplasm usually falls into this category. The presence of highly hyperchromatic nuclei, microfollicular or solid pattern, scanty colloid and necrotic debris suggests a follicular carci-

noma. The diagnosis of follicular neoplasm is an indication for removal of the lobe containing the nodule unless this is contraindicated for medical reasons.

3. Papillary carcinoma, when the characteristic cytoarchitectural features of this tumour type are present, such as straight-edged sheets of cells, nuclear grooves, nuclear pseudoinclusions and, rarely, psammoma bodies (see Figures 20.1 and 20.2). It should be remembered that the optically clear nuclei seen on histological examination are usually not apparent in cytological preparations even when prominent in the tissue sections from the same case, that nuclear pseudoinclusions are not pathognomonic of papillary carcinoma and that cystic degeneration of the tumour may obscure the cell details. In both the classic and follicular variants of this tumour, the colloid often exhibits a peculiar streaking and smearing effect that has been compared with that of bubble gum. The cytological diagnosis of papillary carcinoma is obviously an

indication for therapeutic intervention, normally total thyroidectomy, even if the occasional surgical specimen may show only a papillary *micro*carcinoma (i.e. a lesion for which the need for surgery is debatable).

Various types of thyroiditis can also be identified. Needle aspirate is particularly helpful in the diagnosis of Hashimoto's thyroiditis, when the classic serological changes are not seen or a coexistent neoplasm or progression to lymphoma is suspected. The diagnosis is made by the presence of numerous cytologically reactive lymphoid cells, plasma cells, Hurthle cells and dense colloid.

Head and neck lumps

FNA is of value in the diagnosis and staging of head and neck cancer. It is of dubious value in young adults with lymphadenopathy where lymphoma is considered.

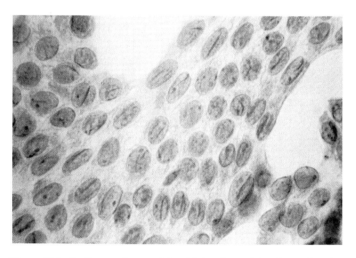

Figure 20.1 Papillary carcinoma of thyroid showing straight edges and nuclear grooves. Pap ×40.

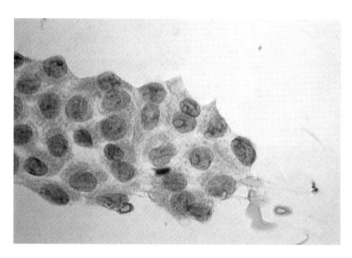

Figure 20.2 Papillary carcinoma of thyroid showing intranuclear pseudoinclusions. Pap ×40.

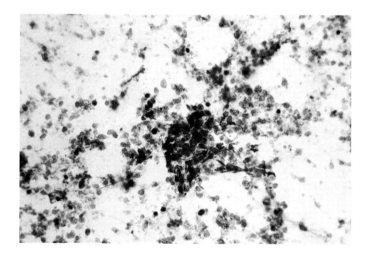

Figure 20.3 Transthoracic FNA of lung lesion showing small cell carcinoma. Pap ×20.

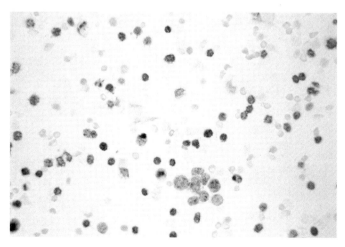

Figure 20.4 Immunohistochemistry on the aspirate showing dot positivity of small cells for cytokeratin. ×20.

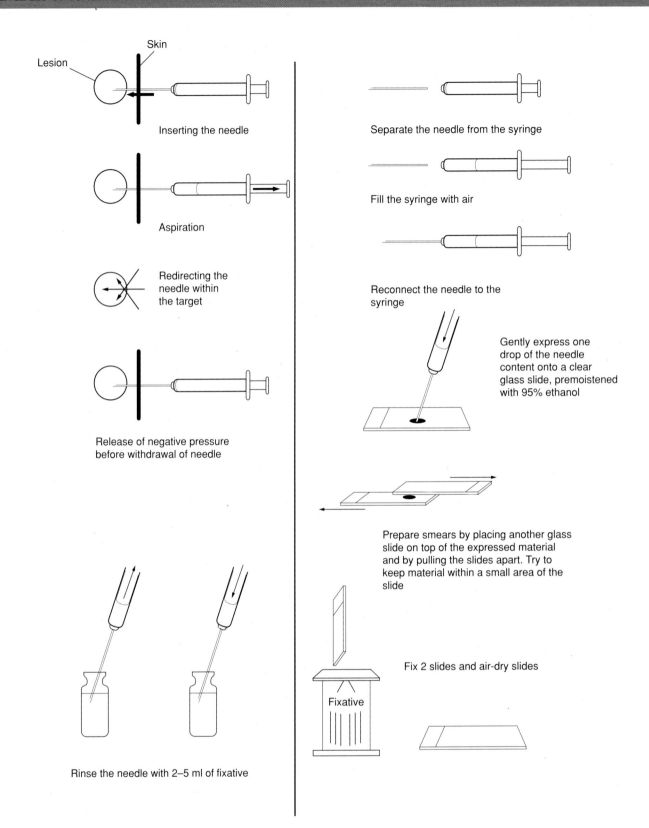

Inserting the needle

Aspiration

Redirecting the needle within the target

Release of negative pressure before withdrawal of needle

Rinse the needle with 2–5 ml of fixative

Separate the needle from the syringe

Fill the syringe with air

Reconnect the needle to the syringe

Gently express one drop of the needle content onto a clear glass slide, premoistened with 95% ethanol

Prepare smears by placing another glass slide on top of the expressed material and by pulling the slides apart. Try to keep material within a small area of the slide

Fixative

Fix 2 slides and air-dry slides

Figure 20.5 Method of fine needle aspiration of a palpable lump.

Respiratory tract cytology

Recent developments in sampling techniques have changed the practice of respiratory tract cytology. Radiological imaging allows FNA sampling of lesions at virtually any site within the thorax and has improved the safety of these procedures. Material is obtained through either the transbronchial or transthoracic approach. The former is useful in the sampling of lesions extrinsic to the bronchus or where surface necrosis would prevent accurate direct sampling. The latter technique is particularly useful in the investigation of lesions that are out of reach of the bronchoscope (see Figures 20.3 and 20.4).

Methods

The aspirated sample is smeared onto slides using a blood film technique or with more pressure if solid particles are present. Some slides should be air-dried for MGG staining and others fixed in alcohol for the Papanicolaou stain. Spare material obtained by rinsing the needle in normal saline or tissue culture medium can be processed as a cell block or made into cytospin preparations for other stains and for immunocytochemistry (see Figure 20.5). Electron microscopy, tumour proliferation studies and cytogenetic analysis are among the additional procedures that can be performed on FNA material.

Advantages

- Quick.
- Cheap.
- Can be carried out in outpatients setting.
- Risk of complications is minimal.

Disadvantages

- Palpable masses. FNA is contraindicated in the case of carotid body tumours, malignant melanoma (subsequent distortion of Breslow thickness assessment), lymphoma (the diagnosis may be possible but not the architectural assessment required for classification) and the necrotic centre of tumours which would provide unsuitable material.

- Non-palpable masses (image detected). Any cystic lesion on the capsule of the liver should be treated with caution as both hepatocellular carcinoma and haemangiomata may bleed. Phaeochromocytomas may release catecholamines on aspiration.

- Unhelpful when differentiation between benign and malignant depends on capsular status or vascular invasion, e.g. follicular neoplasms in thyroid gland.

Complications

- Bleeding (the procedure is relatively contraindicated in patients with a bleeding diathesis).
- Nerve injury.
- Tracheal perforation (thyroid aspiration)
- Tumour implantation, e.g. mesothelioma, pleomorphic salivary adenoma. In fact, this is a rare occurrence and obtaining a diagnosis outweighs the risk of implantation.
- Pneumothorax (lung aspirates).

Exfoliative cytology

Exfoliative cytology is the examination of cells that naturally exfoliate and therefore this can be applied to any organ where this occurs. However, the majority of specimens examined are from the cervix or sputum or urine.

Cytological examination of urine sediment is a simple diagnostic procedure which can reveal evidence of disease anywhere in the urinary tract from the kidneys, ureters and bladder to the urethra and its related structures. This is used as a first-line investigation in patients presenting with haematuria, suspected urinary tract neoplasia and acute interstitial nephritis.

MICROBIOLOGICAL SPECIMENS

A good specimen should be truly representative of the site of infection and be sent in the correct container, arrive in the laboratory promptly or, if delayed, be stored under proper conditions and be accompanied by sufficient relevant clinical detail and patient information to enable the laboratory to process, interpret and return results to the correct ward or doctor.

Pus, swabs, exudate and tissue

Swabs are probably the most common specimens taken from sites of infection or colonisation. It may be necessary to moisten the swab with a little sterile water before use. When possible, the swab should be sent to the laboratory in transport medium. This is designed to improve bacterial survival without encouraging too much growth.

Swabs are not indicated in the following situations:

1. When there is a large amount of pus it is better to take a good sample of fluid rather than dip the swab into the collection as a larger sample may detect organisms present in only small numbers and some rapid diagnostic techniques require a larger volume of fluid.

2. When there is a discharging sinus or any lesion which requires removal of superficial tissue and deep probing is necessary.

Superficial swabs will often fail to detect the relevant pathogen and may provide misleading results.

Sputum

If the patient is on a ventilator a trap specimen of bronchial secretions is a good solution. A sputum sample obtained with the help of the physiotherapist is likely to be of reasonable quality. However, the majority of sputum samples taken by non-invasive means are often only saliva. If the patient is already on antibiotics saliva samples will grow resistant Gram-negative bacilli and as such are rarely significant.

Blood

The patient's skin should be disinfected with alcohol. If a needle and syringe are used, the needle should be changed before blood is put into the bottle. Contamination with skin organisms resulting from poor technique is the biggest problem in blood cultures.

Urine

Urine is the most common specimen sent to the laboratory. Midstream urine (MSU) samples and catheter specimens of urine (CSU) samples are the norm. Too many urine samples are sent as a matter of routine without clinical indication, simply because it is an easy sample to obtain.

Urine is a good bacterial growth medium. With MSU samples the definition of infection depends on the number of bacteria/ml ($>10^5$). Contaminating organisms derived from the periurethral area can easily multiply to this level within a few hours. Therefore urine samples which cannot be sent immediately should be kept at 4°C.

FURTHER READING

1   Bell DA, Hajdu SI, Urban JA, Gaston JP. Role of aspiration cytology in the diagnosis and management of mammary lesions in office practice. *Cancer* 1983; **51**: 1182–1189

2   Frable WJ. Needle aspiration of the breast. *Cancer* 1984; **53**: 671–676

3   Grant CS, Goellner JR, Welch JS, Martin JK. Fine needle aspiration of the breast. *Mayo Clin Proc* 1986; **61**: 377–381

4   Åkerman M, Tennvall J, Biörklund A, Märtensson H, Möller T. Sensitivity and specificity of fine needle aspiration cytology in the diagnosis of tumours of the thyroid gland. *Acta Cytol* (Baltimore) 1985; **29**: 850–855

5   Caraway NP, Sneige N, Samaan NA. Diagnostic pitfalls in fine-needle aspiration. A review of 394 cases. *Diagn Cytopathol* 1993; **9**: 345–350

6   Murthy P, Laing MR, Palmer TJ. Fine needle aspiration cytology of head and neck lesions: an early experience. *Roy Coll Surg Edinb* 1997; **42**: 341–346

21

Cell damage and response to injury

Cell injury
  Reversible cell injury
  Irreversible cell injury
Acute inflammation
  Vascular changes and the formation of fluid
    exudate
  Functions of the fluid exudate
  Cellular accumulation
  Leucocyte migration
  Phagocytosis
  Types of exudate
  Outcomes of acute inflammation
Chemical mediators of inflammation
  Histamine
  The complement system

Kinins
Arachidonic acid metabolites (eicosanoids)
Platelet-activating factor
Nitric oxide
Interleukins and TNF
Chronic inflammation
  The macrophage
  Chronic granulomatous inflammation
  Autoimmune disease
  Abscess formation
Healing
  Healing of a skin wound
  Factors delaying healing

Mark E.F. Smith

CELL INJURY

A wide variety of agents can damage the body's cells including hypoxia, ischaemia, infections, immunological damage, genetic defects and physical agents such as chemicals, drugs, heat or cold. Minor damage results in reversible cell injury whereas more severe damage leads to irreversible cell injury with inevitable cell death.

Reversible cell injury

Cellular insults such as hypoxia readily cause a failure in the cell's energy-making machinery with a resultant decrease in intracellular ATP levels. The cell's sodium pump, which ordinarily pumps sodium ions from an intracellular to an extracellular compartment in exchange for potassium ions, is ATP dependent. Pump failure causes the intracellular accumulation of sodium ions which, with hydration shells larger than those of potassium ions, results in cell swelling, a change which is potentially reversible. (Note: when an ion enters water, water molecules orient themselves around it, forming a hydration shell.)

Fatty change is a further morphological expression of potentially reversible cell damage that is commonly seen in hepatocytes because of their important role in fat metabolism. It may be the consequence of a great variety of insults, principally toxic and metabolic ones. Toxins damage enzymic activity and protein malnutrition results in reduced apoprotein production; these changes inhibit lipoprotein secretion from hepatocytes. Consequently reduced complexing of apoprotein with triglyceride results in fat accumulation within intracytoplasmic vacuoles (Figure 21.1).

Without cell death and inflammation, this reversible change will not jeopardise hepatic structure or function. However, cell death and inflammation, for example as in alcoholic hepatitis, will constitute a risk factor in the progression to cirrhosis.

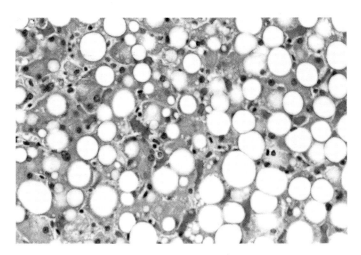

Figure 21.1 Fatty change. Hepatocytes contain large clear fat vacuoles.

Irreversible cell injury

Cell death secondary to irreversible cell injury occurs by one of two mechanisms: necrosis or apoptosis. Necrosis usually results from exogenous damage (e.g. ischaemia) and is characterised by an area of cell death (rather than that of single cells). Necrosis is non-energy dependent and associated with enzymatic cellular digestion and protein denaturation, either of which may be dominant (see coagulative and liquefactive necrosis below). The digestive enzymes are released from lysosomes. Necrosis is associated with characteristic nuclear abnormalities:

- pyknosis (where the nucleus condenses into a shrunken, basophilic mass)

- karyorrhexis (characterised by nuclear fragmentation)

- karyolysis (where the staining of the nucleus fades, a change presumably resulting from DNAase activity).

Necrosis is termed coagulative when the tissue retains substantial structure due to the dominance of the denaturation process. Coagulative necrosis is seen in the infarcts of many organs such as those of the heart and kidney (but not the brain). In liquefactive necrosis tissues are converted into a structureless liquid mass. This form of necrosis is seen where enzymatic digestion is dominant and where the connective tissue support is minimal, particularly in brain infarcts, and in bacterial and fungal infections where the enzymes of the associated inflammatory cells aid the digestive process (e.g. an abscess).

Apoptosis is an energy-dependent form of cell death usually involving individual cells or small groups of cells. It is important in:

- embryogenesis (allowing the resorption of tissues such as the webs between digits)

- normal physiology (e.g. regression of the lactating breast after weaning)

- many pathological states (e.g. the death of tumour cells, cell death induced by viruses or resulting from cytotoxic T cell attack).

In contrast to necrotic cells, apoptotic cells decrease in size through cytoplasmic shrinkage. Ultrastructural examination demonstrates that the structure of their organelles is retained. Peripheral nuclear chromatin condensation is characteristic and may be followed by nuclear fragmentation. Subsequently, apoptotic cells fragment into several membrane-bound bodies which are phagocytosed by adjacent cells. Unlike necrosis, apoptosis does not elicit an inflammatory response. Biochemical changes underlying the structural changes of apoptosis outlined above have been described. The activation of calcium-dependent proteases results in the destruction of nuclear scaffold and cytoskeletal proteins and the triggering of endonucleases which cleave the nuclear DNA.

ACUTE INFLAMMATION

Tissues react to many different types of damage by a stereo-typed response of their microvasculature resulting in acute inflammation. In acute inflammation vascular permeability increases, resulting in the loss of fluid and cells from blood vessels to enter the extravascular interstitial space where they form the fluid and cellular components of the inflammatory exudate. Acute inflammation is accompanied by characteristic clinical signs and symptoms that were described by Celsus in ancient times:

- rubor (redness due to vessel dilatation)

- calor (heat due to increased blood flow)

- tumor (swelling due to the accumulation of the inflammatory exudate)

- dolor (pain).

Though the acute inflammatory response is nearly always beneficial in limiting tissue injury it may occasionally be harmful, as in the swelling it may cause in confined spaces (e.g. an intracranial abscess) or in the obstruction of vital structures such as the airways (e.g. in acute epiglottitis) or perforation of an inflamed viscus, e.g. perforated diverticular abscess.

Vascular changes and the formation of the fluid exudate

Tissue damage is associated with a brief phase of arteriolar vaso-constriction followed by persistent vessel dilatation.

The relaxation of precapillary arteriolar sphincters massively increases the size of the perfused capillary bed. Blood flow within the bed is initially rapid and capillary hydrostatic pressure rises with a consequent increase in solute flow through the capillary walls.

Under the influence of inflammatory mediators such as histamine, platelet-activating factor and leukotrienes, the tight junctions between endothelial cells of postcapillary venules retract, allowing the passage of macromolecules such as plasma proteins into the interstitium. The rise in interstitial osmotic pressure associated with the increased protein content results in the withdrawal of still further fluid from the vascular compartment.

The net effect of these vascular changes is the formation of an interstitial protein-rich exudate. If local damage to blood vessels is very severe (e.g. through toxins, burns or infections) the normal structure and function of all types of vessels may be compromised by direct damage and they may leak in an uncontrolled manner.

Loss of fluid from the vessels in inflammation causes an increase in plasma viscosity, a change which results in the slowing of blood flow. Thus, initially rapid blood flow in acute inflammation gives way to stasis.

Functions of the fluid exudate

The fluid exudate serves to limit cell injury. It dilutes toxins and harmful chemicals and allows immunoglobulins, complement components and antibiotics, all of which have antibacterial properties, access to extravascular sites.

Tissue thromboplastin activates the coagulation pathway, converting plasma fibrinogen to insoluble fibrin. Fibrin may limit the spread of bacteria and aid their removal by phagocytes.

Activation of many plasma enzyme cascades in the interstitium leads to the formation and/or release of inflammatory mediators such as complement components and kinins whose actions maintain the inflammatory focus.

Factor XII of the coagulation pathway, the Hageman factor, has a key role in the activation of several plasma enzyme cascades important in the maintenance and development of an acute inflammatory focus. Hageman factor is activated by diverse stimuli such as exposure to basement membrane components, proteolytic enzymes, bacterial lipopolysaccharide and foreign material. Factor XII activates the fibrinolytic system converting plasminogen to the active enzyme plasmin, so fibrin degradation, a process important in the eventual resolution of an inflammatory focus, starts early in the course of acute inflammation. Plasmin activity also leads to the release of the activated complement components C3a and C5a, both of which are chemical mediators of inflammation. Factor XII also activates the kinin system resulting in the production of the inflammatory mediator, bradykinin.

Cellular accumulation

In inflammatory reactions phagocytic inflammatory cells accumulate in the damaged area. Initially, the neutrophil polymorph is the dominant cell type. Later, macrophages become more prominent. Figure 21.2 shows a prominent cellular exudate filling alveolar spaces in a lobar pneumonia. Both neutrophils and

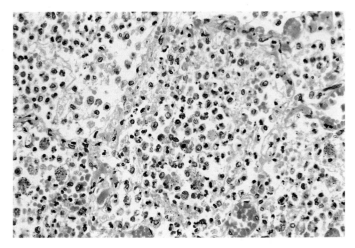

Figure 21.2 Lobar pneumonia. The alveoli are filled with a dense cellular exudate.

macrophages participate in the phagocytosis of foreign material such as microorganisms and debris.

Leucocyte migration

In acute inflammation migration of leucocytes out of blood vessels occurs through the walls of postcapillary venules.

Normally, blood cells are confined to the centre of vessels, avoiding contact with endothelial cells, a feature known as axial flow. In the stasis of acute inflammation, however, leucocytes make contact with endothelial cells. Initial contacts are weak and are mediated between selectin molecules (P- and E-selectins) expressed at high levels on the activated endothelium of an inflammatory focus and sialyl-Lewis X components expressed on the surface membranes of blood leucocytes. These weak interactions limit leucocyte movement to a rolling motion along the endothelial surface.

In the vicinity of activated endothelium, leucocytes are exposed to inflammatory mediators which activate them. Leucocyte activation is associated with conformational changes in their LFA-1 integrin molecules which increases this molecule's avidity for its endothelial receptor, ICAM-1. The inflammatory milieu also results in increased expression of endothelial ICAM-1. Tight binding between endothelial ICAM-1 and activated leucocyte LFA-1 brings leucocyte movement to a halt. The binding of blood leucocytes to endothelium is known as margination.

Leucocytes subsequently migrate between adjacent endothelial cells, temporarily breaking interendothelial bonds such as those mediated between CD31 on adjacent endothelial cells and penetrating the endothelial basement membrane to gain the extravascular interstitial space where their phagocytic role may be fulfilled. This activity occurs in the venules of the systemic vasculature and the capillaries of the lung. Unopposed inappropriate activation contributes to the structural and functional damage of 'shock lung'. Leucocyte migration is controlled by chemotaxins which include bacterial products and inflammatory mediators such as leucotriene B_4 and the C5a complement component. Chemotaxis is defined as the unidirectional movement of cells up a concentration gradient of chemotactic molecules.

Phagocytosis

The immune system of the body produces immunoglobulin molecules which bind foreign antigens such as those of bacteria. This bacterial/immunoglobulin interaction leads to the activation of the complement system. The end result is that bacteria become coated with opsonins such as immunoglobulin and C3b molecules, promoting their phagocytosis through the binding of the opsonins to specific surface receptors present on macrophages and neutrophil polymorphs.

Recognition is rapidly followed by engulfment and the creation of an internal membrane-bound phagocytic vacuole which subsequently fuses with lysosomal granules to form a phagolysosome.

Killing of phagocytosed bacteria is achieved mostly by reactive oxygen metabolites whose production is associated with a sudden increase in oxygen consumption, the respiratory burst. The activation of NADPH oxidase leads to the formation of the superoxide anion (O_2^-) within the phagolysosome. The superoxide anion is subsequently converted to hydrogen peroxide (H_2O_2). Following the fusion of a neutrophil polymorph's specific granules with the phagolysosome, the enzyme myeloperoxidase, in the presence of chloride ions, catalyses the formation of the potent antibacterial product hypochlorous acid (HOCl) from the hydrogen peroxide.

Bacterial killing can also be achieved by oxygen-independent mechanisms. For example, the enzyme lysozyme hydrolyses the muramic acid–N-acetyl-glucosamine bond present in bacterial cell walls.

Types of exudate

Acute inflammatory exudates are variable in nature. They may be:

● serous (with much protein but little fibrin and few cells)

● fibrinous (with much fibrin) (Figure 21.3)

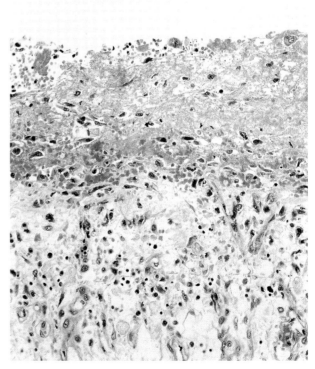

Figure 21.3 Fibrinous exudate. The serosal surface is covered with a thick layer of eosinophilic (pink) fibrin (H&E).

● purulent (with very large numbers of neutrophil polymorphs).

Though the presence of neutrophil polymorphs is characteristic of most acute inflammatory exudates, in rare circumstances, such as viral infections like acute viral hepatitis, the lymphocyte, a cell type more typical of chronic inflammation, may predominate. Eosinophils may be prominent in the cellular reactions to parasite infestations or to certain antigens, e.g. drugs where an allergic element operates.

Outcomes of acute inflammation

Several different outcomes to acute inflammation are possible (Box 21.1). The most satisfactory is its complete resolution with the restoration of the tissues to their previous normal state. This occurs following removal of the inflammatory stimulus and the digestion and removal of inflammatory debris by the fibrinolytic system and by neutrophil and macrophage phagocytes.

Box 21.1 Outcomes of acute inflammation

Resolution, with elimination of stimulus
Fibrosis, with or without elimination of stimulus
Abscess formation, without elimination of stimulus
Chronic inflammation, with or without elimination of stimulus

---

Alternatively, following an acute inflammatory reaction, the acute exudate may be organised by granulation tissue, resulting in fibrosis. This is especially likely if fibrin is prominent in the exudates or the injurious agent is persistent.

Acute inflammation caused by pyogenic bacteria may result in the formation of an abscess, a focus of suppurative necrosis where the lytic enzymes from disintegrating neutrophils in pus cause localised liquefactive tissue necrosis. If they are not drained, abscesses tend to persist due to their poor vascularisation. They are discussed at greater length in the section on chronic inflammation below.

If the body fails to eradicate the agent causing acute inflammation, damage will persist and be associated with prolonged (chronic) inflammation which is associated with attempts to heal, usually in the form of fibrosis.

CHEMICAL MEDIATORS OF INFLAMMATION

Chemical mediators of inflammation are the chemicals whose formation and release lead to the creation of an inflammatory focus (Table 21.1). They are derived either from plasma (usually subsequent to the synthesis of an inactive precursor molecule by the liver) or from cells. The active plasma-derived mediators usually form following proteolytic cleavage at the inflammatory focus. Cell-derived mediators are either stored within granules (e.g. histamine within mast cell and basophil granules) and released when required or are generated *de novo* at the inflammatory site (e.g. prostaglandins). Some of the different groups of mediators are discussed below (see also Table 21.1). Complex mechanisms of inhibition exist to regulate and limit the action of many of the inflammatory mediators.

Histamine

The vasoactive amine histamine is important in initiating inflammation because its storage in the granules of mast cells, basophils and platelets allows its rapid release to the extracellular environment following an appropriate stimulus. Mast cell degranulation may result from a wide variety of stimuli, such as:

● physical injury including trauma, heat and cold

● immune reactions including:
  – the crosslinking with specific antigen of IgE bound to mast cells by their Fc receptors
  – the action of complement anaphylotoxins C3a and C5a and of
  – the cytokines IL-1 and IL-8.

Histamine increases the permeability of postcapillary venules.

Table 21.1 Chemical mediators of inflammation

Mediator	Source	Increased vascular permeability	Leucocyte chemotaxis
Histamine	Mast cells, basophils, platelets	+	–
Bradykinin	Plasma substrate	+	–
C3a	Plasma substrate	+	–
C5a	Plasma substrate	+	+
Leukotriene B$_4$	Leucocytes	–	+
PAF	Leucocytes	+	+
IL-1, TNF	Macrophages	–	+

The complement system

The complement system is a series of 20 plasma proteins that have diverse important functions in the immune response and in inflammation following their proteolytic activation. The critical step in complement activation is the activation of its third component, C3, which may occur via:

- the classic pathway (following the binding of C1 to IgG or IgM that is bound to antigen)

- the alternative pathway which may be activated by a variety of stimuli including exposure to endotoxin.

The end result of complement activation is the formation of a membrane attack complex (C5 through C9) which lyses the cell or microbe on which it is deposited. When C3b is deposited on bacteria following complement activation it acts as an opsonin, increasing the likelihood of bacterial phagocytosis. Activated soluble complement components are also released such as the anaphylotoxins C3a and C5a, which increase vascular permeability both directly and through the induction of histamine release by mast cells. C5a is also a powerful chemotactic agent for neutrophils and monocytes.

Kinins

Activated Hageman factor (factor XII of the intrinsic coagulation system) converts plasma prekallikrein into the active enzyme kallikrein, which in turn cleaves the vasoactive nonapeptide bradykinin from the precursor plasma protein, kininogen. Bradykinin increases vascular permeability. It has a short half-life, being inactivated by kininase.

Arachidonic acid metabolites (eicosanoids)

The eicosanoids, metabolites of arachidonic acid (a 20-carbon polyunsaturated fatty acid), are generated within cells by the actions of two major classes of enzymes:

- the cyclooxygenases which produce prostaglandins and thromboxanes

- lipoxygenases which produce leukotrienes and lipoxins.
The eicosanoids participate in virtually all the components of inflammation. For example, PGI_2 (prostacyclin) is a potent vasodilator and leukotriene B_4 is a potent chemotaxin. The efficacy of cyclooxygenase inhibitors such as aspirin and non-steroidal antiinflammatory drugs in reducing the pain and fever associated with inflammation demonstrates the participation of prostaglandins in these processes.

Platelet-activating factor

PAF is a phospholipid-derived inflammatory mediator that can be produced by many cell types including platelets, basophils, mast cells, neutrophils, monocytes/macrophages and endothelial cells. In addition to platelet activation, PAF participates at many stages in the acute inflammatory response, increasing vascular permeability, leucocyte adhesion and chemotaxis.

Nitric oxide

Nitric oxide (NO) is a soluble gas produced by endothelial cells, macrophages and a subset of neurones through the action of the enzyme nitric oxide synthase (NOS). There are three different types of NOS:

- endothelial (eNOS)

- neuronal (nNOS)

- cytokine inducible (iNOS).

Inducible NOS is expressed by macrophages following their activation with cytokines such as gamma interferon and TNF-alpha. NO has a very short half-life and is active only in the immediate vicinity of the cells which produce it (paracrine effect). NO causes vasodilatation through the relaxation of vascular smooth muscle. Also, overproduction of NO by iNOS reduces leucocyte recruitment in inflammation and acts, therefore, as a counterbalance to the many other inflammatory mediators causing leucocyte recruitment. NO has antimicrobial activity.

Interleukin-1 and tumour necrosis factor

Activated macrophages produce abundant IL-1 and TNF-alpha. Activated T-lymphocytes produce TNF-beta (lymphotoxin). Their secretion is stimulated by:

- endotoxin

- immune complexes

- toxins

- physical injury.

They participate at many levels in the inflammatory and immune responses, including endothelial activation. Their involvement in fibroblast stimulation, increasing fibroblast proliferation and collagen synthesis, gives them an important role in chronic inflammation and healing. IL-1 and TNF also mediate the acute-phase responses associated with inflammation including pyrexia, neutrophilia, elevated corticosteroid levels and elevated acute-phase protein levels.

CHRONIC INFLAMMATION

Acute inflammation is, by definition, shortlived whereas chronic inflammation is prolonged, lasting often weeks, months or even years. Some examples of chronic inflammation represent progression from acute inflammation whereas others, such as granulomatous and autoimmune disease, usually arise insidiously with no clearcut acute inflammatory origin. Chronic inflammation is liable to occur when the body fails to eradicate a harmful agent. This might take the form of an infection, for example with mycobacteria or fungi, or it might result from the contamination of a wound with foreign material that may harbour infection. In autoimmune disease the body's own cells are the stimulus for the formation of a self-destructive and inappropriate immune response.

In all cases the hallmark of chronic inflammation is persistent inflammation in association with continued tissue destruction and attempts at healing, usually in the form of fibrosis.

The dominant inflammatory cell of chronic inflammation is the macrophage (see below). It is usually accompanied by lymphocytes and plasma cells. In parasitic infestations and allergic reactions, eosinophils are common. Although neutrophil polymorphs are the cell type characteristic of acute inflammation, they are frequently present, though usually in reduced numbers, in chronic inflammation. Chronic inflammation is said to be 'active' in their presence, for example in active chronic inflammatory bowel disease. Of course, in chronic suppurative (pus-forming) inflammation such as chronic suppurative osteomyelitis or in a chronic abscess, they are abundant.

The macrophage

The macrophage may be considered the dominant cell type of chronic inflammation, just as the neutrophil polymorph is the dominant cell type of acute inflammation. Macrophages are tissue cells derived from circulating monocytes which in turn take origin from the bone marrow. The half-life of blood monocytes is approximately one day whereas that of tissue macrophages is measured in months.

In acute inflammation monocyte migration from blood vessels into tissues follows that of neutrophil polymorphs. As is the case for neutrophils, monocyte migration is controlled by the interaction between leucocyte and endothelial adhesion molecules. Within tissues monocytes transform into macrophages which possess more abundant cytoplasm. If the causative agent inducing inflammation is not eradicated then chronic inflammation will ensue and, in some circumstances, macrophages become activated. Activation occurs in response to exposure to gamma-interferon (secreted by activated T lymphocytes), endotoxins and extracellular matrix components. It is particularly seen in chronic granulomatous inflammation such as occurs in tuberculosis where groups of activated macrophages form granulomas (see section on chronic granulomatous inflammation below). Activated macrophages have an increased cell size, a more active metabolism and higher levels of lysosomal enzymes and an increased capacity to phagocytose and kill microorganisms.

The activated macrophage may unfortunately damage adjacent normal tissues through its production and release of toxic sub-

stances such as oxygen metabolites and nitric oxide. It may also stimulate fibrosis through the release of peptide growth factors and cytokines such as platelet-derived growth factor (PDGF), fibroblast growth factors (FGFs), transforming growth factor beta (TGF-beta), interleukin-1 (IL-1) and tumour necrosis factors (TNFs).

Cytokines such as macrophage-inhibiting factor immobilise macrophages at the inflammatory focus.

Chronic granulomatous inflammation

Chronic granulomatous inflammation is characterised by the presence of granulomas which are defined as circumscribed collections of activated macrophages. They are of two types, foreign body granulomas and immune granulomas.

Foreign body granulomas form in an attempt to remove non-degradable material. This may be of exogenous origin (e.g. foreign material in a skin wound) or of endogenous origin (e.g. naked hair shafts in a pilonidal sinus). In attempts to engulf larger fragments, some adjacent macrophages fuse to form foreign body giant cells which have multiple and apparently randomly distributed nuclei within their cytoplasm.

Immune granulomas result from a cell-mediated immune response to poorly degradable antigenic material, often of infectious origin. Macrophages complex the processed antigen to self MHC class II antigens, allowing its presentation to T lymphocytes which become activated. Activated T lymphocytes produce interleukin-2, which activates further T lymphocytes, and gamma-interferon which transforms macrophages to an activated epithelioid phenotype. This type of activated macrophage is termed epithelioid because its abundant cytoplasm and apparent cohesion with adjacent macrophages simulates the appearance of epithelium. Granulomas with epithelioid macrophages and Langhans-type giant cells (whose nuclei are arranged at the periphery of the cell) are characteristic of immune-type granulomas (Figure 21.4). They are classically seen in chronic infections such as tuberculosis, syphilis, fungal infections and tuberculoid leprosy as well as diseases of uncertain aetiology such as sarcoidosis. The epithelioid granulomas of tuberculosis characteristically show central caseous necrosis.

Autoimmune disease

Autoimmune disease is a specific subtype of chronic inflammation that arises from a failure of immunological tolerance, allowing immunological attack directed against the body's own tissues. Speculative causes would include alteration of antigen structure by viral infection/integration. It may involve a single organ, as in Hashimoto's thyroiditis (Figure 21.5) or multiple organs as in systemic lupus erythematosus. As an example, in Hashimoto's thyroiditis cytotoxic T lymphocytes destroy thyroid epithelium which is replaced by repair fibrosis and dense chronic inflamma-

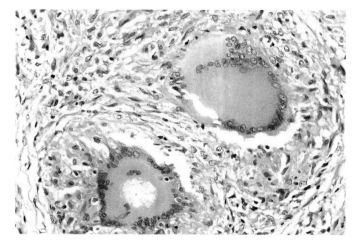

Figure 21.4 An immune granuloma. A circumscribed collection of epithelioid macrophages. Note the Langhans-type giant cells.

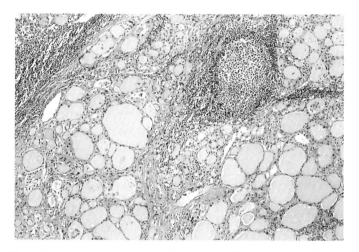

Figure 21.5 Hashimoto's thyroiditis. Thyroid epithelium is replaced by fibrosis. Chronic inflammatory cells (lymphocytes and plasma cells) are prominent.

tory cell infiltrates comprising lymphocytes and plasma cells. The loss of functioning thyroid epithelium causes hypothyroidism.

Abscess formation

An abscess is a focus of suppurative necrosis; in other words, it is an area of pus formation associated with liquefactive tissue necrosis. If abscesses are not drained surgically they have a tendency to become chronic due to the absence of a vascular supply at their centres. In a chronic abscess there is ineffectual healing at its vascular periphery in the form of a fibrotic capsule. Continued suppuration from the vascular periphery of an abscess leads to an increase in pressure within the abscess and this may lead to its rupture, with the extension of pus into surrounding tissues. Discharge of the contents of an abscess may result in the formation of a

blind-ending sinus tract, sometimes communicating with the skin or a mucosal surface, or of a fistula tract which joins skin to a mucosal surface or two mucosal surfaces to each other. Discharge temporarily reduces the pressure within a chronic abscess but eventually continued suppuration leads once more to elevated pressures and the cycle of intermittent discharge repeats itself.

HEALING

Acute inflammation is a process vital to the elimination of agents harmful to the body. Inevitably, it is sometimes associated with the loss or disruption of tissues leading to the formation of a tissue defect. Such defects may also occur directly through trauma, of course. In both circumstances healing, which is defined as the replacement of lost or destroyed tissue by viable tissue, occurs. Healing may occur by:

- regeneration, where the replacement cells are of specialised type (e.g. hepatocytes replacing dead hepatocytes)

- repair where the replacement cells are of non-specialised type (usually fibroblasts which give rise to a fibrotic scar).

Often healing occurs by a combination of regeneration and repair. Undoubtedly, ideal tissue healing occurs in regeneration where the structure and functional capacity of a tissue are regained. Repair, or a mixture of repair and regeneration, are less favourable in that they are inevitably associated with disordered architecture and some reduction in a tissue's functional capacity (e.g. hepatic cirrhosis or scarring in the base of a gastric peptic ulcer which may lead to gastric outlet obstruction). Whether healing occurs by regeneration or by repair is dependent on the proliferative capacity of an organ's specialised cells, on the severity of tissue damage and on the extent of the loss of viable tissue.

Cells differ hugely in their capacity to proliferate.

- *Continually renewing* cell populations include the luminal epithelia of the gut, the epidermis and bone marrow cells.

- *Conditionally renewing* (or stable) populations do not proliferate in normal circumstances but have the capacity to do so following cell loss. The majority of cell types in the body belong to this stable category, including the epithelial cells of solid organs such as liver, kidney, endocrine glands and pancreas and many connective tissue cells such as osteoblasts, smooth muscle and endothelial cells.

- *Permanent* (or static) cell populations such as cardiac muscle cells and neurones do not retain any capacity to proliferate.

Obviously, continually and conditionally proliferating cell populations have the capacity to heal by regeneration (e.g. the regeneration of epithelial tubular cells in acute tubular necrosis) with the restoration of normal tissue structure and function. The loss of permanent cells (e.g. in myocardial and brain infarcts) can only be made good by repair (e.g. gliosis in the brain, fibrosis at other body sites). However, when damage is very severe, as occurs, for

305

example, in a renal infarct destroying all viable cells and the connective tissue framework, healing occurs by repair even in continually and conditionally renewing cell populations.

The healing process is orchestrated by peptide growth factors released by many cell types, e.g. platelets, macrophages and activated endothelium. Single cell types often produce more than one such growth factor (e.g. macrophages secrete many including PDGF, bFGF and TGF-beta which have important roles in fibroblast proliferation and collagen production). Each peptide growth factor usually has several functions, e.g. PDGF participates in the control of monocyte chemotaxis, fibroblast migration and proliferation, and collagen production.

Healing of a skin wound

Healing by first intention

The healing of a cleanly incised wound whose edges have been brought into close proximity is referred to as primary union or healing by first intention. An incision into the dermis severs blood vessels which haemorrhage into the wound space. Bleeding is halted by the formation of platelet plugs and by blood coagulation.

- Epidermal healing occurs by regeneration. Within 24–48 hours epidermal cells begin to migrate from the margins of the wound towards its centre. This epidermal migration is made easier by the decreased expression of the intercellular adhesion molecule E-cadherin by the migrating epithelium, allowing greater freedom of cellular movement. Epidermal migration occurs only over a viable tissue base so the advancing epithelial tongue dips beneath the inert surface scab.

- During the first 24 hours there is a mild acute inflammatory reaction at the wound edges. Plasmin and enzymes released from disintegrating neutrophils initiate the phase of demolition. By the third day neutrophils are scanty in a non-infected wound, the dominant inflammatory cell type now being the macrophage which continues the demolition.

- By day 3 granulation tissue (Figure 21.6), a mixture of new leaky capillaries, fibroblasts and macrophages, grows into the dermal wound site. The blood vessels of granulation tissue reflect new vessel formation (angiogenesis) resulting from the actions of bFGF and vascular endothelial growth factor (VEGF). Many factors stimulate the fibroblast proliferation (e.g. FGFs and PDGF) within granulation tissue. The fibroblastic element of granulation tissue progressively produces collagen which is prominent by the second week. By this stage the wound blood vessels are regressing and by the end of the first month the dermal wound comprises poorly vascular scarring fibrosis. The dermal adnexal structures such as hair follicles that are destroyed by the wound

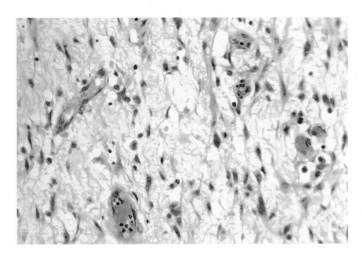

Figure 21.6 Granulation tissue. This comprises fibroblasts, capillaries and spaces occupied by oedema fluid.

are not replaced. The strength of the wound increases over ensuing weeks and months, in part due to structural changes in the collagen such as increased crosslinking.

Healing by secondary intention

The healing of extensive skin defects with separated edges (healing by secondary intention) shares many features with healing by primary intention. However, the greater loss of tissue must be made good by the production of large quantities of granulation tissue, which are eventually replaced by large quantities of fibrotic scar material. Some cells within the granulation tissue named myofibroblasts combine the contractile properties of smooth muscle with the synthetic capability of fibroblasts. It is thought that these cells are responsible for the striking wound contraction seen in the first few weeks of healing by secondary intention. Wound contraction is not seen in healing by primary intention because there is relatively little granulation tissue present.

Factors delaying healing

Healing may be delayed by local and systemic factors. Local factors that delay healing are:

- an inadequate blood supply

- infection

- the presence of foreign or dead material or of extensive haematoma

- excessive movement of the wound margins

- previous local irradiation.

Systemic factors that delay healing include:

- protein malnutrition

- vitamin C deficiency

- the presence of high levels of corticosteroids

- diabetes mellitus (which makes an individual more prone to infection).

Protein malnutrition and vitamin C deficiency both delay wound healing by impairing collagen formation. A normal function of vitamin C is the activation of prolyl- and lysyl-hydroxylases, enzymes essential to the normal maturation of collagen. In severe vitamin C deficiency (scurvy) underhydroxylated collagen is produced which is unstable, poorly transported out of synthesising fibroblasts and susceptible to degradation.

FURTHER READING

1 Cotran RS, Kumar V, Collins T. *Robbins Pathologic Basis of Disease*. Philadelphia: WB Saunders, 1999

22

Blood and circulation

Aneurysms
 Atherosclerotic aneurysms
 Dissecting aneurysms of the aorta
 Infective aneurysms
 Inflammatory aortic aneurysms
 Berry aneurysms
 Charcot–Bouchard microaneurysms
Atherosclerosis
 Morphology of atheromatous plaques
 Epidemiology and risk factors
 Pathogenesis

Haemostasis
 Normal haemostasis
 The coagulation cascade
Thrombosis
 General considerations
 Morphology of thrombi
 Clinical outcome
 Disseminated intravascular coagulation
Embolism
 Pulmonary thromboembolism
 Systemic thromboembolism

Neil Robertson

ANEURYSMS

A true aneurysm is an abnormal localized dilatation of an artery or the heart wall, defined precisely, but perhaps unhelpfully, as having a diameter greater than 50% of the original vessel diameter. The fundamental cause of all aneurysms is the weakening of the normal load-bearing structure of the media. The media can be damaged by a variety of unrelated disease processes of which the two most important are atherosclerosis and inflammation. The usual outcome of significant structural damage is the replacement of normal medial components with fibrous scar tissue which, under the tension created by luminal pressure, gradually stretches to form a localized dilatation. Aneurysms are permanent structures which, if left untreated, slowly but relentlessly enlarge.

A false aneurysm is a saccular bulge that occurs outside the vessel wall and is delineated by adventitia or surrounding connective tissue. It communicates with the lumen of the vessel through a narrow defect in the media. Such aneurysms are usually caused by penetrating trauma, particularly knife wounds.

According to their pathogenesis, several types of aneurysm can be defined: atherosclerotic, dissecting, infective, inflammatory, berry and those of microscopic dimension, e.g. Charcot–Bouchard, those associated with diabetes mellitus.

Atherosclerotic aneurysms

Atherosclerosis is the most common cause of aneurysms. Atherosclerotic aneurysms usually develop after the age of 50 years, are approximately nine times more common in males than females and are more common in smokers and in those with hypertension. They occur most frequently in the abdominal aorta, although involvement of the iliac arteries and the descending thoracic aorta is far from uncommon. Occasionally involvement of the ascending thoracic aorta is seen. It has been estimated that atherosclerotic aortic aneurysms are found in 2–4% of adult autopsies.

Approximately 75% of atherosclerotic aneurysms of the aorta are located below the level of the renal artery ostia and it is not unusual to find in such cases associated smaller aneurysms of the iliac arteries. All these aneurysms are caused primarily by large, usually complicated, intimal plaques, the elastase activity of the plaque macrophages causing medial destruction and thinning. Most aneurysms are fusiform, involving the entire vessel circumference (Figure 22.1), although occasionally they are saccular, involving only part of the vessel circumference. Invariably they are filled with friable atheromatous debris and laminated mural thrombus, which often give rise to emboli that may occlude small arteries in the lower limbs. Occasionally an aneurysm may extend to involve the ostia of the renal, superior mesenteric or inferior mesenteric arteries with consequent luminal occlusion due to direct pressure or concomitant thrombosis.

Atherosclerotic aortic aneurysms may manifest clinically in a variety of ways:

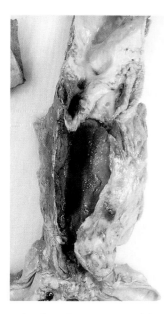

Figure 22.1 Atherosclerotic aortic aneurysm containing atheromatous debris and thrombus.

- rupture into the retroperitoneum, peritoneal cavity or thoracic cavity with massive, and often fatal, haemorrhage

- compression of an adjacent structure, e.g. ureter, or erosion of vertebral bodies

- occlusion of an arterial branch due to compression or mural thrombosis

- embolism from mural thrombus or atheromatous debris

- an abdominal mass, which may be pulsatile.

The larger the aneurysm, the more likely it is to rupture: aneurysms up to 5 cm in diameter rarely rupture, whereas those larger than 6 cm in diameter carry a 50% risk of fatal rupture within a 10-year period of follow-up. So high is the operative mortality in cases of rupture and so acceptable the low mortality of elective surgery that early detection is desirable. As such, some criteria of a screening programme are fulfilled and ultrasound offers the most sensitive detection modality.

Dissecting aneurysms of the aorta

Dissecting aneurysms of the aorta are thought to be caused by a tear in the intima allowing blood to enter the media, usually between its middle and outer thirds. The blood then tracks both proximally and distally for a variable distance before ultimately rupturing outwards through the adventitia or inwards back into the lumen of the aorta. Dissecting aneurysms differ from other types of aneurysm in that they do not often give rise to significant dilatation of the aorta – hence the more favoured terms aortic dissection and dissecting haematoma. They occur most commonly after the age of

311

60 years and are 2–3 times more common in men than women. However, below the age of 40 years the male-to-female ratio falls, owing to the increased occurrence of dissections in pregnancy.

In more than 60% of dissections the intimal tear is located in the ascending thoracic aorta (usually within 10 cm of the aortic valve), in 25% of cases it is located in the descending thoracic aorta, in 10% of cases the aortic arch and in 3% of cases the abdominal aorta. However, cases of aortic dissection in which there is no apparent intimal tear are not rare. When a tear is present it is usually 4–5 cm in length, sharply defined and transverse, although it may be T-shaped or even longitudinal. The intramedial haematoma that develops may extend proximally but more usually tracks distally and often involves the roots of the main branches of the aortic arch. Propagation along the coronary, renal, mesenteric and iliac arteries may also occur.

The most frequently encountered histological lesion is cystic medial degeneration (Figure 22.2), which consists of elastic fibre fragmentation with separation of the elastic and fibromuscular components of the media by small cystic or cleft-like spaces filled with glycosaminoglycans and other ground substance material. Inflammation is not a feature.

Aortic dissections are divided into two groups depending on the location of the primary intimal tear:

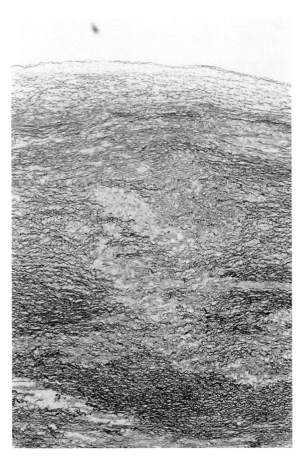

Figure 22.2 Aorta showing cystic medial degeneration. Elastic fibres are stained black.

- type A, or proximal, dissections involve the ascending aorta alone or extend to involve the descending aorta. They are the most common and fatal type.

- type B, or distal, aortic dissections do not involve the ascending aorta and often begin distal to the subclavian artery.

Dissections involving the ascending part of the aorta are much more likely to rupture externally than dissections involving any other part, because the outer wall of the dissection in the ascending aorta is very thin. Rupture leads invariably to massive haemorrhage into the mediastinum, pleural cavities or pericardium with concomitant excruciating chest pain. Death rapidly ensues.

In approximately 10% of dissections a second intimal tear develops distally, thus giving rise to two aortic lumina – the so-called double-barrelled aorta. In time the lining of the false channel may undergo fibromuscular thickening and dystrophic calcification. Alternatively the lumen may become completely occluded by thrombus. Dissections involving the proximal parts of the main branches of the aorta may lead to ischaemia in the tissues supplied. Less than 10% of all acute aortic dissections progress to a healed phase that is compatible with long survival. Occasionally, healed dissections are discovered coincidentally at autopsy, indicating that acute dissections may produce little symptomatology.

The pathogenesis of aortic dissection is complex and much remains to be discovered. More than 80% of dissections occur after the age of 60 years when the only discernible risk factor is systemic hypertension. In patients younger than 40 years of age dissections are strongly associated with genetic defects of connective tissue synthesis, the most well recognized of which is Marfan's disease, an autosomal dominant disease caused by mutations in the fibrillin gene on chromosome 15 and characterized by skeletal, cardiovascular and ocular abnormalities. One of the roles of the fibrillin glycoprotein is to promote the adhesion of elastic fibrils, which is essential for maintaining the normal structural integrity of the aortic media and in particular for resisting the shear stresses created by the blood pressure during systole. The main cardiovascular complications include aortic dissection, dilatation of the aortic root and mitral valve prolapse, any one of which may cause the premature death of a patient with Marfan's disease. Individuals with known Marfan's disease should be monitored, the aortic root diameter determining the timing of valve surgery, often with root and arch replacement.

Cystic medial degeneration is frequently found in patients with Marfan's disease, whereas those with hypertension show a variety of histological changes ranging from focal and mild fragmentation of elastic fibres to well-established cystic medial degeneration, but just how far hypertension contributes to cystic medial degeneration is uncertain. It is well worth remembering, however, that cystic medial degeneration is a frequent incidental finding at autopsy in patients who do not have a dissection.

Aortic dissections used to be almost always fatal but nowadays the prognosis is much better. Early surgical intervention involving plication of the aortic wall, together with early and aggressive antihypertensive therapy, allow the survival of up to 75% of patients.

Infective aneurysms

Infective aneurysms are divided for convenience into two groups: those caused by syphilis and those due to any other infective agent.

Approximately one-third of patients with untreated primary syphilis will develop tertiary syphilis and of these, approximately 80% will have cardiovascular involvement. Syphilitic aortitis, which usually involves a discrete segment of the aorta (most often a band just above the aortic valve), usually begins with inflammation of the adventitia. Inflammation then spreads along the vasa vasorum of the media to produce an obliterative endarteritis in which lymphocytes and plasma cells predominate. Narrowing of the lumina of the vasa vasorum causes ischaemic damage to the media with patchy loss of smooth muscle cells and elastic fibres and their later replacement with collagenous scar tissue. The aorta thus loses its elastic properties and gradually dilates to produce a syphilitic aneurysm, which is often of saccular type. The contraction of fibrous scars may cause wrinkling of intervening areas of non-scarred intima to produce the characteristic 'tree-bark' appearance (Figure 22.3). Syphilitic aortitis may also cause dilatation of the aortic valve ring with subsequent left heart failure. Most syphilitic aneurysms occur in the ascending aorta and arch and in these sites may compress or erode into the right bronchus, superior vena cava or right pulmonary artery. Aneurysms involving the descending part of the thoracic aorta may compress or erode into the trachea or oesophagus.

Mycotic (non-syphilitic) aortic aneurysms are usually well-defined saccular aneurysms that develop after an episode of bacterial endocarditis or septicaemia. They carry a high risk of rupture unless treated surgically. Causative organisms include *Staphylococcus aureus*, pneumococci and *Salmonella typhi*. Their exact pathogenesis is not certain, although it is likely that viable organisms seed the media directly by way of the vasa vasorum or indirectly by intimal adherence of an infected thrombus. Tuberculous aortic aneurysms do occur but are extremely rare.

Inflammatory aortic aneurysms

Giant cell aortitis usually occurs in patients over 50 years of age and is more common in women and black people. It is thought to have an autoimmune aetiology and is present in 10–15% of cases of temporal giant cell arteritis. It can give rise to an aortic aneurysm and even incompetence of the aortic valve. It is characterised histologically by inflammation of the media in which elastic fibres are engulfed by epithelioid macrophages and multinucleate giant cells.

Rheumatoid nodules can occur in the aorta and, particularly in the ascending aorta, may lead to aneurysm formation by causing medial destruction.

Berry aneurysms

Berry aneurysms are small saccular aneurysms that arise at branch points on the circle of Willis at the base of the brain or on the large arteries just beyond. They range in diameter from a few millimetres to 2 or 3 cm and have a thin, translucent wall. They are discovered in approximately 2% of all adult autopsies and in 20–30% of cases they are multiple.

The berry aneurysm is the most common type of intracranial aneurysm (other rare types include atherosclerotic, mycotic, traumatic and dissecting) and a ruptured berry aneurysm is the most frequent cause of clinically significant subarachnoid haemorrhage. Ruptured berry aneurysm is also the fourth most common cerebrovascular disorder – after atherosclerotic thrombotic infarct, thromboembolism and hypertensive intracerebral haemorrhage.

Rupture of a berry aneurysm usually occurs at its apex and gives rise to haemorrhage into the subarachnoid space, brain parenchyma or both. Histologically the wall of the aneurysm is devoid of muscle, being composed only of thickened intima overlaid with adventitia. The risk of rupture relates directly to size: those with a diameter of 10 mm or more have a 50% annual risk of rupture. Rupture is most likely to occur during an acute elevation of intracranial pressure, such as may occur with straining at stool or sexual orgasm. The cardinal symptom of rupture is excruciating headache, followed rapidly by loss of consciousness. Between 25% and 50% of patients will die during the first episode of rupture, but those who recover have a high risk of rebleed.

The pathogenesis of berry aneurysms is not known although there may be congenital absence of medial muscle and elastic fibres at bifurcation points in the circle of Willis. In some cases, genetic factors may play a role, for these aneurysms occur more frequently in patients with inherited systemic disorders, such as autosomal dominant polycystic renal disease, Ehlers-Danlos syndrome type 4, neurofibromatosis type 1, and Marfan's disease.

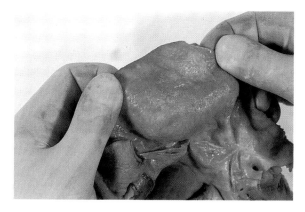

Figure 22.3 Syphilitic aortitis with tree-bark appearance of intima.

They are also associated with fibromuscular dysplasia of extracranial arteries and coarctation of the aorta, and both cigarette smoking and systemic hypertension are accepted predisposing factors for their development.

Charcot–Bouchard microaneurysms

Charcot–Bouchard microaneurysms are minute aneurysms that develop, in the presence of systemic hypertension, in vessels of the brain that are less than 300 µm in diameter. They occur most commonly in the basal ganglia and may rupture to produce catastrophic intracerebral haemorrhage. They account for about 15–20% of cerebrovascular accidents.

ATHEROSCLEROSIS

Arteriosclerosis is the blanket term for two types of arterial disease characterised by mural thickening and loss of elasticity:

- atherosclerosis
- Monckeberg's medial calcification.

Atherosclerosis is by far the most important of the two in terms of impact on human morbidity and mortality and will be discussed in some detail shortly. Monckeberg's medial calcification (Figure 22.4), briefly, is characterised by the deposition of plates or circumferential rings of calcium in the media of medium-sized muscular arteries in middle-aged and elderly people.

Arteriolosclerosis is a disease of small arteries and arterioles and is seen most often in association with hypertension and diabetes mellitus. Two variants, hyaline and hyperplastic, are recognised, both of which cause thickening and loss of elasticity of the vessel wall with luminal narrowing and consequent rise in luminal pressure, thus augmenting any pre-existing hypertension.

The defining lesion of atherosclerosis is the atheromatous or fibro-fatty plaque (Figures 22.5 and 22.6), which forms in the intima, protrudes into the vessel lumen, may weaken the subjacent media and has the potential to undergo a number of clinically significant

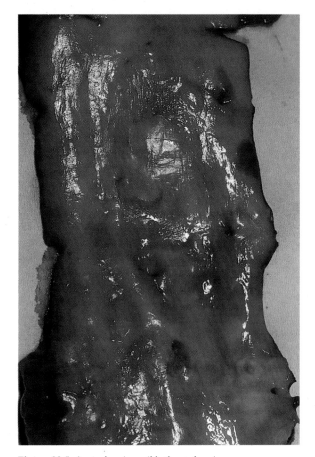

Figure 22.5 Aorta showing mild atherosclerosis.

complications. Atherosclerosis affects elastic arteries, such as the aorta, iliac and carotid, and both large and medium-sized muscular arteries, such as the coronary and popliteal. Atheromatous plaques often appear in childhood and tend to progress slowly through adulthood but do not usually become clinically significant until middle age or later, at which time they are the most important cause of ischaemia in the Western world. Atherosclerosis can affect any organ or tissue in the body, but most symptomatic disease is confined to the arteries supplying the heart, brain, kidneys, lower limbs and small intestine. Myocardial infarction, cerebral infarction and aortic aneurysm are by far the most important clinically significant consequences of atherosclerosis.

Atheromatous plaques in small arteries may by themselves be occlusive and thereby cause ischaemic damage in distant organs and tissues, but plaques can also rupture and induce local thrombosis thus further compromising blood flow. In large arteries enzymes released from plaque macrophages can digest the elastic of the media. Such inflammatory destruction will lead to fibrous repair, thus weakening the vessel wall and predisposing it to the formation of aneurysms or, by altering local blood flow, encouraging thrombosis. Large atheromas can also erupt and shed friable debris into the circulation. Such atheromatous emboli can produce ischaemic damage some distance from their place of origin (Figure 22.7).

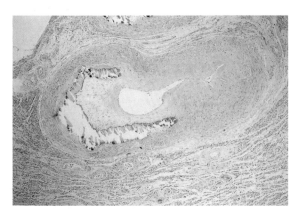

Figure 22.4 Monckeberg's medial calcification.

cytes and small amounts of extracellular lipid. Their only clinical importance is that they may develop into atheromatous plaques.

Atheromatous plaques consist basically of a core of lipid (mostly cholesterol and cholesterol esters) covered with a fibrous cap (Figure 22.8). They vary in size from a few millimetres to 1.5 cm in diameter, are yellowish white and invariably encroach upon the vessel lumen. They can be discrete but often coalesce to form large irregular masses. Their distribution in humans is fairly characteristic. Lesions are usually most numerous and severe in the abdominal aorta and tend to accumulate round the ostia of its main branches. After the abdominal aorta, the most severely affected vessels (in descending order) are the coronary arteries, the popliteal arteries, the descending thoracic aorta, the internal carotid arteries and the arteries of the circle of Willis.

The composition of atheromatous plaques (Figure 22.8) is variable. In general there is a surface cap of dense collagenous tissue (the so-called fibrous cap) in which are embedded smooth muscle cells and leucocytes. Beneath the cap and to its sides there is a cellular zone containing macrophages, smooth muscle cells and lymphocytes and in the core there is an admixture of lipid material (mostly cholesterol and cholesterol esters), cholesterol clefts, cellular debris and foamy (lipid-laden) macrophages. At the periphery of large plaques there may be proliferating small blood

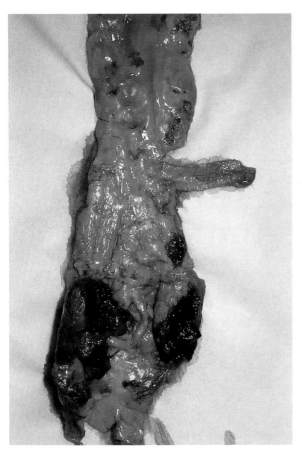

Figure 22.6 Aorta showing marked complicated atherosclerosis with mural thrombus.

Morphology of atheromatous plaques

Fatty streaks are thought to be the forerunners of atheromatous plaques. They occur in the aortas of children and in some cases are present before the age of one year. They first appear as flat, yellow intimal spots, less than 1 mm in diameter, that gradually coalesce to form elongated streaks 1 cm or more in length. They consist of collections of lipid-filled macrophages with associated lympho-

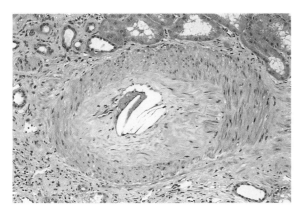

Figure 22.7 Small artery in renal cortex occluded by atheromatous embolus. Note central cholesterol clefts and also intimal thickening due to hypertension.

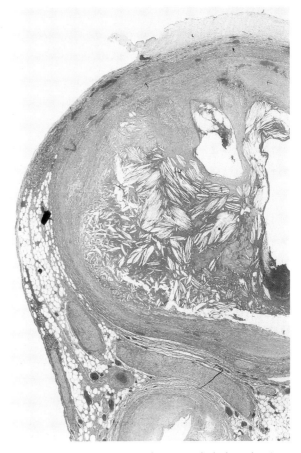

Figure 22.8 Coronary artery showing marked atherosclerosis.

vessels, mostly capillaries. In essence, atheromatous plaques result from persistent endothelial damage (pressure, chemical, immune and infective factors may all operate) in the presence of elevated low-density lipoprotein-related cholesterol, with macrophage uptake of the latter and a variably mature fibrous response.

Atheromatous plaques assume their greatest clinical significance when they become complicated by any of the following processes: rupture or ulceration, intraplaque haemorrhage, thrombosis, and damage to the underlying media. Rupture or ulceration of the luminal surface of a plaque may expose highly thrombogenic substances to the blood, thereby inducing, the formation of a thrombus, or may permit the release of atheromatous debris into the circulation. Haemorrhage may occur into a plaque either from the capillaries that surround it or as a consequence of rupture of the fibrous cap. In either case an intraplaque haematoma will form, which may rupture through the surface of the plaque and induce local thrombosis or atheromatous embolism. As mentioned previously, encroachment of the plaque upon the media may cause medial destruction with consequent formation of an aneurysm.

Epidemiology and risk factors

Atherosclerosis is widely prevalent throughout the populations of Europe, North America, Australia and New Zealand; its prevalence in Central and South America, Africa and Asia is, in contrast, much lower. Atherosclerosis is therefore predominantly a disease of developed countries. Factors that predispose to atherosclerosis are either:

- constitutional (age, sex, genetics) and therefore unchangeable or

- acquired (hyperlipidaemia, hypertension, cigarette smoking, diabetes mellitus) and potentially avoidable or at least amenable to control.

Constitutional

Atherosclerosis is a disease that begins in childhood and progresses slowly throughout adulthood. It is not surprising, therefore, that death rates due to atherosclerotic diseases increase relentlessly with age; for example, between the ages of 40 and 60 years, the incidence of myocardial infarction increases roughly fivefold.

Men are more likely to develop atherosclerosis and its sequelae than are women; between the ages of 35 and 55 years, the death rate from ischaemic heart disease is approximately five times higher in white men than in white women. This is probably because, other things being equal, premenopausal women are protected against atherosclerosis by their natural levels of oestrogen. After the menopause, when oestrogen levels fall, the incidence of atherosclerotic diseases in women rises, until by the seventh or eighth decades it more or less equals that in men.

It is accepted that genetic factors may predispose an individual to atherosclerosis; in some cases well-defined inherited genetic aberrations of lipid metabolism give rise to hyperlipidaemia, whereas in others more nebulous genetic anomalies may serve to increase the risk for the development of hypertension or diabetes mellitus.

Acquired

Hyperlipidaemia, particularly hypercholesterolaemia, is strongly associated with the development of atherosclerosis, but it is the low-density lipoprotein component of total serum cholesterol that carries the biggest risk. The higher the level of low-density lipoproteins, the higher the risk of atherosclerosis, whereas the higher the level of high-density lipoproteins, the lower the risk of atherosclerosis. Diets high in cholesterol and saturated fats raise blood cholesterol levels, whereas diets low in cholesterol and the ratio of saturated to polyunsaturated fats lower blood cholesterol levels. A number of genetic defects in lipoprotein metabolism causing hyperlipidaemia are directly associated with increased rates of atherosclerosis. When levels of serum cholesterol are lowered (or the balance of serum lipoprotein components adjusted in favour of high-density lipoproteins), either by a modification of diet or by drugs, the rate of progression of atherosclerosis falls, some atheromatous plaques may even regress, and both morbidity and mortality from atherosclerotic diseases fall.

Hypertension in all age groups is associated with higher levels of atherosclerosis; middle-aged men with blood pressures exceeding 169/95 mmHg are more than five times as likely to develop ischaemic heart disease than those whose blood pressure is 140/90 mmHg or less. Antihypertensive agents reduce the risk of atherosclerotic diseases, especially ischaemic heart disease and stroke, but the endpoint of any one trial (myocardial infarction or stroke) may include indirect factors, for example thrombosis or haemorrhage, not directly reflecting atheroma.

Cigarette smoking is a well-established risk factor for atherosclerosis in both men and women and diabetes mellitus predisposes to atherosclerosis indirectly by way of hypercholesterolaemia and abnormalities of endothelial function. Elevated levels of plasma homocysteine can induce atherosclerosis through the formation of oxygen free radicals. The reaction to infective agents, for example CMV or chlamydia, may lead to endothelial damage and stimulate plaque growth. Some studies have detected such a relationship, but the contribution of infective agents to the development of disease is not yet established. Other factors, such as a lack of exercise, stressful lifestyle and gross obesity, are also thought to increase the risk of atherosclerosis but their relative contribution in most cases is difficult to quantify. A moderate intake of alcohol appears to be protective.

Pathogenesis

The current hypothesis for atherogenesis – the response to damage hypothesis – regards atherosclerosis as a chronic inflammatory response of the arterial wall to endothelial damage.

1. Endothelial damage, focal and often subtle, is thought to increase both endothelial permeability and leucocyte adhesion.

2. Lipoproteins, mainly low-density lipoproteins and very low-density lipoproteins, enter the intima and undergo oxidation.

3. Blood monocytes (and other leucocytes) adhere to the damaged endothelium before migrating into the intima, where they transform into tissue macrophages and foam cells.

4. Platelets adhere either to the damaged endothelium or to already adherent leucocytes.

5. Activated platelets, macrophages and vascular cells then release chemotactic factors that stimulate the migration of smooth muscle cells from the media into the intima, where they begin to proliferate.

6. Subsequent elaboration of extracellular matrix leads to an accumulation of proteoglycans and collagen fibres.

HAEMOSTASIS

Normal haemostasis involves the rapid formation of a localised haemostatic plug at a site of blood vessel rupture. Thrombosis, on the other hand, involves the inappropriate activation of haemostatic processes (resulting in the formation of a thrombus) in vessels that are intact or only slightly damaged. Both haemostasis and thrombosis depend upon interactions between the blood vessel wall, platelets and the components of the coagulation cascade.

Normal haemostasis

Initial blood vessel damage is followed by transient arteriolar vasoconstriction, mediated by reflex neurogenic mechanisms and endothelin, a potent vasoconstrictor derived from endothelium. Damage to the endothelium exposes highly thrombogenic subendothelial extracellular matrix (of which collagen is the most important constituent) to which platelets adhere via von Willebrand factor (vWF) released by endothelial cells.

The platelets become activated, i.e. they alter their shape and release secretory granules of two types:

● alpha granules, containing fibrinogen, fibronectin, factor V and vWF, platelet factor 4 (a heparin-binding chemokine), platelet-derived growth factor and transforming growth factor-beta

● delta granules, containing adenosine diphosphate (ADP) and triphosphate (ATP), ionised calcium, histamine, serotonin and adrenaline. Calcium is important because it is needed in the coagulation cascade and ADP mediates in platelet aggregation.

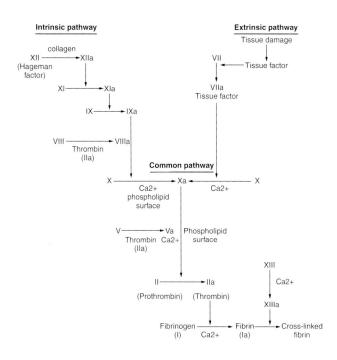

Roman numerals identify coagulation factors. Activated factors are indicated with lower case 'a'. Ca2+ - calcium ion.

Figure 22.9 Coagulation cascade.

Platelet activation also triggers the surface expression of a phospholipid complex, which acts as a nucleation site for the binding of calcium and coagulation factors of the intrinsic clotting pathway. Endothelial cells also liberate inhibitors of plasminogen activator, which depress fibrinolysis.

Platelet adhesion and secretion are followed by platelet aggregation, a process mediated by ADP and thromboxane A2, both derived from platelets. The resultant platelet aggregate is called the primary haemostatic plug.

Thrombin, generated by activation of the coagulation cascade, binds to the platelets and promotes yet more platelet aggregation and following contraction, an irreversibly fused clot of platelets results – the secondary haemostatic plug.

Meanwhile thrombin in the plug converts fibrinogen, a soluble plasma protein, to the insoluble fibrillar protein fibrin, which acts as a mortar to bind the platelets together. Anticoagulant mechanisms, involving tissue plasminogen activator, are then triggered to limit the haemostatic plug to the site of injury.

The coagulation cascade

The coagulation cascade (Figure 22.9) is a series of conversions of inactive proenzymes to activated enzymes resulting in the formation of thrombin, essential for the conversion of fibrinogen to fibrin.

317

Each reaction in the cascade follows the assembly of a complex composed of:

● an enzyme (activated coagulation factor)

● a substrate (proenzyme form of coagulation factor) and

● a cofactor (reaction accelerator)

all held together by calcium ions. The complex is assembled on a phospholipid complex expressed on the surface of activated platelets and endothelial cells.

Traditionally, extrinsic and intrinsic coagulation pathways are described, which converge where factor X is activated. The intrinsic pathway begins with the activation of factor XII (the Hageman factor), whereas the extrinsic pathway is activated by tissue factor, an endothelial lipoprotein released at sites of tissue damage. This clear division into extrinsic and intrinsic pathways is, however, an oversimplification, because interconnections between the two pathways exist, e.g. a tissue factor–factor VIIa complex, in addition to activating factor X in the extrinsic pathway, activates factor IX in the intrinsic pathway.

Coagulation is regulated by three types of naturally occurring anticoagulants:

● antithrombins (e.g. antithrombin III) which inhibit thrombin and factors IXa, Xa, XIa and XIIa

● proteins C and S, two vitamin K-dependent proteins, which inactivate factors Va and VIIIa

● plasmin, derived from circulating plasminogen, which breaks down fibrin and inhibits its polymerisation.

Plasminogen is converted to plasmin either by a factor XII-dependent pathway or by plasminogen activators (PAs), of which two distinct classes exist:

● urokinase-like PA, present in plasma

● tissue-type PA, synthesised predominantly by endothelial cells

Plasminogen is also activated by the bacterial product streptokinase.

THROMBOSIS

General considerations

There are three primary factors that predispose to the formation of thrombi:

● endothelial damage

● stasis or turbulence of blood flow

● blood hypercoagulability.

Collectively these factors are known as Virchow's triad and in any particular clinical setting they may operate independently or in combination to induce thrombosis.

Endothelial damage is the most important component of Virchow's triad and can by itself lead to thrombosis. Clinical settings in which endothelial damage, occurs abound. In the heart it often follows endocardial damage caused by, for example, myocardial infarction or valvulitis. In arteries it is frequently seen over complicated atheromatous plaques, may occur at sites of traumatic damage or vasculitis, and it may result from the haemodynamic stresses associated with hypertension. In veins it can result from direct pressure. Bacterial endotoxins may destroy the endothelium in any vessel type. Whatever the cause of endothelial damage, the result is the same: subendothelial collagen fibres (and other platelet activators) become exposed, platelets adhere to the exposed collagen, and prostacyclin, nitrous oxide and plasminogen activator become locally depleted, the usual antithrombotic endothelial mechanisms being locally lost.

Turbulence in the bloodstream can predispose to thrombosis in one of two ways:

● by damaging endothelium

● by creating pockets of stasis.

Stasis plays an important part in venous thrombosis. Normal blood flow is laminar, i.e. the cellular components of blood flow in the central part of the stream and are generally separated from the endothelium by a cushion of relatively acellular slower moving plasma. Stasis and turbulence upset normal laminar flow and allow platelets and activated clotting factors to come into contact with the endothelium. They also impede the ingress of clotting factor inhibitors, thereby allowing thrombi to grow, and promote endothelial cell activation which further predisposes to local thrombosis.

There are a number of clinical settings in which turbulence and/or stasis play an important part in thrombosis.

● Ulcerated atheromatous plaques contribute to thrombosis not only by exposing highly thrombogenic subendothelial collagen to the blood but also by causing local turbulent blood flow.

● Arterial aneurysms favour thrombosis by causing local stasis.

● Myocardial infarctions contain areas of non-contractile myocardium that are associated with local stasis of blood in the adjacent heart chamber. This predisposes to mural thrombosis.

● Atrial fibrillation leads to stasis within the atria and their appendages and is a frequent precursor of thrombosis within the atrial appendages.

Hypercoagulability states exist when the coagulation pathways change in ways that predispose to thrombosis. They are divided into:

● primary (genetic)

● secondary (acquired) disorders (Box 22.1).

Mutations in the factor V gene are the most common cause of

318

Box 22.1 Hypercoagulable states

Primary (genetic)
Mutations in factor V
Antithrombin III deficiency
Proteins C or S deficiency
Fibrinolysis defects
Homocysteinaemia
Allelic variations in prothrombin levels

Secondary (acquired)
High risk for thrombosis
    Prolonged immobilisation or bed rest
    Myocardial infarction
    Tissue damage from surgery, burns, fracture, etc.
    Malignant tumours
    Prosthetic heart valves
    Disseminated intravascular coagulation
    Heparin-induced thrombocytopaenia
    Antiphospholipid antibody syndrome
Low risk for thrombosis
    Atrial fibrillation
    Cardiomyopathy
    Nephrotic syndrome
    Hyperoestrogenic states
    Oral contraceptives
    Sickle cell anaemia
    Smoking

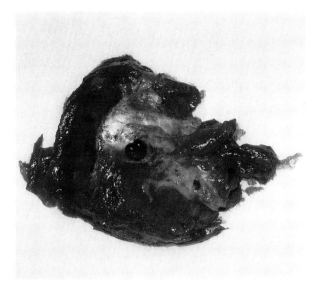

Figure 22.10 Red thrombus occluding a deep vein in a calf muscle.

hereditary hypercoagulability. Between 2% and 15% of the white population carry a factor V gene mutation (known as the Leiden mutation) that results in the amino acid glutamine being substituted for the normal arginine at position 506 in the protein molecule. People who have an inherited lack of anticoagulants, e.g. antithrombin III, protein C or protein S, usually present in adolescence or early adulthood with venous thrombosis and recurrent thromboembolism.

In many clinical settings, however, the pathogenesis of hypercoagulation is complex and multifactorial, e.g. the hypercoagulability associated with oral contraceptives may be due partly to increased hepatic synthesis of a variety of coagulation factors and partly to reduced synthesis of antithrombin III.

Morphology of thrombi

Thrombi can form anywhere in the cardiovascular system. In arteries they usually form at sites of endothelial damage (most commonly due to atheromatous plaques) or where blood flow is turbulent, e.g. at points of bifurcation or round ostia in the aorta. In veins they usually form where there is stasis. They vary in size, shape and colour depending on the circumstances leading to their formation and the sites where they form. Arterial thrombi are often greyish white and friable, due to their consisting of a tangled mesh of fibrin, platelets and red cells; venous thrombi, on the other hand, contain more red cells and consequently appear red (Figure 22.10). From their point of attachment arterial thrombi tend to grow in a retro-

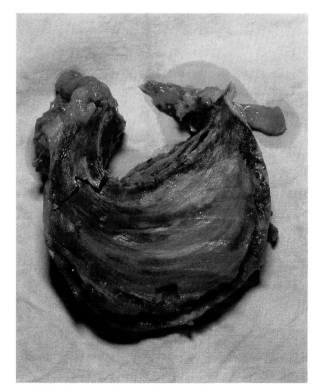

Figure 22.11 Lines of Zahn in a thrombus from an atherosclerotic aortic aneurysm.

grade direction, in contrast to venous thrombi which tend to grow towards the heart in the direction of blood flow.

Thrombi that form in the heart or in large arteries may have macroscopic pale and dark laminations called lines of Zahn (Figure 22.11). These are caused by layers of platelets and fibrin (pale) alternating with layers in which red cells are numerous

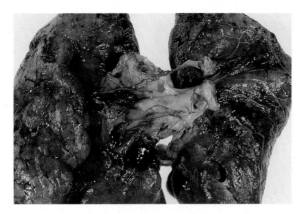

Figure 22.12 Dark red thrombus occluding both main pulmonary arteries at the lung hila.

(dark). Their only significance is that when present, they indicate thrombosis has occurred where blood flow has been relatively quick. Lines of Zahn are rarely visible to the naked eye in venous thrombi.

Thrombi that form in the heart or aorta are usually adherent to the wall and are called mural thrombi. Such thrombi in the heart usually overlie areas of infarction, whereas in the aorta they usually either overlie complicated atheromatous plaques or line aneurysms (see Figures 22.1 and 22.6). Thrombi that form in smaller arteries are usually occlusive. Venous thrombi are almost invariably occlusive and tend to propagate for long distances, forming a cast of the lumen.

Clinical outcome

Once a thrombus has formed there are four possible outcomes:

- it may propagate by the acquisition of more fibrin and platelets and eventually occlude the vessel

- it may give rise to emboli

- it may undergo complete dissolution by fibrinolysis

- it may stimulate inflammation and fibrosis (organisation) with eventual recanalisation or incorporation into the vessel wall.

Thrombi are important for two reasons: they may obstruct arteries and veins and they may give rise to emboli.

Approximately 90% of venous thrombi form in the superficial or deep veins of the lower limbs, although no site is exempt. Superficial thrombi usually involve the saphenous system, especially in the presence of varices, but only rarely do they embolise. They do, however, produce local pain, swelling and tenderness and can give rise to varicose ulceration. Thrombi that form in the large deep veins are, however, much more serious because they are apt to embolise. Deep venous thrombosis is a well-recognised consequence of congestive cardiac failure, major surgery, trauma

or burns and the puerperal and postnatal states but whatever the clinical setting, old age, immobilisation and bedrest all significantly increase its risk.

Arterial thrombi, in addition to causing luminal obstruction, may give rise to emboli capable of lodging in distant sites such as the brain, kidneys, spleen and lower limbs.

Disseminated intravascular coagulation (DIC)

In brief, DIC is characterised by the deposition of fibrin thrombi throughout the microcirculation. It occurs as a secondary phenomenon in a wide variety of pathological states ranging from advanced malignancy to obstetric complications. The microthrombi are not usually visible to the naked eye but are readily seen at light microscopy. With the formation of vast numbers of thrombi there is a concomitant depletion of platelets and coagulation factors and when fibrinolysis begins to take over, what began as a thrombotic problem may rapidly evolve into a life-threatening bleeding disorder.

EMBOLISM

An embolus is a detached intravascular solid, liquid or gaseous mass that is carried by the blood to a site distant from its place of origin. A thromboembolus is a dislodged part of a thrombus. Approximately 99% of all emboli are thromboemboli and therefore, unless otherwise specified, all emboli should be regarded as thromboemboli. Rare types of emboli include atheromatous debris (see Figure 22.7), bubbles of air or nitrogen, droplets of fat and fragments of tumour or bone marrow. Emboli eventually lodge in vessels too small to admit their passage. The clinical consequences of this depend on whether the vessels are in the pulmonary or systemic circulation.

Pulmonary thromboembolism

Pulmonary embolism (Figure 22.12) is responsible for about 200 000 deaths per year in the USA, despite the fact that the rate of fatal pulmonary embolism has dropped from 6% to 2% in the last 25 years. More than 95% of venous emboli arise from deep venous thrombi above the level of the knee. They travel along the femoral vein and inferior vena cava to reach the right side of the heart, whence they enter the main pulmonary trunk. Depending on their size, they may lodge in the main pulmonary trunk, straddle the bifurcation (saddle embolus) or pass along progressively smaller branching arteries and arterioles to reach the lung periphery. Often emboli are multiple and occasionally, showers of tiny emboli become lodged throughout both lungs. When a septal or ventricular defect is present an embolus can pass into the systemic circulation (paradoxical embolism).

Between 60% and 80% of pulmonary emboli are too small to manifest clinically. Most of these are eventually organised and incorporated into the vessel wall but in some cases there remain delicate fibrous bands spanning the vessel lumen. Large emboli may cause sudden death, right heart failure (cor pulmonale) or cardiovascular collapse, particularly if they compromise more than 60% of the pulmonary circulation. Emboli that occlude medium-sized arteries may give rise to pulmonary haemorrhage but do not usually cause infarction owing to the dual blood supply of the bronchi. Infarcts may occur, however, if there is concomitant left heart failure. Cumulative scarring from multiple emboli over a long period of time may lead to pulmonary hypertension and right ventricular failure.

Systemic thromboembolism

The vast majority of emboli in the systemic circulation arise from mural thrombi in the heart (approximately two-thirds of which overlie left ventricular infarcts). Most of the remainder come from complicated atheromatous plaques, aortic aneurysms or fragmented valvular vegetations. The destinations of systemic emboli depend largely on the origin and size of the emboli, although the main sites of arrest are the lower limbs and brain, the kidneys, intestines, spleen and upper extremities being involved to a lesser degree.

FURTHER READING

1   Bick RL, Murano G. Physiology of hemostasis. *Clin Lab Med* 1994; **14**: 677

2   Dammerman M, Breslow JL. Genetic basis of lipoprotein disorders. *Circulation* 1995; **91**: 505

3   Gotto AM. Cholesterol management in theory and practice. *Circulation* 1997; **96**: 4424

4   Lijnen HR, Collen D. Mechanisms of physiological fibrinolysis. *Baillière's Clin Haematol* 1995; **8**: 277

5   Roberts W. Aortic dissection: anatomy, consequences and causes. *Am Heart J* 1991; **101**:195–214

6   SHEP Cooperative Research Group. Prevention of stroke by antihypertensive drug treatment in older persons with isolated systolic hypertension: final results of the Systolic Hypertension in the Elderly Program. *JAMA* 1991; **265**: 3255

23

Infection in surgery

Surgical site infection
  Definition
  Epidemiology and surveillance
  Microbiology
  Prosthetic device infection
  Risk factors
  Prevention
Soft tissue infection
  Surgical wound infection
  Cellulitis
  Necrotising fasciitis
  Pyomyositis
  Breast abscess
  Tetanus
  Toxic shock syndrome
Postoperative pneumonia

Urinary tract infection
Multiresistant Staphylococcus aureus (MRSA)
Clostridium difficile
Viral gastroenteritis
Bloodborne viruses and surgery
  Surgery on BBV carriers
  Surgery by BBV carriers
Infection of intravascular devices
  Aetiology and pathogenesis
  Diagnosis
  Treatment
  Prevention
Antibiotic policies
  Treatment
  Prophylaxis

Richard Cunningham, David Dance

SURGICAL SITE INFECTION

The risk of infection at the site of a surgical procedure, in the worst cases leading to systemic sepsis and death, has always been one of the factors that has limited the development of surgical techniques, particularly those involving intrinsically contaminated sites such as the bowel. A better understanding of the specific risk factors for surgical site infection (SSI) has led to the development of rational preventive techniques that now enable surgeons to undertake procedures that previously were unthinkable. Even so, severe SSI remains a feared complication of any operation. In addition to causing morbidity and death, surgical infections are a substantial drain on resources, since each infected patient has been estimated to stay in hospital an extra 6.5 days on average, doubling the hospital costs.

Definition

Most surgeons think they know when a wound is infected but in practice such judgements are subjective and reflect a continuum from normal wound healing to gross sepsis rather than a simple 'black and white' situation. Key features include purulent discharge from the wound itself and spreading cellulitis of the surrounding skin. Clear and precise definitions are essential for surveillance, particularly when interventions are being evaluated or comparisons are being made between units or individual surgeons, which is likely to be an increasingly important aspect of clinical governance.

A wide range of definitions of SSIs can be found in the literature. Some workers have developed complex scoring systems with abbreviations such as ASEPSIS and SWAS. These are perhaps too complicated to use for routine surveillance. Even the definitions used in routine surveillance (e.g. NNIS in the USA or NINSS in the UK) are complex. These are adapted from those developed by the Centers for Disease Control and classify SSIs into superficial incisional infection, deep incisional infection and organ/space infection.

Epidemiology and surveillance

The incidence and severity of SSIs inevitably vary in place and time but the quality and comparability of data are highly dependent on the surveillance system. A good surveillance scheme must use sound definitions based on direct observation of the wound rather than laboratory records and must stratify infection rates according to risk factors. Another important consideration is post-discharge surveillance, which assumes increasing importance as inpatient stays become ever shorter. Between 12% and 84% of SSIs are now detected after the patient has been discharged from hospital, although most declare themselves within three weeks of the original procedure. Feedback should be provided to the surgeons themselves, who must have confidence in the data. Good surveillance with feedback is an important component of

strategies to reduce SSI risk. Since good surveillance is extremely time consuming, it should be targeted at high-risk procedures and used to answer specific questions.

The greatest experience with SSI surveillance comes from the USA, where the National Nosocomial Infections Surveillance (NNIS) system was established in the 1970s. Many European countries are now following suit. Broadly speaking, the reported incidence of infections found by the various national surveillance schemes is similar for comparable types of surgery. The results of NINSS surveillance in 96 hospitals in England between 1997 and 1999 are shown in Table 23.1. Caution should be used in interpreting these data, since some observations (e.g. cholecystectomy) are based on a very small number of infections.

Table 23.1 Incidence of SSI by surgical procedure (NINSS)

Procedure	Overall infection rate (%)	Proportion (%) of infections classified as:		
		Superficial	Deep	Organ or space
Abdominal hysterectomy	2.5	77.7	9.6	11.7
Bile duct, liver or pancreatic surgery	12.0	53.8	7.7	38.5
Cholecystectomy	2.1	100	0	0
Gastric surgery	10.9	65.0	20.0	15.0
Small bowel surgery	7.5	18.8	43.8	37.5
Large bowel surgery	10.4	55.8	26.9	15.6
Coronary artery bypass graft	3.9	69.1	24.6	5.8
Vascular surgery	8.1	77.6	14.4	8.0
Limb amputation	14.5	62.9	34.3	2.9
Open reduction of long bone fracture	3.4	59.4	12.5	28.1
Hip prosthesis	2.9	75.1	11.2	13.7
Knee prosthesis	2.1	84.0	9.0	6.0

Microbiology

The microbial aetiology of wound infections depends on the nature of the organisms liable to contaminate the surgical field. In all sites, however, the most important cause of SSI is *Staphylococcus aureus*. Although the virulence of *Staph. aureus* is complex and poorly understood, it is clearly well adapted to establish infection in damaged skin and tissues, particularly in the presence of foreign material such as sutures. Unfortunately, an increasing proportion of *Staph. aureus* infections worldwide is caused by strains resistant to multiple antibiotics (MRSA), many of which seem particularly well adapted to spread and persist within hospitals and retain comparable virulence to their antibiotic-susceptible counterparts. These are the so-called epidemic MRSA strains, those designated EMRSA 15 and 16 currently posing the greatest problems in hospitals in the United Kingdom. Deep-seated infections following bowel surgery are likely to be caused by a mixture of endogenous gut flora (i.e. Gram-negative aerobic bacilli such as *Escherichia coli*, anaerobic Gram-negative bacilli such as *Bacteroides fragilis*, capnophilic and anaerobic cocci, including the various species of streptococci comprising the 'milleri' group – *Streptococcus anginosus, Strep. constellatus* and *Strep. intermedius*). However, some of these organisms (*B. fragilis*, 'Streptococcus milleri' group) undoubtedly have greater intrinsic ability to cause infections than others, since they are isolated far more frequently from abscesses than their proportion as a component of gut flora would lead one to expect. The capsule of *B. fragilis* has been shown to be an important virulence factor and stimulates the formation of abscesses. Other organisms, such as *Strep. pyogenes*, are also important causes of severe SSIs. The range of pathogens isolated from SSIs reported to the NNIS scheme is shown in Table 23.2.

The presence or absence of SSI cannot be established on the basis of surface swab culture of the wound itself. Bacteria such as *Staph. aureus* can readily colonise the surface of a wound without causing infection. Furthermore, in the case of deep-seated infections with sinus formation, the flora at the surface may not reflect the flora deep in the wound and treatment based on surface swab cultures may be inappropiate. Quantitative cultures of wound tissue biopsies may give a better indication of infection, the presence of 10^5 bacteria per gram of tissue suggesting clinical infection. In practice, however, such cultures are rarely performed. Studies based simply on non-quantitative surface cultures may thus be misleading.

Table 23.2 Distribution of pathogens isolated from SSIs reported to the NNIS system (USA), 1990–96

Pathogen	Percentage of isolates
Staphylococcus aureus	20
Coagulase-negative staphylococci	14
Enterococcus spp	12
Escherichia coli	8
Pseudomonas aeruginosa	8
Enterobacter spp	7
Proteus mirabilis	3
Klebsiella pneumoniae	3
Other *Streptococcus* spp	3
Candida albicans	3
Group D streptococci	2
Other Gram-positive aerobes	2
Bacteroides fragilis	2

Prosthetic device infection

Prosthetic materials and implants will also influence the micro-organisms likely to cause wound infections. Not only does the presence of such materials lower the number of bacteria needed to initiate an infection but it also enables organisms that are generally considered as harmless commensals, such as coagulase-negative staphylococci (e.g. *Staph. epidermidis*) and other skin flora (e.g.

Corynebacterium spp, *Propionibacterium* spp), to cause significant sepsis. *Staph. epidermidis* produces an extracellular polysaccharide slime that enables it to adhere to plastics, which is an important virulence determinant in this setting.

Unlike *Staph. aureus* infections, those caused by these low-grade pathogens are generally indolent and rarely cause severe systemic sepsis but they may cause much chronic ill health and pain, as in prosthetic joint infections, or even death (e.g. prosthetic valve endocarditis). They are also extremely difficult to diagnose because the organisms involved are normal skin commensals, requiring deep biopsies to establish an aetiological role and to treat, usually necessitating removal of the prosthesis to have any chance of a cure.

Risk factors

Factors that increase the risk of the development of SSI can broadly be categorised into patient factors and operative factors. An understanding of these factors facilitates the analysis of surveillance data, allowing like to be compared with like. It also enables rational preventive strategies to be devised. Some of these factors are listed in Box 23.1. However, not all of these have been proved conclusively to be independent risk factors.

Simple classification of procedures according to the likelihood of bacterial contamination of the wound led to the well-known categorisation of operations as 'clean', 'clean-contaminated', 'contaminated' and 'dirty-infected'. The likelihood of infection in each type of surgery ranges from <2% for 'clean' operations to >30% for 'dirty-infected' procedures. However, more sophisticated stratification of risk is possible by incorporating measures such as duration of the operation and indices reflecting patient morbidity. Perhaps the best known are the SENIC and NNIS risk indices.

Box 23.1 Possible risk factors for SSI

Patient factors	**Operative factors**
Extremes of age	Preoperative skin preparation
Nutritional status	Preoperative shaving
● Malnutrition	Duration of surgical scrub
● Obesity	Skin antisepsis
Smoking	Duration of operation
Diabetes mellitus	Antimicrobial prophylaxis
Systemic steroid use	Operating room ventilation
Altered immune response	Inadequate sterilisation of
Coexistent infections at a	instruments
remote body site	Surgical drains
Colonisation with *Staph. aureus*	Surgical technique
Length of preoperative stay	● Asepsis
Preoperative transfusion	● Haemostasis
	● Failure to obliterate dead
	space
	● Tissue trauma
	Surgical attire and drapes
	Infected/colonised theatre staff
	Postoperative wound care

Prevention

Since the early ground-breaking work of people like Lister and Semmelweiss in the mid 19th century, a wide range of practices has been employed to reduce the risks of SSI. Some are well grounded in evidence and some are not, although many have become so enshrined in surgical ritual that they are unlikely ever to be questioned, let alone abandoned. The evidence base for preventive strategies has recently been comprehensively reviewed and categorised. These recommendations are summarised in Box 23.2. Clearly not all these recommendations are supported by equivalent evidence and some reflect surgical practice in the USA but not the UK.

Box 23.2 Recommendations for prevention of SSI (adapted from reference[2])

Preoperative

Patient
- Treat remote infections wherever possible.
- Do not remove hair unless it will interfere with operation, in which case use clippers immediately before the operation.
- Control diabetes mellitus.
- Encourage patient to stop smoking.
- Do not withhold blood products.
- Antiseptic shower the night before surgery.
- Wash around incision site prior to disinfection.
- Disinfect skin using iodophor, alcohol or chlorhexidine, in concentric circles.
- Keep preoperative stay as short as possible.

Surgical team
- Keep nails short
- Scrub for 2–5 minutes up to elbows, then keep hands up and away from body, dry hands with sterile towel and don sterile gown and gloves.
- Clean under each fingernail before first scrub of the day.
- Do not wear hand or arm jewellery.
- Report infections and develop exclusion policies for infected staff.

Antibiotic prophylaxis
- Give an appropriate antibiotic only when indicated.
- Give intravenously to establish bactericidal concentration when incision is made and continue until, at most, a few hours after the incision is closed.
- Mechanically prepare colon and give non-absorbable antimicrobials prior to bowel surgery. (NB: This reflects practice in the USA but not the UK.)

Intraoperative

Ventilation
- Maintain positive pressure in theatre.
- Maintain at least 15 air changes per hour, at least three of which are fresh air.
- Filter all air.
- Introduce air at ceiling and exhaust near the floor.
- Keep theatre doors closed as far as possible.
- Consider ultraclean air for orthopaedic implant surgery.
- Limit staff in theatre to essential personnel.

Cleaning and disinfection
- Disinfect visibly contaminated surfaces or equipment.
- Do not perform special cleaning after contaminated or dirty operations.
- Wet vacuum the floor after the last operation of the day.

Sampling
- Only sample the environment as part of an investigation, not routinely.

Sterilisation of instruments
- Sterilise all instruments.

Surgical attire and drapes
- Wear a mask that fully covers the mouth and nose throughout the operation.
- Wear a cap or hood to cover hair on head and face.
- Wear sterile gloves if scrub team member.
- Use gowns and drapes that resist liquid penetration.
- Change scrub suits when visibly soiled.

Asepsis and surgical technique
- Adhere to aseptic principles for all invasive procedures, including insertion of cannulas.
- Assemble sterile equipment and solutions immediately before use.
- Handle tissue gently, maintain effective haemostasis, minimise devitalised tissue and foreign bodies and eradicate dead space.
- Used delayed primary closure or leave open heavily contaminated wounds.
- Use closed suction drains only, through a separate incision.

Postoperative
- Protect incisions for 24–48 hours with a sterile dressing.
- Wash hands before and after dressing changes and use sterile technique.
- Educate patient/family about incision care and need to report SSI.
- Conduct surveillance according to recognised system and report to surgical team.

SOFT TISSUE INFECTION

Surgical wound infection

Many of the specific infections described below can complicate the surgical wound, though most infections are minor and may not require antibiotic treatment. Microbial contamination of the wound is inevitable in a small proportion of cases, even with modern aseptic technique and filtered air. A number of factors determine the chance of established infection:

- the patient
- the operation
- the organism
- the use of prophylactic antibiotics.

Local signs of inflammation and a purulent discharge are good indicators of infection. However, many patients will have been discharged from hospital before these are clinically apparent since the incubation period of *Staphylococcus aureus* wound infection is 5–7 days. For this and other reasons, it is difficult to generalise about wound infection rates, though it is likely that high-quality data will soon be available from a multicentre survey in England and Wales. This survey, the Nosocomial Infection National Surveillance Scheme (NINSS), has been established by the Public Health Laboratory Service. It includes a number of prospective studies looking at infections in different types of surgery. Confidential data on local wound infection rates are available to participating centres, together with anonymised overall results. Results are stratified by known risk factors and in some studies give anonymised surgeon-specific rates. Information on this ongoing project is available at the PHLS website.

Management of most surgical wound infections is straightforward. In many cases, drainage of the collection is all that is required. A swab or, ideally, aspirated pus should *always* be sent for culture. This will enable early detection of resistant organisms or cross-infection. Empirical therapy should include flucloxacillin as *Staph. aureus* is the most common cause. If infection complicates bowel surgery then use of an agent active against aerobic Gram-negative organisms should be considered. Antibiotic treatment of common complications of wound infection is summarised in Table 23.3.

Cellulitis

This is an acute, spreading infection of the skin and subcutaneous tissues. The usual local signs of inflammation are present, though the advancing margin of erythema often has an indistinct, impalpable edge. Patients are systemically unwell and septicaemia is common. It is a complication of peripheral oedema, trauma and leg ulcers. The microbiology of cellulitis is straightforward in most cases though immunocompromised patients may be infected with a wide range of uncommon organisms and the advice of a medical microbiologist should be sought prior to starting treatment.

Common causes of cellulitis include:

● *Staphylococcus aureus*

● group A streptococci

● groups C and G streptococci (rarely)

● anaerobes and *Pasteurella multocida* (after bite injuries).

The most useful investigation is blood culture, which must be collected prior to starting antibiotics. Swabs of any wounds may reveal the infecting organism and it is also worth swabbing between the toes of patients with cellulitis of the lower limb, as even very mild athlete's foot can be associated with group A streptococcal cellulitis. Attempts to isolate the causal organism by aspiration from the advancing edge are painful and rarely helpful, though this may be worthwhile if an unusual organism is suspected. Group A streptococcal infection in culture-negative cases may be confirmed by testing paired sera for anti-streptolysin O and anti-DNAase B. Antistaphylococcal antibody testing is too insensitive to be helpful.

Treatment of cellulitis

● Flucloxacillin and benzylpenicillin

● Elevation of the affected limb

Underdosing is common; an adult with normal renal function should be given at least 1 g of flucloxacillin and 1.8 g of benzylpenicillin six hourly. This is because antibiotic levels in the infected tissue will only be a fraction of blood levels. Elevation of the affected limb is crucial, as is adequate analgesia. Treatment of penicillin-allergic patients is difficult and a vague history of penicillin allergy should always be verified with the patient's general practitioner before committing the patient to suboptimal therapy. Erythromycin is often poorly absorbed orally and toxic to veins when given intravenously. Oral clindamycin is well absorbed and

Table 23.3 Empirical antibiotic treatment of soft tissue infection (adult patients with normal hepatic and renal function)		
	First choice	**Penicillin allergic**
Wound infection	Flucloxacillin 500 mg qds	Cephradine 500 mg qds (N.B. small risk of cross-allergy to cephradine)
Cellulitis	Flucloxacillin 1 g qds + benzylpenicillin 1.8 g qds	Clindamycin 300 mg qds
Infection after bites	Co-amoxiclav 1.2 g tds	Clindamycin 300 mg qds
Clostridial cellulitis/ myonecrosis/necrotizing fasciitis	Meropenem 1 g tds + clindamycin 600 mg qds	Meropenem 1 g tds + clindamycin 600 mg qds (N.B. small risk of cross-allergy to meropenem)
Pyomyositis	Flucloxacillin 1 g qds	Clindamycin 300 mg qds
Breast abscess (lactational)	Flucloxacillin 500 mg qds	Erythromycin 250 mg qds
Breast abscess (non-lactational)	Co-amoxiclav 375 mg tds	Erythromycin 250 mg qds + metronidazole 400 mg bd

very effective but is associated with pseudomembranous colitis, particularly in elderly patients. First-generation cephalosporins such as cephradine have good activity against the common causes of cellulitis but may also cause colitis and have a small but definite risk of cross-allergy with penicillin. In severe cases, an intravenous glycopeptide such as vancomycin may be required.

Response to antibiotics in severe cellulitis is slow and incomplete response 3–4 days into the course is not necessarily an indication to change treatment. Marking the edge of the erythema early on provides an objective assessment of response.

Clostridial cellulitis

This is a rare infection of devitalised subcutaneous tissues. It usually occurs following a dirty traumatic wound, especially if debridement is delayed or inadequate. Onset is gradual, systemic features are mild and the characteristic feature is a foul-smelling discharge and crepitus. The findings of Gram-positive rods in the discharge and gas within soft tissues on X-ray support the diagnosis but these investigations should not be allowed to delay surgical exploration, as this is the only reliable way to exclude clostridial myonecrosis (gas gangrene). Provided muscle involvement is excluded at operation, debridement can be limited to the necrotic subcutaneous tissue. Clostridia are highly sensitive to benzylpenicillin or metronidazole, though this is such a devastating infection that the combination of meropenem and clindamycin is advised until a mixed infection is excluded.

Necrotising fasciitis

This is a rapidly progressive necrotising infection of subcutaneous tissue and fascia. It encompasses a wide spectrum of infections, including Fournier's and Meleney's gangrene, though these subdivisions are of little practical importance. It is divided into two types by the causal organisms. Type I is a mixed infection, with anaerobes, Enterobacteriaecae and other organisms. It occurs in patients immunocompromised by age, diabetes or renal failure and may complicate abdominal and pelvic surgery (Figure 23.1). The affected area is extremely tender and the margin of erythema is diffuse. It progresses rapidly and the subcutaneous necrosis extends beneath normal skin. This may lead to thrombosis of small blood vessels with ischaemic necrosis and anaesthesia of skin outside the area of erythema. Patients are markedly systemically toxic and in the early stages this will appear out of proportion to the size of the skin lesions. The mortality is high, up to 43% if the diagnosis is delayed. Immediate surgical debridement down to normal fascia is essential and often has to be repeated after 24 hours. Microscopy and culture of debrided tissue should be performed, though the mixed infection means that full results may not be available for some days. Broad-spectrum antibiotics are used, an appropriate combination being meropenem and clindamycin intravenously until culture results are available. Hyperbaric oxygen therapy is a potential adjunct to surgery and

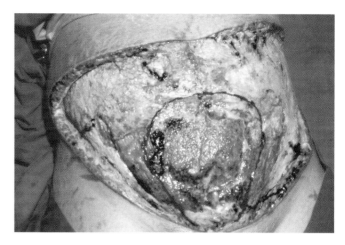

Figure 23.1 Type I necrotising fasciitis in a 17-year-old female after caesarean section. *E. coli* and *Peptostreptococcus anaerobius* were isolated from infected tissue (courtesy of Mr D Hanley, Derriford Hospital, Plymouth).

antibiotics for this condition, though by its nature controlled trials are difficult and unequivocal evidence of benefit is not available. Local experience suggests that it is effective in type I infection.

Type II fasciitis involves group A beta-haemolytic streptococci, either alone or in combination with other organisms. It may affect patients with underlying medical conditions but can also cause a devastatingly rapid infection in young, previously fit people (Figure 23.2). Clusters of infection have been described but these have been found to involve different strains of streptococci and there is no evidence that highly virulent individual strains cause outbreaks of fasciitis in the community. The clinical features are

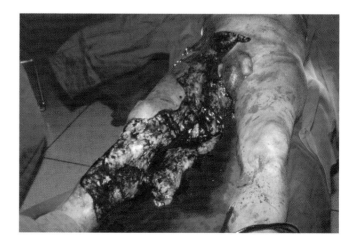

Figure 23.2 Necrotising fasciitis following routine varicose vein surgery. The patient recovered with a good functional and cosmetic result (illustration kindly provided by Professor A Kingsnorth).

similar to type I fasciitis, though it often affects the limbs or head and neck. Bullae are common but not diagnostic. Once again, the mainstay of therapy is complete surgical debridement. Group A streptococci remain highly susceptible to benzylpenicillin and this should be given in combination with clindamycin. Clindamycin is believed to reduce the production of exotoxin by group A streptococci and is more active than penicillin where organisms are multiplying rapidly, at the advancing edge of the lesion. There is no evidence that hyperbaric oxygen therapy affects the outcome, though it is often used if available.

Pyomyositis

This is an acute intramuscular infection, usually caused by *Staph. aureus*, rarely by group A beta-haemolytic streptococci or other organisms. There may be a history indicating local inoculation or contiguous spread, though haematogenous infection can also occur. Haematogenous infection probably requires a local injury or vigorous exercise of the involved muscle in order to become established. It may take 7–10 days before sufficient pus has accumulated to make the diagnosis and clinical signs up to this stage are often non-specific. Surgical drainage and intravenous flucloxacillin should be used until culture results are available.

Clostridial myonecrosis

This is an extension of clostridial cellulitis (see above) and presents in the same way, though severe pain is usual. The crucial difference is the gross appearance of the muscle at operation. Early on the muscle is pale, oedematous and does not bleed. It will not contract on stimulation. Later it becomes friable and discoloured. Antibiotics are used as in clostridial cellulitis but again the mainstay of treatment is surgery. All involved muscle must be excised, with limb amputation if necessary. Hyperbaric oxygen therapy is likely to be helpful if available. This infection may present in the buttocks or abdomen secondary to a mucosal lesion of the colon. This complication of colonic cancer is particularly associated with *Clostridium septicum* and has a high mortality.

Breast abscess

Adult breast abscesses are divided into lactational and non-lactational. Lactational abscesses are most common in the first month after delivery. They may follow a non-infectious mastitis, caused by obstruction of mammary ducts by breastfeeding in an awkward position. Mastitis at this stage can be improved by encouraging drainage of milk from the affected segment, without use of antibiotics. Once an abscess has developed, aspiration or incision and drainage and oral flucloxacillin should be started. Most lactational abscesses are caused by *Staph. aureus*; the few that are caused by anaerobic streptococci are best treated with co-amoxiclav, as metronidazole makes the milk bitter and will inhibit feeding. The above antibiotics and erythromycin are safe in breastfeeding and continued feeding should be encouraged.

Non-lactational infections may affect the periareolar region in young women. This is likely to be a superinfection of preexisting periductal mastitis, exacerbated by smoking. The microbial cause is less predictable in non-lactating women; co-amoxiclav or flucloxacillin with metronidazole are appropriate empirical therapy. Recurrence is not uncommon as antibiotics will not affect the underlying ductal pathology. Peripheral abscesses may also occur, often associated with diabetes or steroid therapy. These abscesses may be multifocal and require repeated aspiration. Pus should be sent for culture prior to starting antibiotics, particularly in recurrent infection. Any residual thickening or persistent refilling of a cystic lesion should be reaspirated and submitted for cytological appraisal as well as culture.

Tetanus

Vaccine coverage for tetanus in the UK is over 95% and consequently this infection is extremely rare, with less than 10 confirmed cases each year. Most cases occur in the elderly or in immigrants who have not been vaccinated, when spores of *Clostridium tetani* become implanted deep into a wound where conditions are anaerobic. A powerful exotoxin is produced which causes muscle spasm, initially apparent at the site of the injury and in the facial muscles but also involving the back, neck, abdomen and extremities. Autonomic dysfunction also occurs and is now the leading cause of death. Most cases occur within two weeks of the injury but cases have been reported after several months. The diagnosis is clinical; microbiological investigations have no role in the initial management.

Treatment of tetanus

- Debridement of the wound
- Intramuscular tetanus immunoglobulin
- Intravenous metronidazole
- Benzodiazepines
- Ventilatory support

Adequate surgical debridement of the wound site is essential to prevent further systemic diffusion of the toxin. There may be no local signs at the site of the injury so an accurate history is crucial. Remarkably, the amount of toxin required to produce these life-threatening symptoms is insufficient to produce immunity and vaccination after recovery is necessary. Immunisation in the UK was introduced in 1961 (1938 for members of the armed forces) and consists of three doses of adsorbed tetanus vaccine one month apart, starting at two months of age. Booster doses are given at school entry and before leaving school. Further booster doses are unnecessary and may cause local reactions. Tetanus-prone wounds include puncture wounds, wounds or burns left unattended for over six hours, wounds with dead tissue, evidence of sepsis or soil contamination. A dose of human tetanus immunoglobulin is recommended if the risk of infection is particularly high or if the patient is not immunised, partially immunised or does not know their status.

Toxic shock syndrome (TSS)

Classically associated with hyperabsorbent tampons, this syndrome also occurs when a burn or a surgical wound becomes colonised by toxin-producing strains of *Staph. aureus*. Invasive infection need not occur; the clinical features are caused by systemic absorption of toxin. The diagnostic criteria are given in Box 23.3. A number of staphylococcal toxins, including TSST-1, and enterotoxins can produce the syndrome, probably by acting as superantigens. Most patients who develop TSS do not have detectable antibody to the toxins before the illness, though 90% of the general adult population do. This suggests that TSS is more a complication of unusual susceptibility in an individual patient than a particularly virulent organism. Routine testing of isolates for toxin production is not necessary and standard infection control procedures are sufficient.

Treatment includes aggressive fluid replacement and flucloxacillin, with removal of colonised dressings or packs. Normal human immunoglubulin contains high levels of neutralising antibody to the toxins and while there is no controlled evidence of benefit, its use in severe cases is logical. A similar condition has been described in group A streptococcal infection, though this is more a complication of invasive infection than absorption of toxin. Again, there is anecdotal evidence of benefit from normal immunoglobulins.

Box 23.3   Diagnostic criteria for toxic shock syndrome

1. Temperature >38.9°C
2. Systolic BP <90 mmHg
3. Rash with subsequent desquamation, especially on palms and soles

Together with three or more of the following:
- diarrhoea or vomiting
- myalgia or raised CK
- hyperaemia of mucous membranes
- renal impairment
- abnormal liver enzymes
- thrombocytopenia
- confusion

POSTOPERATIVE PNEUMONIA

Pneumonia is the leading cause of infectious mortality in hospitalised patients. Surgery and prolonged intubation are the main predisposing factors; others include age, depressed level of consciousness, nasogastric tubes and underlying medical illnesses. Aspiration is the main method of entry of organisms into the lower respiratory tract. Many reports, particularly from US studies, suggest that aerobic Gram-negative bacilli and *Staph. aureus* are the predominant causes.

Defining the aetiology of postoperative pneumonia is extremely difficult, as many patients are unable to produce an adequate sputum sample. The preponderance of Gram-negatives may merely reflect colonisation of the oropharynx and the lingering effects of prophylactic antibiotics. Antibiotics should be started after blood cultures and, if possible, a sputum sample should be collected in patients who are pyrexial with no other focus, with new infiltrates on chest X-ray or clinical signs of consolidation. The choice of agent depends on previous antibiotics and local resistance data; our local recommendation is either oral levofloxacin or intravenous co-amoxiclav. Cephalosporins such as cefotaxime are widely used in this situation but carry a significant risk of *C. difficile* colitis.

Legionnaire's disease has caused major outbreaks in hospitals in the past. However, this should no longer be a major risk with adequate maintenance of water supplies and cooling towers.

Aspiration pneumonitis is a sterile inflammatory response to gastric acid aspiration. It may be complicated by infection but there is no evidence to support the use of antibiotics in the acute stage.

Selective decontamination of the digestive tract (SDD) is a strategy which aims to prevent pneumonia in intubated patients. It involves prophylactic use of a cephalosporin for three days after admission with concurrent application of a mixture of non-absorbed, broad-spectrum antibiotics to eliminate aerobic gut organisms. Its use remains controversial and is limited to centres with a particular interest in this area.

URINARY TRACT INFECTION

This is one of the most common hospital-acquired infections. Predisposing factors postoperatively include immobility and indwelling catheters. Bacteriuria develops in up to 27% of catheterised patients within five days and is almost universal after 10 days. Colonising organisms include *Enterobacteriacae, Enterococci, Staphylococci* and *Candida spp*, often in mixed growth. The conventional criterion of >10^5 colony-forming units/ml for significant growth in ambulant patients is meaningless when a catheter is present. The main purpose served by a CSU result is to provide susceptibility data in case the patient later develops septicaemia. Asymptomatic patients with colonised catheters should not be treated, as recurrence of resistant strains is inevitable unless the catheter is removed. If a patient remains bacteriuric following catheter removal a three-day course of appropriate oral therapy should be considered, remembering that asymptomatic bacteriuria in the elderly is common and usually harmless. Prophylaxis prior to urological surgery in the presence of bacteriuria is essential as there is a significant risk of septicaemia if it is inadvertently omitted. A single dose of gentamicin is widely used and highly effective. There are situations where this is inadequate, e.g. if the urine is colonised with MRSA. This is unlikely in a patient admitted from the community but should be considered prior to surgery on a patient from a ward involved in an outbreak.

MULTIRESISTANT *STAPHYLOCOCCUS AUREUS* (MRSA)

The term MRSA was initially used to describe strains resistant to methicillin which was a precursor of flucloxacillin and is no longer used. The importance of methicillin resistance is that it predicts resistance to all beta-lactam antibiotics (notably flucloxacillin) and also all cephalosporins. Most strains of MRSA have acquired resistance to other classes of antibiotic and may also express virulence factors which lead to rapid dissemination within a hospital. A typical example is the strain EMRSA-16, which caused a major outbreak in Kettering in 1991 and has since spread to most hospitals in the UK.

A typical susceptibility profile of EMRSA-16 is as follows.

- All penicillins   Resistant
- All cephalosporins   Resistant
- Erythromycin   Resistant
- Quinolones   Resistant
- Gentamicin   Resistant (varies according to strain)
- Mupirocin   Resistant (varies according to strain)
- Vancomycin   Susceptible
- Teicoplanin   Susceptible
- Fucidic acid   Susceptible (never use as single agent)
- Rifampicin   Susceptible (never use as single agent)

MRSA strains are no more virulent than sensitive *Staph. Aureus*; their importance lies in the difficulty of treating them when infection does occur. The only oral therapy possible for many strains of MRSA is the combination of rifampicin with fusidic acid. This combination is hepatotoxic and should not be given for more than five days without monitoring of hepatic enzymes. Vancomycin is the most widely used intravenous treatment for MRSA. It must be infused over at least one hour, is usually given twice daily and needs regular monitoring of predose levels. Monitoring of postdose levels is not necessary. It is inherently less active than flucloxacillin and penetrates poorly into abscesses, infected bone and CSF. The main mode of spread of MRSA is on the hands of those caring for colonised patients. This hand carriage is usually transient and the chain of infection is broken by hand washing between each patient. MRSA can survive for hours on hard surfaces, so maintaining a clean clinical environment is also important.

A great deal of guidance is available on control of MRSA infection, though the efficacy of most measures is unproven. Guidelines endorsed by the Hospital Infection Society are available on their website. The local infection control team should always be consulted about specific issues as national guidelines can only represent a consensus view, which may not always be appropriate. Standard preoperative prophylaxis may need to be modified when a patient is known to carry MRSA. For orthopaedic or cardiac surgery, a glycopeptide is a suitable replacement for cephalosporin. It is often impractical to administer vancomycin by infusion in the preoperative period so a single bolus dose of teicoplanin may be the best option. This will not protect against later wound infection, so obsessional attention to aseptic technique when changing dressings is essential.

CLOSTRIDIUM DIFFICILE

Diarrhoea caused by overgrowth of toxin-producing strains of *C. difficile* is an increasing problem in surgical patients. The causative organism is carried by up to 14% of acute elderly patients and diarrhoea usually follows the use of antibiotics, though occasional cases have been precipitated by chemotherapy or immunosuppressants. There is wide variation in the relative risk of *C. difficile* diarrhoea for different antibiotics but unfortunately cefotaxime and co-amoxiclav are highly associated with this complication. Metaanalysis has been used to rank antibiotics for *C. difficile* diarrhoea risk. Tetracyclines are the least associated agents while cefotaxime had the strongest association.

The risk of *C. difficile* diarrhoea is minimised by avoiding unnecessary antibiotics, using narrow-spectrum agents wherever possible and implementing standard isolation procedures for patients with diarrhoea. *C. difficile* diarrhoea is diagnosed by detection of toxin, either by ELISA or its cytopathic effect in cell culture. This is a relatively expensive test and few laboratories are able to test every inpatient specimen. It is essential to inform the laboratory that the patient has had antibiotics to ensure appropriate investigations are performed. Repeat testing is not helpful as toxin may be detectable in stool for weeks after the illness has resolved. Many cases will resolve with withdrawal of the precipitating antibiotic; if not, the treatment of choice is oral metronidazole. Oral vancomycin is equally effective but expensive and may be associated with development of vancomycin-resistant enterococci. Patients who cannot take oral medication should be treated with intravenous metronidazole as intravenous vancomycin does not reach effective levels in the gut. Relapse after initially successful treatment occurs in up to 37% of cases, though many of these are due to reinfection rather than recurrence. Antimotility agents have been associated with worsening of *C. difficile* diarrhoea, presumably because of accumulation of toxin in the gut lumen. The evidence base for this is not strong and antimotility agents may have a role in less severe cases.

VIRAL GASTROENTERITIS

The most important cause of viral gastroenteritis is the small round structured viruses, often loosely referred to as Norwalk virus, though in fact a number of distinct strains occur. They circulate widely in the community and are a frequent cause of hospital outbreaks with a winter seasonality. Their main importance to surgical practice is the disruption they cause if introduced to a surgical ward. The illness is characterised by projectile vomiting and diarrhoea and the secondary attack rate among staff and patients is extremely high. The incubation period is usually about 48 hours and closure of the ward is usually necessary to control the outbreak. Patients and staff from an affected ward should not be transferred to other wards or units until the outbreak is over. In practice, this is usually at least 72 hours after the last symptomatic case. The ward environment must be thoroughly cleaned before admitting new susceptible patients if another wave of cases is to be avoided. A crucial aspect of infection control, often forgotten by surgical trainees, is the need to stop work immediately if GI symptoms develop. The inconvenience this causes to colleagues is negligible compared with the consequences of a member of staff vomiting billions of infectious virus particles on the ward or theatre coffee room! The pattern of the illness allows a reliable clinical diagnosis and confirmation is by electron microscopy of faeces or PCR.

BLOODBORNE VIRUSES AND SURGERY

Bloodborne viruses (BBV), particularly HIV, hepatitis B (HBV) and hepatitis C (HCV), are an increasing hazard of surgical practice. Not only may they cause serious illness to surgeons who acquire them occupationally, they may also bring a surgical career to a premature end. Guidance on the ability of surgeons who carry BBV to practise surgery is under constant review and up-to-date recommendations are available on the UK Department of Health website and summarized in Table 23.4. The following is general guidance on avoiding infection with or transmission of these agents.

Surgery on BBV carriers

The prevalence of these viruses varies enormously in different ethnic and social groups and in general, preoperative screening is not performed. This is because of the practical difficulty of obtaining informed consent, the issue of false negatives and, more frequently, false positives and the use of universal precautions whether the patient is a BBV carrier or not. At the time of writing there are about 16 000 known HIV-positive people in England and Wales, over 600 newly diagnosed cases of acute hepatitis B and over 3000 new reports of hepatitis C each year. The mortality from HIV has plummeted with the use of effective antiretroviral therapy and its prevalence is likely to increase substantially. It should also be remembered that most cases of hepatitis B and C are asymptomatic and reported cases are only a fraction of the true prevalence.

Exposure-prone procedures (EPP)

These are defined as procedures where there is a risk that injury to the worker may result in exposure of the patient's open tissues to the blood of the worker. These procedures include those where the worker's gloved hands may be in contact with sharp instruments, needle tips or sharp tissues (spicules of bone or teeth) inside a patient's open body cavity, wound or confined anatomical space where the hands or fingertips may not be completely visible at all times. Examples and more detailed guidance are available on the UK Department of Health's website.

Vaccination against BBV

All surgeons carrying out exposure-prone procedures should be immunised against HBV and have their response checked. This covers virtually all surgery, with the possible exception of some endoscopic procedures. Following a case where a carrier surgeon submitted another person's blood sample for analysis, this is now performed by the hospital occupational health department. Current guidance is that those who produce an anti-HBs level greater than 100 IU should have a single booster five years later. Further immunisation of those whose level is between 10 IU and 100 IU is complex and should be discussed individually. Non-responders must be tested for natural HBV infection. Most of these will have cleared the virus (HBsAg negative) and can practise normally. If they are HBsAg positive the sample should be tested urgently for HBeAg. This is a marker of high infectivity and surgeons positive for this marker are not allowed to continue doing EPP. Current guidance suggests that HBsAg-

Table 23.4 Ability of BBV-carrying surgeons to practise	
Status of surgeon	Restriction of surgical practice (as of October 2000)
Anti-HIV +	Cannot perform exposure-prone invasive procedures
HβsAg +, HβeAg +	Cannot perform exposure-prone invasive procedures
HβsAg +, HβeAg − or indeterminate	Can practise normally if HBV viral load is < 10³ copies/ml
HβsAg −, anti-HBc +	No restriction of practice (immune from past infection)
Anti-HCV +	Can practise normally unless shown to have transmitted HCV to a patient

positive, HBeAg-negative surgeons can continue to practise if their HBV viral load is less than 10^3 copies/ml. Outbreaks of hepatitis B from carriers with this serological profile are well described and it is likely that the guidance may be modified in the future. Effective vaccines against HCV and HIV are probably many years away, as both of these are RNA viruses, with a high rate of mutation.

Risk reduction strategies

Most surgical injuries are caused by sharp suture needles, usually to the non-dominant index finger. A high proportion are caused to the assistant by the operator. The rate varies between procedures: the rate of percutaneous injury has been quoted as 10% for abdominal and 21% for vaginal hysterectomies. Double gloving reduces the rate of inner glove puncture and may also reduce the risk of viral transmission by wiping the external surface of the needle. Blunt-tipped needles and staples are the safest option where their use is appropriate.

General management of inoculation injuries

All UK health authorities and NHS trusts are required to have a designated doctor and local policy for the management of blood exposure incidents. The detail of where to seek advice, availability of testing and postexposure prophylaxis will vary between centres. Surgeons should familiarise themselves with their local arrangements as uncertainty about the need for prophylaxis after an incident is stressful and may be extremely dangerous.

Immediately following an exposure, the wound should be washed liberally with soap and water but without scrubbing. Exposed mucous membranes should be irrigated copiously. Puncture wounds should be gently encouraged to bleed but not sucked. Our local practice is for the injured member of staff to go to the accident and emergency department where a blood sample is collected for long-term storage. Another doctor or nurse will seek consent from the patient for urgent hepatitis B surface antigen and hepatitic C antibody testing in all cases. It is exceptional for this request to be refused. It is not considered necessary for UK surgeons to cease operating pending serological follow-up after an exposure to bloodborne viruses, though they should not donate blood or carry an organ donor card and consideration should be given to safe sex procedures.

Potential HIV exposure

If the patient is in an at-risk group for HIV infection, it is crucial that postexposure prophylaxis is made available as soon as possible, ideally within one hour. It is not usually possible to HIV test the source patient within this timeframe, so in most cases the

injured health-care worker will need to decide whether to start antiretroviral therapy on the basis of incomplete information. Guidelines on the management of this dilemma have been drawn up by the Expert Advisory Group on AIDS. These suggest the use of zidovudine, lamivudine and indinavir for four weeks. This combination causes significant nausea and vomiting and about a third of recipients discontinue the drugs early as a result. This combination may not be optimal if the exposure is from a patient who has been on antiretroviral therapy and who may have selected out a resistant virus, in which case prompt advice from a local expert is required.

HBV exposure

In contrast to HIV, management of hepatitis B exposure is straightforward. All surgeons should know their HBV immune status and known responders to the vaccine are usually given a booster dose as a precaution, though there is no evidence that this is necessary. Non-responders will require intramuscular hepatitis B immunoglobulin as soon as possible after the injury.

HCV exposure

At present there is no postexposure prophylaxis for hepatitis C. Our local policy is to test any anti-HCV positive source patients by PCR. If this is negative, the risk of transmission is infinitesimal. If the source patient is PCR positive, the health-care worker is tested by PCR six weeks after the injury and for anti-HCV at six months. The aim is to detect transmission of HCV as early as possible. This is because there is some evidence that interferon treatment early in the course of HCV infection is more effective at eradicating the virus.

Surgery by BBV carriers

Detailed advice on the management of surgeons who are or may be HIV infected is available on the Department of Health's website. In essence, any surgeon who thinks they might have been exposed to HIV infection should seek confidential advice from a specialist occupational health physician. They must not rely on their own assessment of the risk they pose to patients. At present, UK health-care workers are not permitted to carry out exposure-prone invasive procedures if they are HIV or hepatitis B e antigen (HBeAg) positive. Surgeons with chronic hepatitis C are permitted to continue operating unless they are shown to have transmitted infection to a patient. This is extremely rare, with only one proven case in the UK. Likewise, carriers of hepatitis B who are e antigen negative must have their HBV viral load measured as some HBeAg-negative carriers are highly infectious carriers of what is called a precore mutant virus. Such carriers are best detected by PCR for HBV DNA, a test which is only available in specialist reference laboratories.

INFECTION OF INTRAVASCULAR DEVICES

Aetiology and pathogenesis

Many of the considerations mentioned above in relation to prosthetic device infections also apply to infections of intravascular devices (IVD). These devices, with the exception of totally implantable systems, breach one of the body's most efficient defence systems, the skin, giving a variety of organisms direct access to the bloodstream. Furthermore, they are foreign bodies which act as a nidus for infection, permitting relatively avirulent organisms to gain a foothold and rendering eradication of pathogens extremely difficult.

Staphylococci are the most common causes of intravascular line infections. *Staph. aureus* infections are usually associated with more pronounced signs of inflammation at insertion sites and more profound systemic disturbance than those caused by coagulase-negative staphylococci. A wide range of other organisms, including Gram-negative bacilli (Enterobacteriaceae, *Pseudomonas* spp, *Acinetobacter* spp and other environmental bacteria), Gram-positive bacilli and cocci (including streptococci, *Corynebacterium* spp and *Propionibacterium* spp) and yeasts may also infect IVDs. Central venous cannulas, which are usually left *in situ* for longer periods of time, become infected more frequently than peripheral cannulas, although the latter are the most common source of hospital-acquired *Staph. aureus* bacteraemia. Yeast infections are particularly associated with the use of total parenteral nutrition.

Diagnosis

Infection of an IVD should be considered in any febrile patient in whom a line is or has recently been present. The single most important investigation is a blood culture, although obviously even a positive blood culture does not prove that a line is the source of the bacteraemia. Cultures of exit sites are also potentially helpful if the site is inflamed, although the presence of skin organisms (e.g. coagulase-negative staphylococci) in such sites is difficult to interpret. Paired blood cultures from both the IVD and a peripheral vein may be helpful, particularly if a quantitative technique is used, although these are not employed routinely in many centres. Removal of the IVD and culture of the tip, usually semiquantitatively, allows retrospective diagnosis but by definition means that the vascular access has been lost and so techniques such as intraluminal brush culture, which permit retention of non-infected lines, are gaining in popularity.

Treatment

If a line is no longer required, it should obviously be removed immediately. In some situations (e.g. infection with relatively avirulent bacteria, such as coagulase-negative staphylococci), this may be all that is needed for complete resolution of the infection. In other situations (e.g. where vascular access is still necessary), the position is more difficult. Some success in salvaging lines infected with organisms of low virulence has been achieved through the use of relatively long courses (usually at least two weeks) of antibiotic therapy. Since these organisms are often resistant to several antibiotics, treatment should be guided by susceptibility patterns and frequently involves the use of glycopeptide agents such as vancomycin. If the infection fails to resolve, if severe systemic disturbance is present or if the infection is caused by organisms that are known to be difficult to eradicate (e.g. Gram negatives, Candida *spp*), then removal of the line is mandatory.

Prevention

National guidelines for the prevention of infection associated with IVDs were produced in the USA in the mid 1990s and similar guidelines are being prepared in the UK by the EPIC project. Recommendations for the prevention of infection related to central venous cannulas are given in Box 23.4.

Box 23.4 Recommendations for the prevention of infections associated with the use of central venous catheters (CVCs)

- Use single lumen catheter if possible.
- Use an exclusively designated catheter for TPN.
- Use a tunnelled or implantable device if long-term access (> 30 days) is anticipated.
- If possible use subclavian lines or peripherally inserted catheters, in preference to jugular or femoral lines.
- Use aseptic technique, including sterile gown, gloves and drapes, during insertion.
- Disinfect the insertion site with chlorhexidine or povidone iodine.
- Disinfect the catheter hub as above before accessing the system.
- Use either a sterile gauze or transparent dressing on the insertion site.
- Replace gauze dressings if damp, loose, soiled or removed for inspection of the site.
- Do not use antimicrobial ointments routinely on the insertion site.
- Routinely flush catheters with anticoagulant.
- Do not routinely replace non-tunnelled CVCs as a prophylactic measure.
- If infection is suspected but there is no evidence of insertion site infection, replace catheter over guidewire.
- If infection is proven, replace catheter at a different site.
- Replace all tubing when a CVC is replaced.
- Replace tubing and stopcocks no more frequently than 72 hourly unless clinically indicated.
- Replace tubing used to administer blood, blood products or lipid emulsions at the end of the infusion or within 24 hours of starting the infusion.
- Do not use routine systemic antibiotic prophylaxis before insertion or during use of CVC.

ANTIBIOTIC POLICIES

Treatment

There is increasing concern about both the rising incidence of hospital-acquired infection and the growing prevalence of antibiotic-resistant bacteria. Rational use of antibiotics is a vital component of control measures for both of these problems. The ecological benefits of avoiding the unnecessary use of antibiotics, both in hospital and the community, seem self-evident. Antibiotic use in an individual patient may also render them more likely to acquire infection with bacteria resistant to one or more antimicrobials and is an essential prerequisite for infection with some nosocomial pathogens, such as *Clostridium difficile*.

Consequently, greater emphasis is being given to the development and enforcement of policies and guidelines for antibiotic use in hospitals and the community. It is beyond the scope of this chapter to give details of a policy for the use of antibiotics in all possible clinical situations. Furthermore, local variations in the aetiology of hospital-acquired infection and resistance patterns make this inappropriate. However, readers should familiarise themselves with the policy in their own institution. At the very least, doctors should develop the habit of asking themselves a few key questions before prescribing an antibiotic.

- Are this patient's signs/symptoms likely to be due to bacterial infection?

- If so, where and what are the likely infecting species?

- Would measures other than antibiotic therapy (e.g. removal of invasive devices, surgical drainage) help to avoid a need for antibiotics?

Similarly, the continued need for antibiotic therapy should be reviewed daily in all patients undergoing treatment including, where appropriate, consideration of a less invasive mode of administration (e.g. oral or rectal in preference to intravenous or intramuscular).

Prophylaxis

The appropriate use of prophylactic antibiotics has been a key development in the prevention of surgical infections. Again, it would be inappropriate to give detailed advice in a book such as this and readers are referred to the guidelines in their own hospitals. It is worth noting when reading the literature that there are considerable differences in practice from country to country, both in the choice of agents (e.g. cefazolin, widely recommended in the USA, is not available in the UK) and in the mode of administration (e.g. the use of non-absorbed intraluminal agents for colonic surgery, which has been recommended in the USA but rarely adopted in the UK). A few important principles should also be borne in mind when prescribing surgical prophylaxis.

- The agent(s) chosen should be active against the organisms likely to contaminate the operative field.

- They should be present at appropriate concentrations in the tissues at the time when contamination is most likely to occur. In most situations this can be achieved by giving the first dose with induction of anaesthesia. In prolonged operations further doses may need to be given after 1–2 half-lives of the agent concerned.

- There is little evidence that further doses are necessary after the operation has finished. At the very most, only one or two postoperative doses should be given.

Prophylaxis is generally considered as indicated in the following situations.

- Procedures that entail entry into the gastrointestinal tract.
- Head and neck procedures that entail entry into the oropharynx.
- Abdominal and lower extremity vascular procedures.
- Craniotomy.
- Orthopaedic procedures with hardware insertion.
- Cardiac procedures with median sternotomy.
- Hysterectomy.
- Caesarean section.
- Other prosthetic implants.

Prophylaxis is considered optional in the following circumstances.

- Breast and hernia procedures.
- Other clean procedures considered to be at high risk of infection.
- Clean procedures in which contamination takes place.
- Low-risk gastric and biliary procedures.

Finally, one simple measure that may increase compliance with agreed policies for surgical prophylaxis is the printing of sticky labels giving a limited choice of 'approved' regimens, which can be affixed to prescription charts.

FURTHER INFORMATION

1 PHLS website: http://www.phls.co.uk/

2 Department of Health website. http://www.doh.gov.uk/dhhome.htm

3 DoH. *Guidance on Postexposure Prophylaxis for Health-care Workers Occupationally Exposed to HIV*. PL/CO(97)1. London: Department of Health, 1999

4 UK Health Departments. *AIDS/HIV Infected Health Care Workers: Guidance on the Management of Infected Health Care Workers and Patient Notification*. London: UK Health Departments, 1998

5 Mandell G, Bennett J, Dolin. *Principles and Practice of Infectious Diseases*, 4th edn. New York: Churchill Livingstone, 1995

6   Ayliffe G, Babb J, Taylor L. *Hospital-acquired Infection*, 3rd edn. Oxford: Butterworth Heinemann, 1999

7   DoH *Hepatitis B Infected Health Care Workers*. HSC 2000/020 London: Department of Health, 2000

8   Plowman R, Graves N, Griffin M et al. *The Socio-economic Burden of Hospital-acquired Infection*. London: Public Health Laboratory Service, 2000

9   Pearson A, Wilson J, Ward V. *Surveillance of Surgical Site Infection in English Hospitals 1997–1999*. London: Public Health Laboratory Service, 2000

Index

Note: references to figures are indicated by '(f)', references to tables by '(t)', and boxes by '(box)' when they fall on a page not covered by the text reference.

A

abdomen
  diagnostic radiology 30–2, 33(f)
  incisions 53
    Gridiron 56, 57(f)
    Kocher's 55
    Lanz 56, 57(f)
    lower midline 53–4
    McEvedy's 55
    paramedian 54–5
    Pfannenstiel 56
    upper midline 53, 54(f)
abscess
  anorectal 79–81
  breast 44–6, 330
  formation 305
acetylcholine, at neuromuscular junction 234–7
acetylcholine receptor 235–6
acetylcholinesterase 236
  antagonists, reversal of neuromuscular blockade 239–40
acid–base balance
  buffering systems 181–2
  disturbances of 182–4
  interpretation of changes 184–5
acquired gastric outlet obstruction (pyloric stenosis) 218
action potentials 233–4, 237
acute renal failure, and fluid balance 186–8
adrenal insufficiency 256–7
aeseptic technique 5–6
age, and cancer incidence 280
ageing, of cells 287–8
agenesis 277
airway obstruction, from foreign bodies 126–7
albumin, for transfusion 207
alcohols, as antiseptics 5
allergies 209–10
alloreactivity 210
aminoglycosides, effect on neuromuscular system 241
amyloid 286–7
anaemia
  deficiency of haematinics 193–4
  haemoglobin level and surgery 196
  haemolytic 194–5
anal fissure 77–9
analgesia, methods
  cordotomy 248

epidural 247–8
local anaesthetic blocks 247
patient-controlled analgesia 248
transcutaneous electrical nerve stimulation (TENS) 248
analgesics
  clonidine 246
  ketamine 247
  local anaesthetics 244–5
  mechanisms of action 242–4
  non-steroidal antiinflammatory drugs (NSAIDs) 246
  opiates 245–6
  tramadol 247
aneurysms
  atherosclerotic 311
  berry 313–14
  Charcot–Bouchard 314
  definition 311
  dissecting aneurysms of the aorta 311–13
  infective 313
  inflammatory aortic 313
angioedema 210
anion gap, and metabolic acidosis 183
anorectal abscess
  clinical features 79–80
  incision and drainage 80–1
anorectal fistula
  clinical features 81
  operative procedures 81–2
antibiotics, policies on 336
anticholinesterases, reversal of neuromuscular blockade 239–40
anticoagulants 203
  and surgery 197, 198(box)
antidiuretic hormone (ADH) 178–9
antiphospholipid syndrome, and thrombosis 202
antiseptics 5
antithrombin deficiency, and thrombosis 201
aplasia 277
aponeuroses, handling techniques 7
apoptosis 299
  and tumour development 281
appendiectomy 57–8
arachidonic acid metabolites, and inflammation 302(t), 303
areolar tissue, handling techniques 6–7
arterial system, interventional radiology 36–7
arterial thrombosis 200

arteriosclerosis, definition 314
aspiration cytology *see* fine needle aspiration cytology (FNAC)
aspirin, for thrombosis treatment 203
atherosclerosis
  aneurysms 311
  atheromatous plaques, morphology 315–16
  characteristics 314, 315(f)
  epidemiology and risk factors 316–17
  pathogenesis 317
atrophy 278
autoimmune disease 304–5

B

benign tumours
  classification 283
  definition 264–5
Bier's block 11
biliary system
  biliary fistulas 222
  contrast radiology 28
  imaging 32
  interventional radiology 35–6
biopsy specimens
  fine needle aspiration cytology 292–5
  fixation and transport 291–2
  frozen sections 291
  microbiological specimens 295–6
  procedures for 291
bleeding disorders
  congenital 197
  patient assessment 200
blood
  components 193
  donation 204
  loss
    assessment 18–19
    and fluid balance 185–6
  microbiological specimens 296
  transfusion 19
    autologous transfusion 208
    blood costs 207
    blood products 206–7
    blood substitutes 20, 208
    complications 19–20, 207–8
    crossmatching 204–5
    effects on coagulation and bleeding 198
    and haemoglobin level 196
    hospital committees 208
    in Jehovah's Witness patients 209

blood – *continued*
  transfusion – *continued*
    ordering schedules 205–6
    serious hazards of transfusion (SHOT)
      scheme 208
blood gas analysis, interpretation of 184–5
bloodborne viruses
  surgery by carriers 334
  surgery on carriers 333–4
body water *see* fluid balance
bone, handling techniques 7–8
bone marrow failure, and anaemia 195–6
botulism, neuromuscular effects 241
bowel *see* large bowel; small bowel
breast tissue
  abscess 330
    incision and drainage 45–6
    needle aspiration 44–5
  carcinoma, TNM classification 267,
    268(box)
  cysts, needle aspiration 41–2
  mass
    excision 46–7
    fine needle aspiration cytology 42–3
  needle core biopsy 43–4
  reconstructive surgery 167–70
bronchoscopy 127–9
bypass grafting, saphenous vein harvesting
  132–3

C
calcification 285
calcium
  effect on neuromuscular system 241
  and muscle contraction 237
castration 92–3
cells
  cell cycle 275–6
  cellular accumulations 284–6, 300–1
  growth potential 275
  injury 299
  senescence 287–8
cellular adaptation 275(f), 276
  atrophy 278
  dysplasia 279
  hyperplasia 277
  hypertrophy 276–7
  hypoplasia 277
  metaplasia 278–9
cellulitis 328–9
central venous catheters
  infection 335
  insertion 129–30
chest drains, insertion 131–2
chlorhexidine, as antiseptic 5
cholinergic receptor 235–6
chronic renal failure, and fluid balance
  188–9
circumcision 89–90
clonidine 246
clostridial myonecrosis 330
Clostridium difficile infection 332
clotting factors 196
  for transfusion 207
coagulation cascade 196, 317–18
coagulation disorders, acquired 197–9

coagulation inhibitors 199
  abnormalities 200–2
coagulopathy, correction of 19
cobalamin (vitamin B$_{12}$) deficiency 194
Colles' fracture 139–42
colostomy 62–4
coma 147
complement system, and inflammation 302(t),
  303
computed tomography (CT) 29
  of gastrointestinal system 30–2, 33(f)
connective tissue, handling techniques 6–7
Conn's syndrome 256
continuous sutures, technique 13(f), 14
contrast radiology
  biliary 28
  contrast media 26
  gastrointestinal 26–7
  renal 27–8
  vascular 28
cordotomy 248
cricothyroidotomy 123–4
cryoprecipitate, for transfusion 207
cystoscopy 97

D
death certification 269–70
deep vein thrombosis (DVT) 203–4
denervation injury, muscle effects 241–2
depressed skull fracture 151–2
diagnostic radiology
  abdomen 30–2, 33(f)
  computed tomography (CT) 29
  contrast radiology 26–8
  head and neck 34
  magnetic resonance imaging (MRI)
    29–30
  musculoskeletal system 34
  radiation dose 25–6
  radiographs 26
  radionuclide radiology 30
  thorax 33–4
  ultrasound 29
  urinary tract 33
  vascular system 33
diarrhoea, causes and treatment 220–1
diathermy 9–11
differentiation, of tumours 265, 282–3
digital subtraction angiography (DSA) 28
diseases
  classification 263, 264(f), 267–8
  staging 266–7, 268(box)
dislocation, shoulder 142–4
disseminated intravascular coagulation (DIC)
  198, 320
distal radial fracture 139–42
diuresis 178–9
DNA repair, and cancer risk 281
drains 16
  removal 18
  specialist uses 17–18
  types of 16–17
dressings, types of 15–16
Dukes' staging system 266
duodenal ulcer, perforated 59–60
duodenum, diagnostic radiology 31

dysplasia 279
  definition 265

E
eicosanoids, and inflammation 302(t), 303
electrolyte disorders 179–81
electrolytes
  problems after surgery 185–9
  requirements 185
embolism 320–1
endocrine control 251
endoscopic surgery, urological *see* urological
  endoscopic surgery
endotracheal intubation 121–3
endplate potential 237
epidemiology
  death certification 269–70
  incidence, definition 268
  mortality data 270–1
  prevalence, definition 268
  screening programmes 269
epididymal cysts, excision 92
epidural analgesia 247–8
erythrocytes
  membrane disorders 194
  for transfusion 206
excitable tissue, properties 233–4
exfoliative cytology 295
extradural haematoma 147–9

F
factor V Leiden, and thrombosis 201
fasciotomy 116–17
fatty change, of cells 284–5, 299
femoral hernia 67–8, 69(f)
fibrinolytic drugs 202, 203(box)
fibroadenoma, of the breast, excision 46–7
fine needle aspiration cytology (FNAC)
  advantages and disadvantages 295
  of breast mass 42–3
  complications 295
  methods 294(f), 295
  uses 292–3, 295
fixatives, for tissue specimens 291–2
fluid balance. *see also* gastrointestinal system,
  fluid loss
  acid–base balance 181–5
  body water distribution 177
  diuresis 178–9
  electrolyte disorders 179–81
  fluid and electrolyte requirements 185
  oedema 189
  problems after surgery 185–9
  renal function 177–8
  third compartment 217
folate deficiency 193, 194(box)
foreign bodies, removal from airways
  126–7
foreskin surgery
  circumcision 89–90
  congenital abnormalities 87
  dorsal slit 88–9
  frenuloplasty 87–8
  general considerations 87
  paraphimosis 90
  urethral stricture 87

fractures
Colles' 139–42
skull 151–2
splints and plaster casts 137–9
frenuloplasty 87–8
fresh frozen plasma (FFP), for transfusion
206–7

G

gallbladder, interventional radiology 36
ganglia, excision 141(f), 142
gastroenteritis, viral 333
gastrointestinal system
contrast radiology 26–7
diagnostic radiology 30–2, 33(f)
fluid loss 185(box), 186
biliary fistulas 222
diarrhoea 220–1
gastric outlet obstruction 217–18
ileostomy 221, 222(t)
intestinal fistulas 222
intestinal obstruction 218–20
pancreatitis (acute) 222
gastric outlet obstruction 217–18
secretions, volume and composition 217,
218(t)
genes, and cancer development 280–2
glomerular filtration rate (GFR) 177
glucose-6-phosphate dehydrogenase (G6PD)
deficiency 194
glyceryl trinitrate (GTN), for anal fissure
treatment 78
grading, of tumours 265–6
granulomas 304, 305(f)
Graves' disease 251–2
Gridiron incision 56, 57(f)
groin surgery
orchidectomy 92–3, 95
varicocele ligation 95
growth factors, and tumour growth 281

H

haematinics, deficiency 193–4
haematoma, intracranial 147–51
haemoglobin level, and surgery 196
haemoglobinopathies 194–5
haemolytic anaemia 194–5
haemophilia 197
haemorrhage, venous 113–14
haemorrhoids
clinical features 73–4
haemorrhoidectomy 75–7
injection sclerotherapy 74–5
rubber band ligation 75
haemostasis 317–18
head and neck, diagnostic radiology 34
head and neck lumps, aspiration cytology 293,
295
head injury
coma 147
depressed skull fracture 151–2
intracranial clots 147–51
raised intracranial pressure 147
and spinal fracture 152
healing process 305–7
Henderson–Hasselbalch equation 182

heparin, thrombosis treatment 202–3
hepatic failure 227–9
hepatitis, and surgery 333–4
hereditary angioedema 210
heredity, and cancer incidence 280
hernia
femoral 67–8, 69(f)
inguinal 65–7
umbilical 69–70
histamine, as inflammatory mediator 302
HIV, and surgery 333–4
Hodgkin's disease 210–11
homocystinuria, and thrombosis 201
human leucocyte antigen (HLA) system, and
transplantation 210
hyaline change 285–6
hydrocele, excision 91–2
hyperaldosteronism 256
hypercalcaemia 253–4
hyperhomocysteinaemia, and thrombosis 201
hyperkalaemia 181
hypernatraemia 180
hyperplasia, of cells 277
hypertension
hypertensive crisis 254–5
hypertensive encephalopathy 255
phaeochromocytoma 255–6
hyperthermia, malignant 242
hyperthyroidism 251–2
hypertrophic scars 164–6
hypertrophy, of cells 276–7
hypocalcaemia
after thyroid surgery 252
effect on neuromuscular system 241
hypokalaemia 181, 182(box)
hyponatraemia 180–1
hypoplasia, of cells 277
hypospadias, surgery 87

I

ileostomy, fluid loss 221, 222(t)
immune response 209
immunocompromised patients 209
and tumour development 281–2
immunoglobulins, for transfusion 207
incidence of a disease, definition 268
incisions, abdominal see abdomen, incisions
infantile hypertrophic pyloric stenosis (IHPS)
217–18
infection
immune response 209
of soft tissue see soft tissue infection
of surgical site see surgical site infection
(SSI)
of urinary tract 331–2
inferior vena caval filter, interventional
radiology 37
inflammation
chemical mediators 302–3
chronic 303–5
and pain 242–3
tissue changes 300–2
inguinal hernia 65–7
injection sclerotherapy
haemorrhoids 74–5
varicose veins 109–10

interleukin-1, and inflammation 302(t), 303
International Classification of Diseases (ICD)
267–8
interrupted sutures, technique 13(f), 14
interventional radiology 34
percutaneous biliary procedures 35–6
percutaneous biopsy and drainage
procedures 35
uroradiology 37–8
vascular procedures 36–7
intestinal fistulas, fluid loss 222
intestinal obstruction
in adults 219–20
in neonates 218–19
intracerebral haematoma 151
intracranial clots 147–51
intracranial pressure, raised 147
intravascular devices
infection 335
interventional radiology 36
intravenous fluids, and fluid balance 185
intubation, endotracheal 121–3
iodophores, as antiseptics 5
iron deficiency anaemia 193

J

jaundice 225–7
joints, aspiration and injection 137
juxtaglomerular apparatus 177–8

K

keloid scars 164–6
Kessler suture 7, 8(f)
ketamine 247
kidney function see renal failure; renal system
kinins, and inflammation 302(t), 303
Kocher's incision 55

L

Lanz incision 56, 57(f)
large bowel
contrast radiology 27
diagnostic radiology 31
laryngeal carcinoma, TNM classification 266,
267(box)
latex, allergy to 209
leucocytes, and inflammation 301
Lichtenstein technique, for inguinal hernia
repair 65–7
liver
bleeding disorders 197–8
diagnostic radiology 32
local anaesthetics 244–5
anaesthetic blocks 247
lupus anticoagulant, and thrombosis 202
lymph nodes, biopsy 48–9, 213
lymphatic function 189
lymphomas
classification 210, 212(box)
Hodgkin's disease 210–11
non-Hodgkin's lymphoma 211–13

M

macrophages, and inflammation 304
magnesium, effect on neuromuscular system
241

magnetic resonance imaging (MRI) 26(f), 29–30
major histocompatibility complex (MHC), and transplantation 210
malignant hyperthermia 242
malignant lymphomas *see* lymphomas
malignant tumours
  classification 283
  definition 264
malnutrition, in hospitalised patients *see* nutritional failure
mattress sutures, technique 13(f), 14
maximum blood-ordering schedules (MBOS) 205–6
Mayo operation, for umbilical hernia 69–70
McEvedy's incision 55
median sternotomy 131
membrane potential 233–4
metabolic acidosis 183
metabolic alkalosis 183–4
metaplasia 278–9
metastases
  genetic factors 282
  and tumour classification 283–4
MHC (major histocompatibility complex), and transplantation 210
microbiological specimens 295–6
microsurgery, principles 20
Milligan–Morgan technique, for haemorrhoidectomy 75–7
Monckeberg's medial calcification 314
mortality data 270–1
motor unit 233–7
multiresistant *staphylococcus aureus* (MRSA) 332
muscle
  action potential 237
  contraction 237
  handling techniques 7
musculoskeletal system, diagnostic radiology 34
myasthenia gravis 242
myasthenic syndrome 242
myonecrosis, clostridial 330

N

necrosis 299
necrotising fasciitis 329–30
needle aspiration
  of breast abscess 44–5
  of breast cysts 41–2
needle core biopsy (NCB), of breast tissue 43–4
neoplasia
  aetiology 280–2
  definition 279
  tumour classification 282–4
Nernst equation 233
nerve fibres 234
nerve stimulators, and use of neuromuscular-blocking drugs 239
neuromuscular-blocking drugs
  indications 238
  mechanisms of action 237–8
  monitoring of blockade 238–9
  onset of action 239

pharmacodynamics 239
  reversal of blockade 239
  risks 240–1
neuromuscular transmission 233–7
nicotinic receptor 235–6
nitric oxide (NO), and inflammation 302(t), 303
nociceptive pathways 242–4
non-Hodgkin's lymphoma 211–13
non-steroidal antiinflammatory drugs (NSAIDs) 246
nuclear medicine, definition 30
nutritional failure
  causes 222–3, 223–5
  functional consequences 223
  nutritional support 225

O

obstructive jaundice 227
oedema 189
oesophagus, diagnostic radiology 31
oncogenes 281
opiates, analgesic actions 245–6
orchidectomy 92–3, 95

P

pain transmission 242–4
pancreas, diagnostic radiology 32, 33(f)
pancreatitis (acute), fluid loss 222
paralytic ileus 220
paraphimosis 90
parathyroid gland, and thyroid lobectomy 104
pathology
  disease staging 266–7
  disease types 263, 264(f)
  International Classification of Diseases (ICD) 267–8
  tumour classification 264–6
patient-controlled analgesia 248
percutaneous procedures
  interventional radiology 35–6
  transhepatic cholangiogram 28
peritoneal cavity, fluid loss after surgery 185(box), 186
Pfannenstiel incision 56
pH, regulation 182
phaeochromocytoma 255–6
phagocytosis, and inflammation 301
plaques, atheromatous 315–16
plasma
  loss, and fluid balance 185–6
  for transfusion 206–7
plaster casts, application 137–9
plastic surgery
  breast reconstruction 167–70
  hypertrophic and keloid scars 164–6
  wound closure methods
    basic principles 155
    direct closure 155–6
    serial excision 156
    skin flaps 160–4
    skin grafts 157–60
    tissue expansion 157
platelet-activating factor (PAF), as inflammatory mediator 302(t), 303

platelets
  disorders of 199
  for transfusion 206
pneumonia 331
pneumothorax 131–2
poliomyelitis, neuromuscular effects 241
potassium
  and action potential generation 233–4
  hyperkalaemia 181
  hypokalaemia 181, 182(box)
  regulation 181
prevalence of a disease, definition 268
primary hyperaldosteronism 256
proctoscopy 73
programmed cell death 299
  and tumour development 281
prosthetic devices, infection 326
protein C deficiency, and thrombosis 201
protein S deficiency, and thrombosis 201
prothrombin abnormality, and thrombosis 201
pulmonary thromboembolism 320–1
pyloric stenosis (acquired gastric outlet obstruction) 218
pyomyositis 330
pyrexia, and fluid balance 185(box), 186

R

radiology *see* diagnostic radiology; interventional radiology
raised intracranial pressure 147
red blood cells
  membrane disorders 194
  for transfusion 206
Reed–Sternberg cells, in Hodgkin's disease 210, 211(f)
renal failure
  effects on coagulation and bleeding 198
  and fluid balance 186–9
renal system
  contrast radiology 27–8
  functions 177–8
renin–angiotensin system 177–8
respiratory acidosis 182(box), 183
respiratory alkalosis 183
respiratory tract lesions, aspiration cytology 295
Rigler's sign, abdominal radiograph 30
running paratenon suture 7, 8(f)

S

saphenous vein, harvesting 132–3
scars 164–6
sclerotherapy
  haemorrhoids 74–5
  varicose veins 109–10
screening programmes 269
scrotal surgery
  epididymal cyst excision 92
  hydrocele excision 91–2
  incision and closure 90–1
  orchidectomy 92–3, 95
  for testicular torsion 93–4
  vasectomy 94–5
'scrubbing up' 5
senescence, of cells 287–8
septicaemia, and fluid balance 185(box), 186

shoulder, dislocation 142–4
sickle cell anaemia 194–5
sigmoidoscopy 73
silicone breast implants 170
skin flaps, for plastic surgery 160–4
skin grafts, for plastic surgery 157–60
skin infections, management 47–8
skin lesions, excision 49–50
skin wounds
    healing process 306
    management 47
skull fracture 151–2
small bowel
    contrast radiology 27
    diagnostic radiology 31
    fistulas, fluid loss 222
    resection 60–2
sodium
    and action potential generation 233–4
    gains and losses 179–80
    hypernatraemia 180
    hyponatraemia 180–1
    regulation 180
soft tissue infection
    breast abscess 330
    cellulitis 328–9
    necrotising fasciitis 329–30
    pyomyositis 330
    superficial skin infections 47–8
    surgical wound infection 327–8
    tetanus 330–1
    toxic shock syndrome (TSS) 331
spinal cord
    descending pathways, and pain 243–4
    pharmacology, and pain 243
spinal fracture, and head injury 152
splenectomy 209
splints, application 137–9
sputum, microbiological specimens 296
Staphylococcus infection
    multiresistant Staphylococcus aureus (MRSA)
        332
    of skin, management 47–8
Starling equilibrium 189
sterilisation, of instruments, methods 6
sternotomy 131
stomach, diagnostic radiology 31
Streptococcus infection, of skin 47–8
subcutaneous lateral internal sphincterotomy
        (SLIS) 78–9
subcuticular sutures, technique 13(f), 14
subdural haematoma 149–51
submandibular gland, excision 105–6
surgical site infection (SSI)
    definition 325
    epidemiology and surveillance 325
    microbiology 325–6
    prevention 327
    prosthetic device infection 326
    risk factors 326
surgical skills workshops 20–2
sutures 11–12
    alternatives to 14–15
    bowel 8–9
    cartilage 7
    connective tissue 6–7

materials for 12–14
muscle 7
techniques 13(f), 14
tendon 7
swabs, microbiological specimens 295–6

T

tendon, handling techniques 7, 8(f)
TENS (transcutaneous electrical nerve
        stimulation) 248
testicular torsion 93–4
testicular tumour 95
tetanus 330–1
    neuromuscular effects 241
thalassaemias 194–5
third (fluid) compartment 217
thoracotomy 130–1
thorax, diagnostic radiology 33–4
thrombocytopenia 199
thromboembolism 320–1
thrombosis
    arterial 200
    clinical outcome 320
    disseminated intravascular coagulation
        (DIC) 320
    morphology of thrombi 319–20
    predisposing factors 318–19
    prevention 203–4
    specialist tests 202
    thrombophilia 200–2
    treatment 202–3
    venous 200, 201(box)
thyroid disorders
    aspiration cytology 292–3
    thyroid carcinoma, TNM classification 266,
        267(box)
    thyrotoxicosis 251–2
thyroid lobectomy
    hazards 104–5
    postoperative management 105
    preparation 101
    procedure 101–4
tissue expansion, for plastic surgery 157
tissue handling
    bone 7–8
    bowel 8–9
    cartilage 7
    connective tissue 6–7
    muscle 7
    tendon 7, 8(f)
tissue sections
    fixation and transport 291–2
    frozen sections 291
TNM classification system 266–7, 268(box)
tourniquets 11
toxic shock syndrome (TSS) 331
tracheostomy 124–6
tramadol 247
transcellular fluid 217
transcutaneous electrical nerve stimulation
        (TENS) 248
transplantation 210
tumour necrosis factor (TNF), and
        inflammation 302(t), 303
tumour suppressor genes 281
tumours

aetiology 280–2
classification 282–4
disease staging 266–7, 268(box)
terminology 264–6

U

ultrasound imaging 29
umbilical hernia 69–70
ureterography 97–8
urethral stricture, surgery 87
urinary tract
    diagnostic radiology 33
    infection 331–2
urine, microbiological specimens 296
urological endoscopic surgery
    cystoscopy 97
    instruments 95–7
    retrograde ureterography 97–8
    ureteric stent placement 98
uroradiology, interventional radiology 37–8

V

varicocele ligation 95
varicose veins
    sclerotherapy 109–10
    surgical treatment 110–13
vascular surgery
    fasciotomy 116–17
    varicose veins 109–13
    vascular suture 114–15
    venous haemorrhage 113–14
vascular system
    abnormalities causing bleeding 199–200
    contrast radiology 28
    diagnostic radiology 33
    interventional radiology 36–7
vasectomy 94–5
veins, harvesting for bypass surgery 132–3
venous catheters
    infection 335
    insertion 129–30
venous system
    haemorrhage 113–14
    interventional radiology 37
    thromboembolism 203–4
    thrombosis 200, 201(box)
viral gastroenteritis 333
Virchow's triad, and thrombosis 318–19
vitamin B$_{12}$ (cobalamin) deficiency 194
vitamin K antagonists, thrombosis treatment
        203
vitamin K, deficiency, and coagulation
        disorder 197
Von Willebrand's disease 197

W

warfarin
    and surgery 197, 198(box)
    thrombosis treatment 203
wounds
    cleaning agents 16
    closure methods
        adhesives 14–15
        stapling devices 15
        sutures see sutures
    surgical wound infection 327–8